Chemical Composition and Activity of Natural Products

Chemical Composition and Activity of Natural Products

Guest Editors

Stela Dimitrova
Ana M. Dobreva
Petko Denev

MDPI

Basel • Beijing • Wuhan • Barcelona • Belgrade • Novi Sad • Cluj • Manchester

Guest Editors

Stela Dimitrova
Department of Bioorganic Chemistry
Medical university of Plovdiv
Plovdiv
Bulgaria

Ana M. Dobreva
Institute for Roses and Aromatic Plants
Agricultural Academy
Kazanlak
Bulgaria

Petko Denev
Laboratory of Biologically Active Substances
Bulgarian Academy of Sciences
Plovdiv
Bulgaria

Editorial Office

MDPI AG
Grosspeteranlage 5
4052 Basel, Switzerland

This is a reprint of the Special Issue, published open access by the journal *Molecules* (ISSN 1420-3049), freely accessible at: https://www.mdpi.com/journal/molecules/special_issues/WI249VOQY2.

For citation purposes, cite each article independently as indicated on the article page online and as indicated below:

Lastname, A.A.; Lastname, B.B. Article Title. *Journal Name* **Year**, *Volume Number*, Page Range.

ISBN 978-3-7258-6430-0 (Hbk)
ISBN 978-3-7258-6431-7 (PDF)
https://doi.org/10.3390/books978-3-7258-6431-7

Contents

About the Editors

Stela Dimitrova

Stela Dimitrova is an associate professor in the Department of Bioorganic Chemistry, Faculty of Pharmacy, Medical University of Plovdiv. She graduated with a Master's degree in Chemistry from the University of Plovdiv "Paisiy Hilendarski". She majored in Theoretical Foundations of Medicinal Chemistry. She completed her PhD studies on the topic "Identification and Antioxidant Activity of Isoprenoids from Biomass of Psychrophilic Yeasts". Her research interests include substances of natural origin, methods for their isolation and analysis, biotechnological methods for production, studies of their activity, and their application as food additives. She currently serves as the Head of the Department of Bioorganic Chemistry.

Ana Dobreva

Ana Dobreva is an Associate Professor/Director in the Institute for Roses and Aromatic plants, Agricultural Academy and lecturer at Thrakia University in Bulgaria. She has expertise with the processing of the oil-bearing and medicinal plants - including distillation extraction and all their multitude of new research methods. Her main research interests include essential oils and other aromatic products (concretes, absolutes, extracts, ets.) their chemical composition, their application and safety. She is also dedicated to utilization of the biowastes, their benefits and properties, with a particular focus on oil-bearing roses.

Petko Denev

Petko Denev is a full professor in Bioorganic chemistry and chemistry of physiologically active substances at the Institute of Organic Chemistry with Centre of Phytochemistry, Bulgarian Academy of Sciences and holds a PhD degree in "Technology of biologically active substances". His research interests are directed for extraction, purification, isolation and characterization of biologically active phytosubstances and their application in the development of nutraceuticals and functional foods. He is author of 113 research papers (Scopus), 3 book chapters, 1 patent and 1 utility model. His works have been cited more than 2800 times with a Hirsch index of 27. In 2013, prof. Denev was awarded with the National Science Award "Pythagoras", for young scientist, presented by the Bulgarian Ministry of Education and Science.

molecules

MDPI

Article

Biological Potential of *Asphodelus microcarpus* Extracts: α-Glucosidase and Antibiofilm Activities In Vitro

Sonia Floris [1], Francesca Pintus [1], Antonella Fais [1,*], Benedetta Era [1], Nicola Raho [2], Chiara Siguri [3], Germano Orrù [4], Sara Fais [4], Carlo Ignazio Giovanni Tuberoso [1], Stefania Olla [3,*] and Amalia Di Petrillo [2]

[1] Department of Life and Environmental Sciences, University of Cagliari, SS 554-Bivio per Sestu, Cittadella Universitaria, 09042 Monserrato, Italy; s.floris@unica.it (S.F.); fpintus@unica.it (F.P.); era@unica.it (B.E.); tuberoso@unica.it (C.I.G.T.)

[2] Gastroenterology Unit, Department of Medical Science and Public Health, University of Cagliari, Cittadella Universitaria, 09042 Monserrato, Italy; nicola.raho@unica.it (N.R.); amalia.dip@unica.it (A.D.P.)

[3] Institute for Genetic and Biomedical Research (IRGB), The National Research Council (CNR), 09042 Monserrato, Italy; chiara.siguri@irgb.cnr.it

[4] Department of Surgical Sciences, University of Cagliari, Cittadella Universitaria, 09042 Monserrato, Italy; orru@unica.it (G.O.); sarafais79@gmail.com (S.F.)

* Correspondence: fais@unica.it (A.F.); stefania.olla@irgb.cnr.it (S.O.)

Abstract: Type 2 diabetes (T2D), characterized by insulin resistance and β-cell dysfunction, requires continuous advancements in management strategies, particularly in controlling postprandial hyperglycemia to prevent complications. Current antidiabetics, which have α-amylase and α-glucosidase inhibitory activities, have side effects, prompting the search for better alternatives. In addition, diabetes patients are particularly vulnerable to yeast infections because an unusual sugar concentration promotes the growth of *Candida* spp. in areas like the mouth and genitalia. *Asphodelus microcarpus* contains bioactive flavonoids with potential enzyme inhibitory properties. This study investigates α-amylase and α-glucosidase inhibitory activities and antioxidant and antimycotic capacity of ethanolic extracts from different parts of *A. microcarpus*. Results show that extracts significantly inhibit α-glucosidase, with the IC_{50} value being up to 25 times higher than for acarbose, while exerting low α-amylase activity. The extracts also demonstrated strong antioxidant properties and low cytotoxicity. The presence of phenolic compounds is likely responsible for the observed biological activities. Molecular docking analysis of 11 selected compounds identified emodin and luteolin as significant inhibitors of α-glucosidase. Additionally, the extracts demonstrated significant antibiofilm action against an MDR strain of *Candida albicans*. These findings suggest that *A. microcarpus* is a promising source of natural compounds for T2D management.

Keywords: *Asphodelus microcarpus*; α-glucosidase; α-amylase; molecular docking

1. Introduction

Diabetes, a significant global health concern, impacts millions of individuals worldwide, underscoring the need for continuous advancements in effective management strategies [1]. While type 1 diabetes primarily necessitates insulin therapy due to pancreatic β-cell dysfunction, type 2 diabetes (T2D) is characterized by insulin resistance and a progressive decline in β-cell function [2]. Managing T2D requires comprehensive strategies to control blood glucose levels and minimize the risk of complications. A critical component of T2D management is the regulation of postprandial hyperglycemia, which is essential in averting long-term vascular complications [3]. Currently, several antidiabetic drugs, such as acarbose, inhibit α-amylase (EC 3.2.1.1) and α-glucosidase (EC 3.2.20). α-Amylase hydrolyzes starch into smaller molecules, while α-glucosidase is an exoenzyme that cleaves disaccharides and oligosaccharides into glucose in the small intestine [4]. Excessive inhibition of α-amylase is associated with side effects, such as gastrointestinal discomfort [5], highlighting the need for more tolerable and efficacious alternatives.

Beyond glucose management, diabetes patients are also predisposed to infections due to compromised immune function. Among the most common are fungal infections, particularly those caused by *Candida albicans*. Individuals with diabetes, especially those with poorly controlled blood glucose levels, are at a higher risk of candidiasis, as hyperglycemia fosters an environment conducive to fungal overgrowth [6]. *C. albicans* is an opportunistic pathogen that causes infections ranging from superficial mucosal involvement to invasive, life-threatening infections in diabetic patients. Managing such infections is crucial to prevent further complications, as fungal overgrowth can exacerbate inflammation and damage in vulnerable tissues [7].

Research has shown that several plants contain substances that can inhibit the activity of α-amylase and α-glucosidase enzymes [8,9]. Flavonoids are revealed to be of particular interest in the inhibition of these enzymes [10,11]. Genus *Asphodelus* spp., renowned for its historical use in folk medicine, has emerged as a novel research domain, courtesy of its prospective bioactive properties, such as antimicrobial and antimycotic activity [12]. *A. microcarpus*, a significant plant in the Liliaceae family, is utilized in traditional medicine for treating local inflammation, with its roots employed against white spots and specifically for ear pain. Various studies have validated the antioxidant, antimelanogenic, anti-inflammatory, and antimicrobial activities of *A. microcarpus*, corroborating its ethnopharmacological applications and providing a scientific basis for its usage in folk medicine [13,14]. Furthermore, *A. microcarpus* is known for its rich phenolic content, and its flowers are laden with antioxidant molecules like luteolin and its derivatives. A high concentration of flavonoids in aerial parts of *A. microcarpus* was also detected in our previous study [13,15]. In particular, the extracts presented luteolin and its glycosylated derivates in high concentrations. These extracts also showed good antioxidant activities. As reported by Kim and coworkers [16] luteolin and some glycosylated derivates showed potent inhibitory activity against α-amylase and α-glucosidase.

Considering these findings, our study aims to investigate the potential of *A. microcarpus* as a valuable source of natural compounds capable of efficiently inhibiting enzymes like α-amylase and α-glucosidase. This exploration is intended to unlock the therapeutic potential of *A. microcarpus* in the context of natural medicine, further contributing to our understanding of its health-promoting properties, particularly regarding diabetes management and infection control.

2. Results

2.1. Enzymatic Inhibition

The prepared extracts, as described in the Materials and Methods, were evaluated for their inhibitory activity against α-glucosidase and α-amylase. The extracts were tested at a concentration of 100 μg/mL and the results are presented in Table 1.

Table 1. Inhibition (%) of *A. microcarpus* ethanolic extracts (EEs) at 100 μg/mL against the enzymes α-glucosidase and α-amylase.

Extract	α-Glucosidase	α-Amylase
Stems	97.6 ± 2.8	13.5 ± 0.3
Leaves	88.8 ± 5.1	20.6 ± 0.6
Flowers	92.3 ± 4.2	14.6 ± 0.4
Tubers	98.2 ± 3.7	20.2 ± 0.9

Our results demonstrated that the EE of *A. microcarpus* completely inhibited α-glucosidase enzyme at the dose tested, while showing relatively low activity towards the α-amylase enzyme.

Based on these results, we calculated the IC_{50} values only for the α-glucosidase enzyme. As shown in Table 2, all extracts exhibited an IC_{50} value statistically lower than that of acarbose ($p < 0.0001$). The extracts were up to 25 times more effective than the standard inhibitor.

Table 2. IC_{50} value of *A. microcarpus* EE against α-glucosidase.

Extract	IC_{50} (μg/mL)
Stems	4.3 ± 0.5
Leaves	3.8 ± 0.4
Flowers	4.6 ± 0.4
Tubers	3.6 ± 0.1
Acarbose	90 ± 7.3

These preliminary results indicate that the extracts of *A. microcarpus* show interesting potential as inhibitors of the α-glucosidase enzyme.

2.2. Antimycotic Activity

The results obtained using the microplate procedure displayed an antibiofilm activity for some ethanol extracts. Furthermore, none of the formulations inhibited the planktonic form of Candida albicans at the tested concentrations (MIC > 4 mg/mL). According to Table 3, ethanol base formulations made from stems, leaves, and flowers exhibited the lowest minimum biofilm inhibitory concentration (MBIC) values when compared to ethanol-extracted tubers; the first cited formulations showed an MBIC equal to 1.3 mg/mL.

Table 3. Antibiofilm pattern of *A. microcarpus* EE against an MDR strain of *C. albicans*.

Extract	MIC (mg/mL)	MBIC (mg/mL)
Stems	>4 mg/mL	1.3 mg/mL
Leaves	>4 mg/mL	1.3 mg/mL
Flowers	>4 mg/mL	1.3 mg/mL
Tubers	>4 mg/mL	4 mg/mL

2.3. Cell Viability and Cellular Antioxidant Activity

As previously reported, the EEs of *A. microcarpus* exhibited good antioxidant activity [13] on ABTS and DPPH assay. Therefore, we investigated their potential to inhibit H_2O_2-induced ROS generation in a cellular model.

First, we checked if the extracts could affect cell viability, using Caco-2 cells as a cellular model. EEs from flowers, stems, leaves, and tubers were tested at concentrations from 0.1 to 10 μg/mL. The results showed that none of the extracts was cytotoxic since the cell viability remained over 84% in all samples (Figure 1). In particular, all the extracts had no effect at 0.1 and 1 μg/mL, with leaves and tubers exerting no effect up to the higher concentrations tested. Only a slight decrease was observed for flower and stem extracts at concentrations of 2.5, 5, and 10 μg/mL with percentages of viability above 91% for flowers and from 91.2 to 84.4% for stems. These values are, however, not statistically significant, except for the stems at the concentrations of 5 ($p < 0.01$) and 10 μg/mL ($p < 0.0001$).

In the cellular antioxidant assay, ROS levels in Caco-2 cells were evaluated before and after H_2O_2-induced oxidative stress and upon treatment with extracts at different concentrations (0.1–10 μg/mL). Figure 2 shows that the treatment with only H_2O_2 significantly increased ROS levels (T vs. NT cells; $p < 0.0001$). All tested extracts demonstrated a significant cellular antioxidant activity reducing fluorescence emission in dose-dependent manner. The reduction in fluorescence emission indicates a decrease in ROS levels on cells treated with the extracts. This effect can be attributed to the action of phenolic compounds present in the extracts, which have been shown to possess antioxidant capabilities. All samples reduced fluorescence emission by about 50% at a concentration of 10 μg/mL. Considering each concentration, the greatest intracellular ROS inhibition was provided by leaf extract (Figure 2).

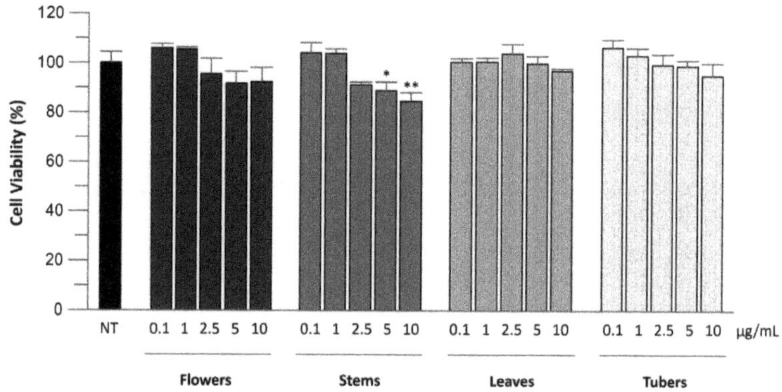

Figure 1. Effect of EEs from flowers, stems, leaves, and tubers of *A. microcarpus* on Caco-2 cell viability. After 24 h of incubation with samples at different concentrations (0.1–10 μg/mL), cell viability was evaluated by the MTT assay. Asterisks indicate statistically significant differences between non-treated (NT) cells and stem samples at concentrations of 5 μg/mL (* $p < 0.01$) and 10 μg/mL (** $p < 0.0001$).

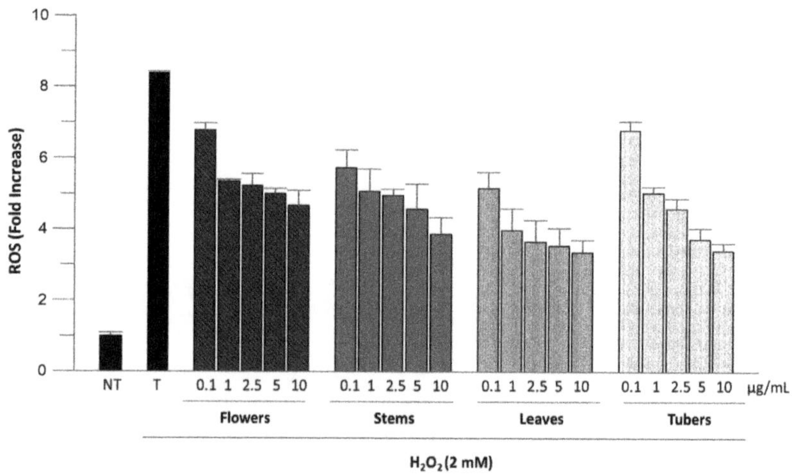

Figure 2. Inhibition of H_2O_2-induced ROS generation by ethanolic extracts of *A. microcarpus* on Caco-2 cells. NT, non-treated cells; T, cells treated with H_2O_2 only. All H_2O_2-treated samples were statistically different from cells treated with H_2O_2 only ($p < 0.0001$).

2.4. (HR) HPLC-ESI-QToF MS and (HR) HPLC-ESI-QToF MS/MS Analysis of A. microcarpus *Extracts*

The EEs obtained from *A. microcarpus* leaves, stems, flowers, and tubers were qualitatively analyzed by (HR) HPLC-ESI-QToF MS/MS in negative ion mode, and the profile showed the presence of various compounds (Table 4), mainly belonging to the classes of polyphenols, anthrones/anthraquinones, and furanocoumarins. Figure 3 reports the LC-ESI-Orbitrap-MS of *A. microcarpus* stem (SEE) and tuber ethanol extract (TEE) (chromatograms of FEE and LEE extracts were previously published [13,15]). Several phenolic compounds, namely 3-O-caffeoylquinic acid (2), 5-O-caffeoylquinic acid (5), luteolin 6-C-glucoside (10), luteolin O-acetylglucoside (13), and luteolin (18), were previously detected in *A. microcarpus* FEE and LEE [13,15]. Compound 7 with molecular ion at *m/z* [M−H]⁻ 337.0938, corresponding to a molecular formula of $C_{16}H_{18}O_8$ and main fragment ion at *m/z* 191.0560 was attributed to coumaroyl quinic acid [17]. Luteolin-6-C-glucoside was the most abundant peak in *A. microcarpus* SEE, LEE, and FEE, while no traces were found in TEE. Also, aloesin (1), a C-glycosylated chromone previously detected in *A. microcarpus* TEE [18], was detected for the first time in the other studied parts of *A. microcarpus*. Several anthraquinones were found in TEE, as well as emodin (4), aloinoside A/B (16), and laccaic acid (19). Emodin was already detected in *A. microcarpus* tubers [19], while aloinoside A/B and laccaic acid were found in Aloe species [20] and Asphodelus species [21], respectively. Compound 15 showed a molecular ion at *m/z* [M−H]⁻ 577.1577, corresponding to a molecular formula of $C_{27}H_{30}O_{14}$ and main fragment ion at *m/z* 253.0507. Taking into account the presence of chrysophanol in *A. microcarpus* tubers [19], the compound was tentatively identified as a chrysophanol diglucoside [22]. Other anthrones and anthraquinones were reported in *A. microcarpus* tubers [18,19], but they were not found in the extracts obtained in this experimentation.

Table 4. Compound identification by (HR) HPLC-ESI-QToF MS/MS in *A. microcarpus* extracts (X, present; -, absent).

Peak N°	R_t	[M−H]⁻ *m/z*	Molecular Formula	Δ mDA	MS/MS *m/z* (%)	Tentative Identification	SEE	LEE	TEE	FEE	References
1	9.29	393.1203	$C_{19}H_{22}O_9$	1.225	273.0774 (100)/ 245.0807 (52)	Aloesin	X	X	X	X	[18,21]
2	9.69	353.0888	$C_{16}H_{17}O_9$	1.68	179.0341 (27)/ 191.0561 (67)	3-O-caffeoylquinic acid	X	X	-	X	[13,15]
3	10.77	351.1307	$C_{14}H_{24}O_{10}$	1.77	101.0598 (100)	Alkyl glycoside	X	X	-	-	[22]
4	10.81	269.0469	$C_{15}H_{10}O_5$	−0.98	225.0571 (100)	Emodin	-	-	X	-	[19]
5	11.23	353.0888	$C_{16}H_{17}O_9$	1.68	179.0352 (33)/ 191.0561 (85)	5-O-caffeoylquinic acid	X	X	-	X	[13,15]
6	11.78	509.1684	$C_{24}H_{30}O_{12}$	0.88	257.0827 (100)	Unknown	-	-	X	-	[22]
7	12.36	337.0938	$C_{16}H_{18}O_8$	1.22	191.0560 (77)	Coumaroyl quinic acid	X	X	-	-	[17]
8	13.04	335.0778	$C_{16}H_{16}O_8$	1.43	179.0341 (86)/ 135.0447 (100)	5-O-Caffeoilshikimic acid	X	-	-	-	[21]
9	14.41	399.1668	$C_{16}H_{18}O_8$	1.81	175.1115 (100)	Alkyl glycoside	X	X	-	-	[22]
10	15.49	447.0948	$C_{21}H_{20}O_{11}$	1.70	357.0626 (100)/ 327.0515 (88)	Luteolin 6-C-glucoside	X	X	-	X	[13,15]
11	18.20	461.1107	$C_{22}H_{22}O_{11}$	1.56	254.0560 (100)	Unknown	X	X	-	-	
12	19.06	475.0899	$C_{22}H_{20}O_{12}$	1.65	431.0982 (100)	Unknown	X	X	-	-	
13	19.25	489.1054	$C_{23}H_{22}O_{12}$	1.38	429.0790 (25)/ 327.0562 (100)	Luteolin acetyl glucoside	X	X	-	X	[13,15]
14	20.51	539.1794	$C_{25}H_{32}O_{13}$	0.01	215.0714 (100)	Unknown	-	-	X	-	[22]
15	22.70	577.1577	$C_{27}H_{30}O_{14}$	0.01	253.0507 (100)	Chrysophanol diglucoside	-	-	X	-	[22]
16	23.93	563.1778	$C_{27}H_{32}O_{13}$	0.01	239.0712	Aloinoside A/B	-	-	X	-	[20]
17	26.06	949.2811	$C_{40}H_{54}O_{26}$	−3.87	859.2484 (100)	Unknown	-	-	X	-	[22]
18	26.15	285.0406	$C_{15}H_{10}O_6$	0.10	-	Luteolin	X	X	-	X	[13,15]

Table 4. *Cont.*

Peak N°	R_t	$[M-H]^-$ *m/z*	Molecular Formula	Δ mDA	MS/MS *m/z* (%)	Tentative Identification	SEE	LEE	TEE	FEE	References
19	29.66	313.0358	$C_{16}H_{10}O_7$	1.46	269.0456 (100)	Laccaic acid	X	-	-	-	[21]
20	30.07	933.2841	$C_{47}H_{50}O_{20}$	−3.38	843.2480 (100)	Unknown	-	-	X	-	[22]
21	30.81	961.2789	$C_{41}H_{54}O_{26}$	4.01	533.1256 (75)/ 490.1066 (100)	Unknown	-	-	X	-	[22]
22	31.91	327.2189	$C_{18}H_{32}O_3$	−1.08	239.1312 (56)	Unknown	X	X	X	-	[21]
23	32.65	933.2820	$C_{47}H_{50}O_{20}$	−1.22	843.2517 (100)	Unknown	-	-	X	-	[22]
24	32.86	242.1763	$C_{13}H_{25}NO_3$	0.15	225.1512 (100)/181.1594 (88)	Amino-oxotridecanoic acid	X	X	X	-	[22]

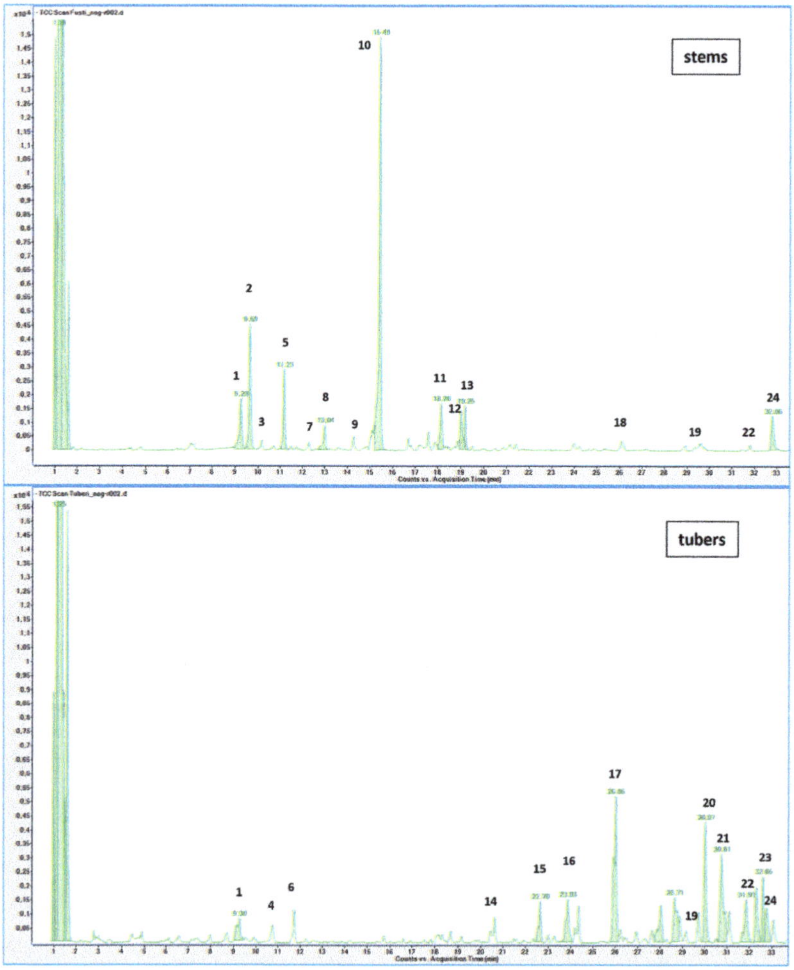

Figure 3. LC-ESI-Orbitrap-MS chromatograms of extracts obtained from the stems and tubers of *A. microcarpus*.

2.5. Molecular Docking

To identify the compounds in EE responsible for inhibiting α-glucosidase, we docked 11 compounds. Our selection of these 11 compounds was strategic. We included aloesin, a compound consistently found in all four ethanol extracts (SEE, LEE, TEE, and FEE). Additionally, we incorporated four compounds that were present in extract T and six compounds that were common across extracts S, L, and T. This comprehensive selection aimed to cover the most likely candidates responsible for the observed inhibitory activity.

Table 5 shows the structures and results of all 11 selected compounds docked in the α-glucosidase enzyme. The results indicate that the most promising compounds exhibiting the best binding affinity for α-glucosidase are emodin (−6.14 kcal/mol) and luteolin (−6.65 kcal/mol), whereas all others display energies inconsistent with enzyme binding affinity, suggesting a lack of activity. Our findings are supported by literature data, which report the in vitro activity of both emodin and luteolin [23,24].

Table 5. Graphical representation and results of docked compounds and their provenance in *A. microcarpus*.

Compounds	Name	Binding Affinity Kcal/mol	Identified in *A. microcarpus* Extracts
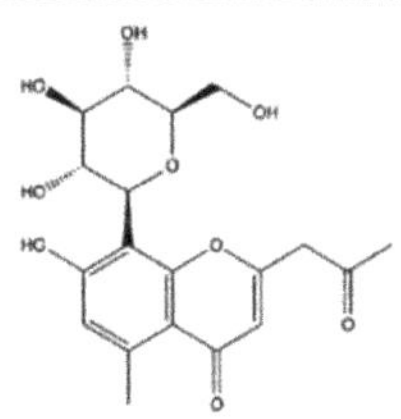	Aloesin	−4.70	ALL
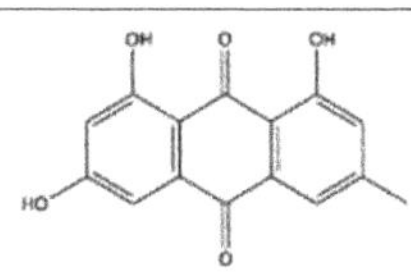	Emodin	−6.14	TEE
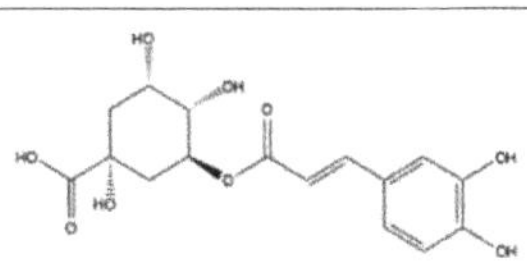	3-*O*-caffeoylquinic acid	−4.87	SEE; LEE; FEE
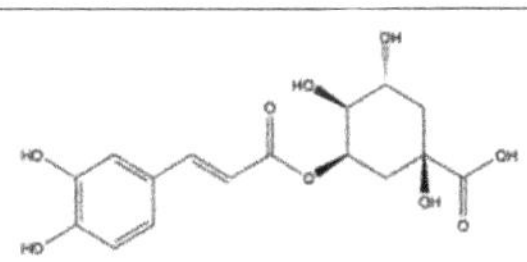	5-*O*-caffeoylquinic acid	−4.15	SEE; LEE; FEE
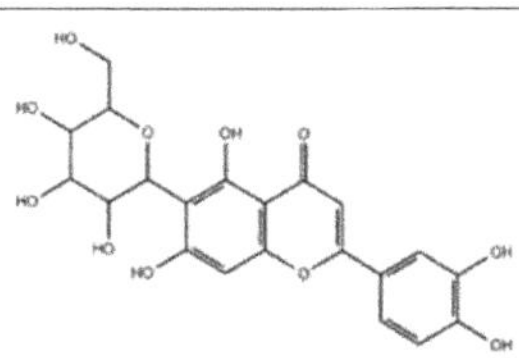	Luteolin 6-C-glucoside	−3.82	SEE; LEE; FEE

Table 5. *Cont.*

Compounds	Name	Binding Affinity Kcal/mol	Identified in *A. microcarpus* Extracts
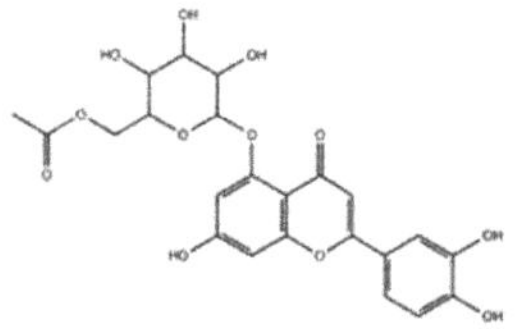	Luteolin 5-*O* acetyl glucoside	−4.11	SEE; LEE; FEE
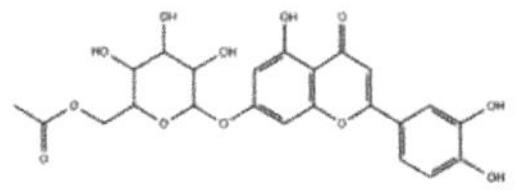	Luteolin 7-*O* acetyl glucoside	−4.63	SEE; LEE; FEE
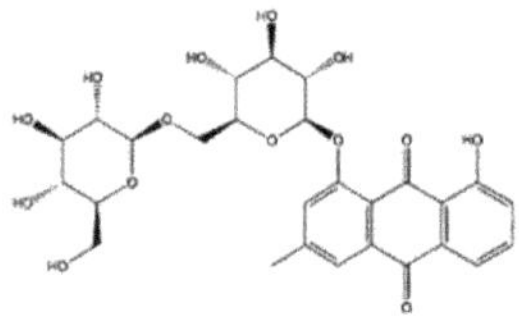	Chrysophanol diglucoside	−2.09	TEE
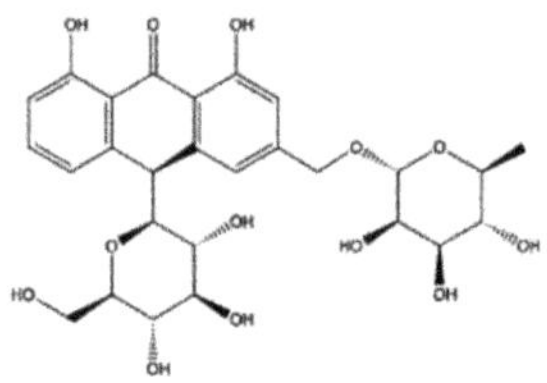	Aloinoside A	−4.57	TEE
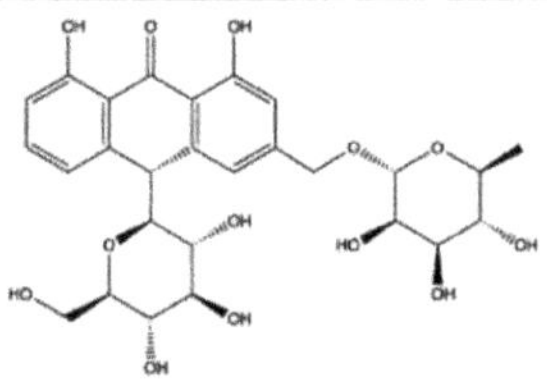	Aloinoside B	−3.43	TEE
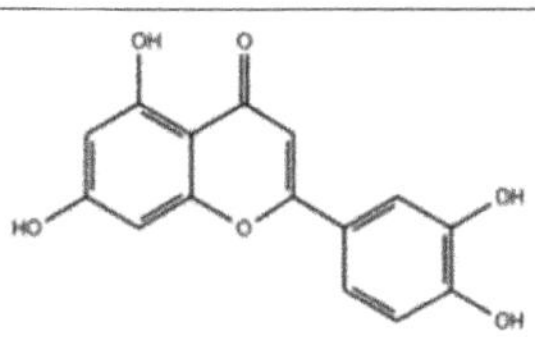	Luteolin	−6.65	SEE; LEE; FEE

Luteolin and emodin exhibit binding in the same pocket (see Figure 4B); luteolin forms hydrogen bonds with Pro131, Asp83, Phe90, and Ser88, whereas emodin interacts with Phe90 and Ser88 (Figure 4B). Additionally, three other compounds—aloesin, lututeolin 6-c glucoside, and aloinoside B—also bind to the same pocket as luteolin and emodin, while no compound binds in the acarbose binding site.

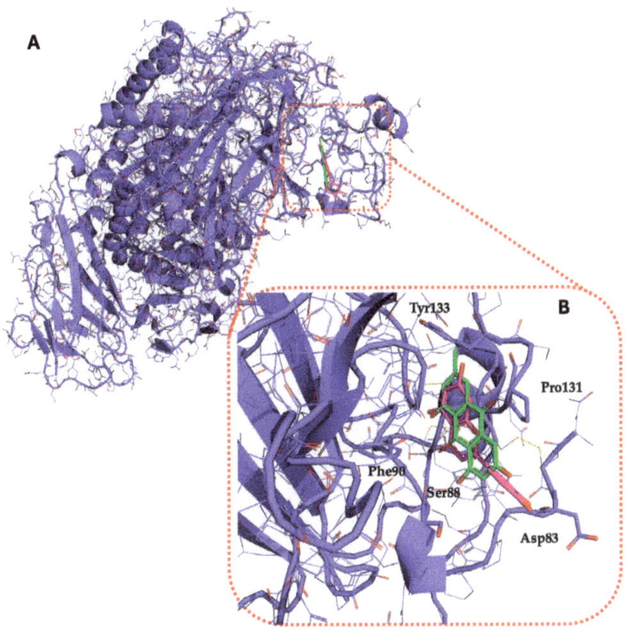

Figure 4. (**A**) Representation of luteolin (magenta) and emodin (green) in α-glucosidase (blue); (**B**) Luteolin (magenta) and emodin (green) show overlapping binding at the α-glucosidase binding site. The highlighted amino acids interact with two compounds.

3. Discussion

The findings from this study demonstrate the significant potential of *A. microcarpus* extracts in inhibiting the enzyme α-glucosidase. The EE exhibited strong inhibitory effects on α-glucosidase while showing minimal inhibition of α-amylase. This selective inhibition is beneficial as it aligns with the therapeutic goal of managing postprandial hyperglycemia in T2D without the gastrointestinal side effects associated with excessive α-amylase inhibition.

The inhibitory activity against α-glucosidase observed in the EE indicates a promising avenue for further development of *A. microcarpus* as a natural antidiabetic agent. The IC_{50} values for the EE are significantly lower than those of acarbose, a commonly used antidiabetic drug, suggesting that *A. microcarpus* extracts are highly potent inhibitors of α-glucosidase.

Additionally, the cell viability assays using Caco-2 cells confirmed that the EEs are not cytotoxic at concentrations up to 10 μg/mL, with cell viability remaining above 84%. The antioxidant activity and antimycotic assays further support the therapeutic potential of these extracts. The significant reduction in H_2O_2-induced ROS levels in Caco-2 cells treated with *A. microcarpus* extracts highlights their ability to mitigate oxidative stress, a common complication in diabetes.

The presence of phenolic compounds, particularly luteolin and its derivatives, is likely responsible for the observed biological activities [24]. Previous studies have shown that luteolin has strong inhibitory effects on both α-glucosidase and α-amylase, as well as potent antioxidant properties. The high concentrations of these compounds in the EE of *A. microcarpus* correlate well with the observed enzyme inhibition and antioxidant effects. Subsequently, we aimed to identify the specific compounds within the EE responsible for the inhibitory activity against α-glucosidase. Using molecular docking, we analyzed the interactions of 11 carefully selected compounds. These compounds included aloesin, which is present in all four ethanol extracts (S, L, T, and F), along with four compounds found in extract T and six compounds common to extracts S, L, and F. This selection ensured a comprehensive evaluation of potential inhibitors. The docking results revealed that only emodin, present in the T extract, and luteolin, present in three extracts (S, L, and F), exhibited significant binding affinity with α-glucosidase, suggesting their potential as inhibitors. The consistent presence of aloesin across all extracts had initially suggested its possible key role in the inhibition mechanism. However, this was not confirmed by the molecular docking studies and in vitro experiments.

In conclusion, this study underscores the therapeutic potential of *A. microcarpus* extracts in the management of T2D. The strong inhibitory effects on α-glucosidase, coupled with the antioxidant properties and lack of cytotoxicity, make these extracts promising candidates for further development as natural antidiabetic agents. On the other hand, these formulations have also demonstrated the ability to hinder the development of pathogenic *C. albicans* biofilm. This outcome is intriguing to contemplate, given that Candida infection frequently qualifies as a "biofilm-related infection". It is a condition that is particularly difficult to treat because it frequently escapes antimitotic treatments and it is especially common in diabetic patients.

Future research should focus on the isolation and characterization of individual bioactive compounds, their pharmacokinetics, and in vivo efficacy to fully elucidate the therapeutic potential of *A. microcarpus*.

4. Materials and Methods

4.1. Plants Materials

Samples of *A. microcarpus* subsp. *microcarpus* Salzm. et Viv., including stems, leaves, flowers, and tubers (S, L, F, and T), were collected. After identification, a voucher specimen (number 1405/16) was archived in the Herbarium of the Life and Environmental Sciences Department, CAG. Following collection, the plant materials were thoroughly cleansed with deionized water. To preserve their integrity and constituents, the samples were immediately frozen at a temperature of −80 °C. Subsequently, they were lyophilized in their original form to ensure the preservation of their natural structure and composition. The lyophilized plant material was pounded, and one gram was used for each extraction process. The materials were extracted using ethanol (ethanol extract, EE) for 24 h at room temperature, ensuring constant stirring to maximize efficiency. The extracts were then filtered and lyophilized to obtain dry powders. Before use, 1 mg of dried powders was dissolved in DMSO (1 mL) for EE.

4.2. α-Amylase Inhibitory Activity

α-Amylase inhibitory activity of extracts was evaluated using 2-chloro-4-nitrophenyl-α-D-maltotrioside (CNPG3) as a synthetic substrate. The assay mixture comprised 60 µL of 50 mM sodium phosphate buffer (pH 7.0), 20 µL of 1 M NaCl, and 40 µL of α-amylase from porcine pancreas (concentration 1 mg/mL). The mixture was incubated at 37 °C for 10 min in the absence or presence of extract. Acarbose was used as a standard inhibitor for comparison. After incubation, 80 µL of CNPG3 solution (2.5 mM) was added. The release of 2-chloro-nitrophenol, due to enzymatic hydrolysis, was monitored spectrophotometrically at 405 nm [25].

4.3. α-Glucosidase Inhibitory Activity

The procedure to assess the inhibitory activity of α-glucosidase consisted of 120 µL 0.1 M phosphate buffer (pH 6.8) and 40 µL of *Saccharomyces cerevisiae* enzyme solution (0.125 U/mL) extract (20 µL) at various concentrations mixed and incubated for 15 min at 37 °C. Then, 20 µL of the substrate p-nitrophenyl α-D-glucopyranoside (pNPG), at a concentration of 5 mM in 0.1 M phosphate buffer, was added and the mixture was incubated again under the same conditions. The reaction was halted by adding 50 µL of 0.2 M sodium carbonate. The *p*-nitrophenol produced in the reaction was quantified at 405 nm using a 96-well microplate reader. DMSO was used as a control, ensuring its final concentration stayed below 8% *v*/*v* to avoid any impact on enzyme activity. Acarbose again served as a positive control. The IC_{50} value, indicating the concentration needed to inhibit 50% of α-glucosidase activity, was determined under the assay conditions.

4.4. Antimycotic Activity

A multidrug-resistant (MDR) isolate of *C. albicans* (CA97) was used for the antifungal susceptibility test by using the microplate dilution method. On this strain we have evaluated the minimum inhibitory concentration (MIC) and minimum biofilm inhibitory concentration (MBIC) of *A. microcarpus* extracts.

The MIC protocol was performed following the Clinical and Laboratory Standards Institute (CLSI) by using the broth microdilution procedure [26,27]. Briefly: the experiment was performed in sterile 96-well microplates (Corning, CLS3788 Merck KGaA, Darmstadt, Germany) containing (1:2) serial dilutions of *A. microcarpus* extract (200 μL) diluted in Sabouraud dextrose broth (BD, Maryland, USA), and the final concentration ranged from 4 to 1.9×10^{-3} mg/mL. Therefore, we added to each well a suspension of *C. albicans* until we reached a final concentration of 10^5 CFU/mL in each well. The microplate was incubated at 37 °C in air. After 48 h of incubation, the plates were read with a microplate reader at 620 nm (Multiskan FC, Thermo Scientific, Monza, Italy). The MIC was the lowest concentration of an antimicrobial that showed the same turbidity value of the negative control (i.e., *Candida* suspension without formulate).

The biofilm protocol: We performed the evaluation of MBIC according to the modified crystal violet staining protocol, as previously reported [27]. *C. albicans* inoculum and the dilution formulation procedures were the same as those already described for the MIC experiments [27]. After 48 h of incubation time, the wells were gently washed three times with 150 μL of 0.9% saline solution. We then left the plate to dry for 30 min at 20 °C in a sterile laminar flow cabinet. Next, 200 μL of 20% acetic acid solution (Sigma) was added to each well, and biofilm was detached by vigorous pipetting. We conducted the experiment using three replicates and six wells serving as the negative control, containing only the growth medium. The plates were read with a microplate reader at 620 nm (Multiskan FC, Thermo Scientific) at 450 nm. The MBIC represented the lowest concentration of formula able to interfere with biofilm formation; in other words, the dilution showed the same absorbance value as the negative control.

4.5. Cell Viability

The MTT assay technique on Caco-2 cells was employed to assess cell viability. Caco-2 cells were maintained in standard conditions, with 5% CO_2, 95% relative humidity, and a temperature of 37 °C. The culture medium used was Dulbecco's modified Eagle's medium, enhanced with 1% penicillin/streptomycin (Euroclone, Milan, Italy) and supplemented with 10% fetal bovine serum (Gibco, Grand Island, NY, USA).

The cells were plated in 96-well plates at a density of 5×10^3 cells per well, treated with extracts at different concentrations (0–10 μg/mL) and then incubated for 24 h. Subsequently, an MTT solution (0.5 mg/mL) was added to cells and incubated for 3 h at 37 °C. The formazan crystals formed were dissolved in DMSO and the absorbance was measured at 590 nm to assess cell viability.

4.6. Dichlorofluorescein (DCF) Assay (or Intracellular ROS Levels)

The 2′,7′-dichlorofluorescein diacetate (DCFH-DA) method was used to measure intracellular reactive oxygen species (ROS) levels and evaluate the antioxidant activity of the extracts. Caco-2 cells were treated with the extract at various concentrations (0–10 μg/mL) for 24 h. Following this, the cells were incubated with 10 μM DCFH-DA at 37 °C for 30 min. After incubation, 2 mM H_2O_2 was added to each well. The fluorescence intensity of DCF was then measured at the excitation wavelength of 485 nm and emission wavelength of 530 nm. The fluorescence data were recorded over 60 min to evaluate the antioxidant activity of the samples.

4.7. (HR) HPLC-ESI-QToF MS and (HR) HPLC-ESI-QToF MS/MS Analysis of A. microcarpus Extracts

For the qualitative assessment of the plant extracts, the method outlined by Di Petrillo et al. [13] with some modifications [28] was used. Briefly, the analytical setup included an advanced ion mobility QToF LC/MS system equipped with a 1290 Infinity II UPLC and a 6560 IM-QToF (Agilent Technologies Inc., Palo Alto, CA, USA) and experiments were conducted using an electrospray ionization (ESI) source, set to operate in negative ion mode. Data acquisition and processing were performed using the Agilent MassHunter Workstation Acquisition software v. B.09.00 (Agilent Technologies, Palo Alto, CA, USA). ESI/QToF MS data were then analyzed using the MassHunter Workstation Qualitative Analysis software v. 10.0 (Agilent Technologies) and the MassHunter METLIN metabolite PCDLdatabase v. B.08.00 (Agilent Technologies) and Sirius® software v. 4.7.4 were used for the tentative identification of the metabolites and predict fragmentation and molecular formulae [22,29], along with comparing experimental MS/MS spectra with fragmentation patterns reported in the literature or with spectra reported in a public repository of mass spectral data (KNApSAcK Core System, n.d.).

4.8. Statistical Analyses

Statistical differences were evaluated using GraphPad software Version 8 (GraphPad Software, San Diego, CA, USA). Comparison between groups was assessed by one-way ANOVA followed by the Tukey test. The values with $p < 0.05$ were considered significant.

4.9. In Silico Studies

4.9.1. Protein and Ligand Preparation

The crystal structure of α-glucosidase 5NN4 [30] was selected from Protein Data Bank (RCSB PDB) [31]. Co-crystallized ligands were removed, and the resulting structure was prepared using the Protein Preparation Wizard (Schrödinger Release 2022-3), all hydrogen atoms were added, bond orders were adjusted, and formal charges were assigned. The appropriate ionization state was determined at pH 7.4 using the PROPKA tool. The protein minimization by OPLS4 force field to fix all molecular overlaps and strains was then performed. The restrained minimization was terminated when the average root mean square deviation (RMSD) of the non-hydrogen atoms was converged to 0.3 Å.

The compounds for docking were selected based on the results of compound identification in *A. microcarpus*. Specifically, aloesin, present in all extracts, eight compounds present in S, L, and F extracts, and emodin found solely in the T extract were chosen for further analysis. All ten compounds were subjected to conformational analysis using Quantum Mechanic (QM) Conformer and Tautomer Prediction by Jaguar (Schrödinger Release 2022-3) [32]. The best conformations obtained were prepared using LigPrep (Schrödinger Release 2022-3) preserving the specified chiralities, employing the OPLS4 force field.

4.9.2. Molecular Docking

Gasteiger charges [33] were assigned and the grids were generated using AutoGrid4.2 using whole protein. For AutoDock4.2 [34], docking experiments were carried out using the Lamarckian genetic algorithm [35,36], a total of 250 runs were performed with a population size of 250 individuals, and maximum numbers of evaluations were set at 2,500,000. Other parameters were kept as default.

5. Conclusions

This study highlights the promising potential of *Asphodelus microcarpus* extracts as effective natural inhibitors of α-glucosidase, a critical enzyme in the management of T2D. The findings demonstrate that the ethanolic extracts of *A. microcarpus* exhibit strong inhibitory activity on α-glucosidase, with IC_{50} values lower than that of acarbose, the standard antidiabetic drug. Conversely, the extracts showed minimal inhibition of α-amylase, indicating a beneficial selectivity that could help mitigate the gastrointestinal side effects commonly associated with excessive α-amylase inhibition.

Additionally, the extracts displayed antioxidant properties and were found not to be cytotoxic. This suggests that *A. microcarpus* not only holds potential for glycemic control but also may contribute to the reduction of oxidative stress, a significant factor in the complications of diabetes.

Further molecular docking studies identified luteolin and emodin as significant binders to the α-glucosidase enzyme, hinting at their roles as key bioactive components contributing to the observed enzyme inhibition. Although aloesin, present in all extracts, initially appeared relevant, it did not demonstrate the same binding affinity, indicating that the therapeutic potential lies more strongly with luteolin and emodin. Furthermore, these formulations have proven to effectively inhibit the growth of pathogenic *C. albicans* biofilm.

In summary, *A. microcarpus* represents a valuable source of natural compounds with potential application in T2D management, offering safer and effective alternatives or adjuncts to conventional treatments.

Author Contributions: Conceptualization, A.D.P. and S.F. (Sonia Floris); methodology, A.D.P., S.F. (Sonia Floris), G.O., S.F. (Sara Fais), C.S., S.O., C.I.G.T., and B.E.; software, C.S. and S.O.; validation, N.R.; formal analysis, C.S., S.O., N.R., and F.P.; investigation, A.D.P., S.F. (Sonia Floris), C.S., C.I.G.T., and S.O.; resources, A.F. and F.P.; data curation, B.E. and F.P.; writing—original draft preparation, A.D.P. and S.F. (Sonia Floris); writing—review and editing, A.F., A.D.P., S.F. (Sonia Floris), G.O., S.F. (Sara Fais), C.S., S.O., C.I.G.T., B.E., N.R., and F.P.; supervision, A.F.; project administration, A.D.P. and A.F. All authors have read and agreed to the published version of the manuscript.

Funding: This research received no external funding.

Institutional Review Board Statement: Not applicable.

Informed Consent Statement: Not applicable.

Data Availability Statement: The data underlying this article are available in the article.

Acknowledgments: We acknowledge the Centro Servizid'Ateneo per la Ricerca (CeSAR) core facility of the University of Cagliari (Italy) for the experiments performed with Agilent 6560 IM-QTOF, Giulio Ferino for assistance with the generation of LC-MS data, Alan Miho for technical support, and Eduardo Araujo de Oliveira for assistance with the hot plate test data and statistical analysis.

Conflicts of Interest: The authors declare no conflicts of interest.

References

1. Kumar, M.; Dev, S.; Khalid, M.U.; Siddenthi, S.M.; Noman, M.; John, C.; Akubuiro, C.; Haider, A.; Rani, R.; Kashif, M.; et al. The Bidirectional Link Between Diabetes and Kidney Disease: Mechanisms and Management. *Cureus* **2023**, *15*, e45615. [CrossRef] [PubMed]
2. Cerf, M.E. Beta Cell Dysfunction and Insulin Resistance. *Front. Endocrinol.* **2013**, *4*, 37. [CrossRef] [PubMed]
3. Nyenwe, E.A.; Jerkins, T.W.; Umpierrez, G.E.; Kitabchi, A.E. Management of Type 2 Diabetes: Evolving Strategies for the Treatment of Patients with Type 2 Diabetes. *Metab. Clin. Exp.* **2011**, *60*, 1–23. [CrossRef] [PubMed]
4. Wu, Z.G.; Jiang, W.; Nitin, M.; Bao, X.Q.; Chen, S.L.; Tao, Z.M. Characterizing Diversity Based on Nutritional and Bioactive Compositions of Yam Germplasm (*Dioscorea* spp.) Commonly Cultivated in China. *J. Food Drug Anal.* **2016**, *24*, 367–375. [CrossRef]
5. Mattio, L.M.; Marengo, M.; Parravicini, C.; Eberini, I.; Dallavalle, S.; Bonomi, F.; Iametti, S.; Pinto, A. Inhibition of Pancreatic α-Amylase by Resveratrol Derivatives: Biological Activity and Molecular Modelling Evidence for Cooperativity between Viniferin Enantiomers. *Molecules* **2019**, *24*, 3225. [CrossRef]
6. Rasoulpoor, S.; Shohaimi, S.; Salari, N.; Vaisi-Raygani, A.; Rasoulpoor, S.; Shabani, S.; Jalali, R.; Mohammadi, M. *Candida albicans* Skin Infection in Patients with Type 2 Diabetes: A Systematic Review and Meta-Analysis. *J. Diabetes Metab. Disord.* **2021**, *20*, 665–672. [CrossRef]
7. Dadar, M.; Tiwari, R.; Karthik, K.; Chakraborty, S.; Shahali, Y.; Dhama, K. *Candida albicans*—Biology, Molecular Characterization, Pathogenicity, and Advances in Diagnosis and Control—An Update. *Microb. Pathog.* **2018**, *117*, 128–138. [CrossRef]
8. Kumar, S.; Narwal, S.; Kumar, V.; Prakash, O. α-Glucosidase Inhibitors from Plants: A Natural Approach to Treat Diabetes. *Pharmacogn. Rev.* **2011**, *5*, 19–29. [CrossRef]

9. Floris, S.; Fais, A.; Medda, R.; Pintus, F.; Piras, A.; Kumar, A.; Kuś, P.M.; Westermark, G.T.; Era, B. *Washingtonia filifera* Seed Extracts Inhibit the Islet Amyloid Polypeptide Fibrils Formations and α-Amylase and α-Glucosidase Activity. *J. Enzym. Inhib. Med. Chem.* **2021**, *36*, 517–524. [CrossRef]
10. Proença, C.; Freitas, M.; Ribeiro, D.; Oliveira, E.F.T.; Sousa, J.L.C.; Tomé, S.M.; Ramos, M.J.; Silva, A.M.S.; Fernandes, P.A.; Fernandes, E. α-Glucosidase Inhibition by Flavonoids: An in Vitro and in Silico Structure–Activity Relationship Study. *J. Enzym. Inhib. Med. Chem.* **2017**, *32*, 1216–1228. [CrossRef]
11. Proença, C.; Freitas, M.; Ribeiro, D.; Tomé, S.M.; Oliveira, E.F.T.; Viegas, M.F.; Araújo, A.N.; Ramos, M.J.; Silva, A.M.S.; Fernandes, P.A.; et al. Evaluation of a Flavonoids Library for Inhibition of Pancreatic α-Amylase towards a Structure–Activity Relationship. *J. Enzym. Inhib. Med. Chem.* **2019**, *34*, 577–588. [CrossRef] [PubMed]
12. Dioguardi, M.; Campanella, P.; Cocco, A.; Arena, C.; Malagnino, G.; Sovereto, D.; Aiuto, R.; Laino, L.; Laneve, E.; Dioguardi, A.; et al. Possible Uses of Plants of the Genus Asphodelus in Oral Medicine. *Biomedicines* **2019**, *7*, 67. [CrossRef] [PubMed]
13. Di Petrillo, A.; González-Paramás, A.M.; Era, B.; Medda, R.; Pintus, F.; Santos-Buelga, C.; Fais, A. Tyrosinase Inhibition and Antioxidant Properties of *Asphodelus microcarpus* Extracts. *BMC Complement. Altern. Med.* **2016**, *16*, 453. [CrossRef] [PubMed]
14. Mayouf, N.; Charef, N.; Saoudi, S.; Baghiani, A.; Khennouf, S.; Arrar, L. Antioxidant and Anti-Inflammatory Effect of *Asphodelus microcarpus* Methanolic Extracts. *J. Ethnopharmacol.* **2019**, *239*, 111914. [CrossRef]
15. Di Petrillo, A.; Fais, A.; Pintus, F.; Santos-Buelga, C.; González-Paramás, A.M.; Piras, V.; Orrù, G.; Mameli, A.; Tramontano, E.; Frau, A. Broad-Range Potential of *Asphodelus microcarpus* Leaves Extract for Drug Development. *BMC Microbiol.* **2017**, *17*, 159. [CrossRef]
16. Kim, J.S.; Kwon, C.S.; Son, K.H. Inhibition of Alpha-Glucosidase and Amylase by Luteolin, a Flavonoid. *Biosci. Biotechnol. Biochem.* **2000**, *64*, 2458–2461. [CrossRef]
17. Jaiswal, R.; Deshpande, S.; Kuhnert, N. Profling the Chlorogenic Acids of Rudbeckia Hirta, Helianthus Tuberosus, Carlina Acaulis and Symphyotrichum Novae-Angliae Leavesby LC-MSn. *Phytochem. Anal.* **2011**, *22*, 432–441. [CrossRef]
18. Abosedera, D.A.; Emara, S.A.; Tamam, O.A.S.; Badr, O.M.; Khalifa, S.A.M.; El-Seedi, H.R.; Refaey, M.S. Metabolomic Profile and in Vitro Evaluation of the Cytotoxic Activity of *Asphodelus microcarpus* against Human Malignant Melanoma Cells A375. *Arab. J. Chem.* **2022**, *15*, 104174. [CrossRef]
19. Ghoneim, M.M.; Ma, G.; El-Hela, A.A.; Mohammad, A.E.I.; Kottob, S.; El-Ghaly, S.; Cutler, S.J.; Ross, S.A. Biologically Active Secondary Metabolites from *Asphodelus microcarpus*. *Nat. Prod. Commun.* **2013**, *8*, 1117–1119. [CrossRef]
20. El Sayed, A.M.; Ezzat, S.M.; El Naggar, M.M.; El Hawary, S.S. In Vivo Diabetic Wound Healing Effect and HPLC–DAD–ESI–MS/MS Profiling of the Methanol Extracts of Eight Aloe Species. *Rev. Bras. Farmacogn.* **2016**, *26*, 352–362. [CrossRef]
21. Lazarova, I.; Zengin, G.; Sinan, K.I.; Aneva, I.; Uysal, S.; Picot-Allain, M.C.N.; Aktumsek, A.; Bouyahya, A.; Mahomoodally, M.F. Metabolomics Profiling and Biological Properties of Root Extracts from Two Asphodelus Species: *A. albus* and *A. aestivus*. *Food Res. Int.* **2020**, *134*, 109277. [CrossRef] [PubMed]
22. Hoffmann, M.A.; Nothias, L.F.; Ludwig, M.; Fleischauer, M.; Gentry, E.C.; Witting, M.; Dorrestein, P.C.; Dührkop, K.; Böcker, S. High-Confidence Structural Annotation of Metabolites Absent from Spectral Libraries. *Nat. Biotechnol.* **2022**, *40*, 411–421. [CrossRef] [PubMed]
23. Yang, D.; Zhao, J.; Liu, S.; Song, F.; Liu, Z. The Screening of Potential α-Glucosidase Inhibitors from the *Polygonum multiflorum* Extract Using Ultrafiltration Combined with Liquid Chromatography-Tandem Mass Spectrometry. *Anal. Methods* **2014**, *6*, 3353–3359. [CrossRef]
24. Yan, J.; Zhang, G.; Pan, J.; Wang, Y. α-Glucosidase Inhibition by Luteolin: Kinetics, Interaction and Molecular Docking. *Int. J. Biol. Macromol.* **2014**, *64*, 213–223. [CrossRef]
25. Delogu, G.L.; Era, B.; Floris, S.; Medda, R.; Sogos, V.; Pintus, F.; Gatto, G.; Kumar, A.; Westermark, G.T.; Fais, A. A New Biological Prospective for the 2-Phenylbenzofurans as Inhibitors of α-Glucosidase and of the Islet Amyloid Polypeptide Formation. *Int. J. Biol. Macromol.* **2021**, *169*, 428–435. [CrossRef]
26. Scano, A.; Mereu, E.; Cabras, V.; Mannias, G.; Garau, A.; Pilloni, M.; Orr, G.; Scano, A.; Ennas, G. Green Preparation of Antimicrobial 1D-Coordination Polymers: $[Zn(4,4'\text{-}bipy)Cl_2]_\infty$ and $[Zn(4,4'\text{-}bipy)_2(OAc)_2]_\infty$ by Ultrasonication of Zn(II) Salts and 4,4′-Bipyridine. *Molecules* **2022**, *27*, 6677. [CrossRef]
27. Manca, M.L.; Usach, I.; Peris, J.E.; Ibba, A.; Orrù, G.; Valenti, D.; Escribano-Ferrer, E.; Gomez-Fernandez, J.C.; Aranda, F.J.; Fadda, A.M.; et al. Optimization of Innovative Three-Dimensionally-Structured Hybrid Vesicles to Improve the Cutaneous Delivery of Clotrimazole for the Treatment of Topical Candidiasis. *Pharmaceutics* **2019**, *11*, 263. [CrossRef]
28. De Luca, M.; Lucchesi, D.; Tuberoso, C.I.G.; Fernàndez-Busquets, X.; Vassallo, A.; Martelli, G.; Fadda, A.M.; Pucci, L.; Caddeo, C. Liposomal Formulations to Improve Antioxidant Power of Myrtle Berry Extract for Potential Skin Application. *Pharmaceutics* **2022**, *14*, 910. [CrossRef]
29. Dührkop, K.; Fleischauer, M.; Ludwig, M.; Aksenov, A.A.; Melnik, A.V.; Meusel, M.; Dorrestein, P.C.; Rousu, J.; Böcker, S. SIRIUS 4: A Rapid Tool for Turning Tandem Mass Spectra into Metabolite Structure Information. *Nat. Methods* **2019**, *16*, 299–302. [CrossRef]
30. Roig-Zamboni, V.; Cobucci-Ponzano, B.; Iacono, R.; Ferrara, M.C.; Germany, S.; Bourne, Y.; Parenti, G.; Moracci, M.; Sulzenbacher, G. Structure of Human Lysosomal Acid α-Glucosidase-A Guide for the Treatment of Pompe Disease. *Nat. Commun.* **2017**, *8*, 1111. [CrossRef]

31. Berman, H.M.; Westbrook, J.; Feng, Z.; Gilliland, G.; Bhat, T.N.; Weissig, H.; Shindyalov, I.N.; Bourne, P.E. The Protein Data Bank. *Nucleic Acids Res.* **2000**, *28*, 235–242. [CrossRef] [PubMed]
32. Bochevarov, A.D.; Harder, E.; Hughes, T.F.; Greenwood, J.R.; Braden, D.A.; Philipp, D.M.; Rinaldo, D.; Halls, M.D.; Zhang, J.; Friesner, R.A. Jaguar: A High-Performance Quantum Chemistry Software Program with Strengths in Life and Materials Sciences. *Int. J. Quantum Chem.* **2013**, *113*, 2110–2142. [CrossRef]
33. Gasteiger, J.; Marsili, M. A New Model for Calculating Atomic Charges in Molecules. *Tetrahedron Lett.* **1978**, *19*, 3181–3184. [CrossRef]
34. Augusto, M.; Sallem, S.; de Sousa, S.A.; e Silva, F.J.d.S. AutoGrid: Towards an Autonomic Grid Middleware. In Proceedings of the 16th IEEE International Workshops on Enabling Technologies: Infrastructure for Collaborative Enterprises (WETICE 2007), Evry, France, 18–20 June 2007; pp. 223–228. [CrossRef]
35. Moitessier, N.; Englebienne, P.; Lee, D.; Lawandi, J.; Corbeil, C.R. Towards the Development of Universal, Fast and Highly Accurate Docking/Scoring Methods: A Long Way to Go. *Br. J. Pharmacol.* **2008**, *153*, 7–26. [CrossRef]
36. Meng, X.Y.; Zhang, H.X.; Mezei, M.; Cui, M. Molecular Docking: A Powerful Approach for Structure-Based Drug Discovery. *Curr. Comput.-Aided Drug Des.* **2011**, *7*, 146–157. [CrossRef]

molecules

MDPI

Article

The *n*-Butanol Extract Obtained from the Inner Bark of *Tabebuia rosea* (Bertol.) DC, Specioside, and Catalposide Induce Leukemia Cell Apoptosis in the Presence of Apicidin

Nancy Yadira Guerrero-Pepinosa [1,2], Luz Angela Veloza [3] and Juan Carlos Sepúlveda-Arias [1,*]

1 Grupo Infección e Inmunidad, Facultad de Ciencias de la Salud, Universidad Tecnológica de Pereira, Pereira 660003, Colombia; nancygue@unicauca.edu.co
2 Facultad de Ciencias Naturales, Exactas y de la Educación, Programa de Biología, Universidad del Cauca, Popayán 190001, Colombia
3 Grupo Polifenoles, Facultad de Tecnologías, Escuela de Química, Universidad Tecnológica de Pereira, Pereira 660003, Colombia; lveloza@utp.edu.co
* Correspondence: jcsepulv@utp.edu.co

Abstract: The cell signaling pathways involved in the antiproliferative activities of *T. rosea* inner bark remain unexplored. This study evaluated the apoptotic effects of two iridoids from the inner bark of *T. rosea* and apicidin on THP-1 cells. The cytotoxic effects of the extract and the pure compounds on THP-1 and Jurkat cells were also evaluated using the MTT assay. The apoptotic effect was determined by measuring the mitochondrial membrane potential. The expression of mRNA and MAPK kinase, Bax, and Bcl-2 proteins was detected by Western blotting and RT–qPCR, respectively. The extract and the compounds evaluated increased the percentage of apoptotic cells. Depolarization of the mitochondrial membrane was observed, and the number of cells in the G0/G1 phase increased. Catalposide and specioside significantly increased p38 protein expression, mostly in cells pretreated with apicidin. The p38 MAPK signaling pathway is at least one of the pathways by which the *n*-butanol extract obtained from *Tabebuia rosea*, catalposide, and specioside exerts its apoptotic effect on THP-1 cells, and this effect generates a response in the G0/G1 phase and subsequent cell death. In addition, there was depolarization of the mitochondrial membrane, an effect that was related to the participation of the proapoptotic protein Bax.

Keywords: *Tabebuia rosea*; catalposide; specioside; apicidin; iridoids; cytotoxicity; apoptosis; cancer; antineoplastic agents

1. Introduction

Currently, cancer is a significant public health problem in terms of morbidity and mortality in developing countries; leukemia is a frequent cancer type and is among the fifteen most common news cases and deaths [1,2]. The most common cancer in children is leukemia, accounting for 30% of cases [3]. Worldwide, in children under 15 years of age, cancer does not represent more than 3% of all malignancies, but it has high mortality rates, especially acute pediatric leukemia [2]; this cancer is characterized by an increase in several abnormal white blood cells that can be either lymphoid or myeloid in origin. Chemoresistance in cancer cells and nonselective cytotoxic effects are troublesome treatments because they decrease the quality of life of leukemia patients. Therefore, research into novel therapeutic agents is essential for effectively treating leukemia.

Ethnopharmacological knowledge about the use of plants to treat diseases has facilitated the identification of therapeutic agents against many diseases, such as cancer. Approximately 75% of the drugs used for cancer treatment are derived from or inspired by plants [4,5]. Various plant extracts have a strong potential to modulate apoptotic pathways [6]. Indeed, the World Health Organization (WHO) reported that various plant fractions and their active constituents are used as traditional medicines by a large part of the population [7,8].

The Bignoneaceae family is considered the second most abundant family of woody plant species in Neotropical dry forests [9] and includes 100 genera and 827 species [10,11]. In addition, indigenous cultures in South America traditionally use some of the Bignonaceae genus for different medical purposes, such as depurative, laxative, blood dysfunction, and leukemia, as well as for cultural practices, such as dyeing in ritual body paintings and protecting the skin against sunlight or repelling insects [12–14]. Plants of the genus *Tabebuia* (*Handroanthus*) belong to the Biognonaceae family and are Neotropical trees and shrubs that are distributed mainly in Central and South America, with relatively low contributions to African, Malagasy and Southeast Asian tropical forests [15]. There is some evidence supporting the ethnobotanical and traditional use of the genus *Tabebuia* as antimicrobial, anti-inflammatory, and anticancer agents [16–18], and several in vitro and in vivo studies have demonstrated its antiproliferative, anti-inflammatory, antioxidant, and antiparasitic activities [19–23].

Tabebuia rosea (Bertol.) DC, commonly called a pink trumpet, rosy trumpet tree, or guayacan, is an evergreen tree; this plant has several molecules with antiproliferative activity, such as naphthoquinones and iridoids [24–26]. Iridoids are naturally occurring heterocyclic monoterpenoids, such as catalposide and specioside. Several molecules with antiproliferative activity can destroy cancer cells through apoptosis, activating proapoptotic proteins such as Bax. Abnormalities in apoptotic mechanisms are hallmarks of cancer cells, and agents that activate programmed cell death could be valuable in cancer therapeutics [27]. Cell cycle control is one of the central regulatory mechanisms of cell growth. The MAPK family, which comprises serine/threonine protein kinases, is involved in the extracellular signal-regulated kinase (ERK), c-Jun-N-terminal kinase (JNK), and p38-MAPK signaling pathways; these proteins may participate in diverse cellular programs, such as the differentiation and arrest of cell cycle checkpoints, leading to apoptotic processes [28]. Indeed, p38 MAPK is a popular target in the pharmaceutical industry [29].

A promising field in current therapies based on plant-derived compounds is the study of their synergistic activity when they are administered in combination with other molecules with anticancer potential [30]. Thus, in this study, a histone deacetylase inhibitor (HDCi) was used in combination with the inner bark extract obtained from *Tabebuia rosea* as well as with two iridoids (Specioside and Catalposide) isolated previously from *T. rosea* to observe whether there was an increase in the number of apoptotic cells; apicidin (APC) is a potent HDACi that selectively binds to class I histone deacetylases (HDACs) and interferes with the deacetylation process. This process remodels chromatin and modifies the expression of genes related to apoptotic processes [31,32]. Notably, combination therapy is a strategy for overcoming resistance to anticancer drugs [33].

2. Results and Discussion

2.1. Phytochemical Analysis

A preliminary phytochemical analysis of extracts prepared from the inner bark of *T. rosea*, including the *n*-butanol extract, revealed the presence of flavonoids, lignans, terpenes, aldehydes, ketones, and unsaturated fatty acids. The results are supplied in the Supplementary Materials (Table S1).

2.2. Effect of the n-Butanol Extract on Cell Viability

Recently, drugs of a natural origin, due to their lower side effects, have been considered essential for treating several human diseases [34]. When evaluating compounds with antitumor potential, it is necessary to conduct tests to determine the selectivity of the compounds toward tumor cell lines of interest to strengthen the preclinical tests required for validation as pharmacological agents [35]. The *n*-butanol extract obtained from the inner bark of *Tabebuia rosea* and the evaluated compounds (catalposide and specioside) presented concentration-dependent cytotoxic effects on THP-1 and Jurkat cells, mainly after 24 h of treatment. Compared with that of the control cells, the viability of the THP-1 cells treated with the extracts at concentrations ranging from 10, 50, 100, and 200 μg/mL was significantly lower ($p < 0.05$) (Figure 1). Similar results were obtained with extracts from the inner bark of *Tabebuia pallida* in Ehrlich ascites carcinoma (EAC) cells, where viability was inhibited below 50% at 24 h at concentrations of 8–120 μg/mL [36]. The IC_{50} values for the *n*-butanol extract, catalposide, and specioside at 24 h were 44.7, 43.9, and 40.3 μg/mL, respectively (Table 1). These concentrations are similar to those reported by Rahman et al. for the inner bark extract of *T. pallida* [36]. According to Kuete and Effath (2015), the compounds evaluated in that study have moderate cytotoxicity since, at 24 h of exposure, the IC_{50} was in the range of 20–50 μg/mL [37].

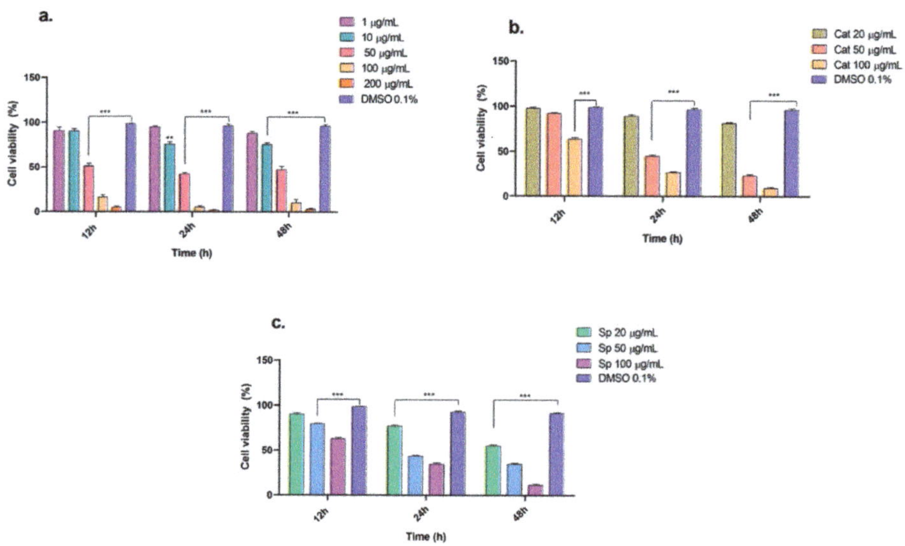

Figure 1. Viability of THP-1 cells in presence of (**a**) *n*-butanol extract, (**b**) catalposide, and (**c**) specioside at different incubation times (12, 24 and 48 h). ** $p \leq 0.01$, *** $p \leq 0.001$. ANOVA, Bonferroni post hoc correction.

Table 1. IC_{50} (μg/mL) and SI of the *n*-butanol extract of *T. rosea*, catalposide, specioside, and doxorubicin in THP-1 and Jurkat cells (median ± SD, $n = 3$).

Time		12 h			24 h			48 h	
Cell Line	**Jurkat**	**THP-1**	**PBMC**	**Jurkat**	**THP-1**	**PBMC**	**Jurkat**	**THP-1**	**PBMC**
Extract	314.8 ± 2.2	35.3 ± 3.2	340.5 ± 2.22	189.5 ± 0.5	44.7 ± 4.082	123.64 ± 5.2	354.3 ± 0.1	36.44 ± 1.4	99.4 ± 4.7
SI	1.08	**9.64**		0.65	**2.77**		0.28	**2.72**	
Catalposide	106.74 ± 5.3	121.6 ± 3.3	125.67 ± 2.8	92.77 ± 1.5	43.86 ± 2.2	87.7 ± 3.1	71.16 ± 2.8	30.16 ± 1.67	43.4 ± 3.4
SI	1.18	1.03		0.94	1.99		0.61	1.44	
Specioside	137.66 ± 1.3	47.25 ± 2.3	165.25 ± 3.1	81.71 ± 3.5	40.32 ± 1.3	70.66 ± 3.7	68.86 ± 2.1	26.33 ± 6.8	54.22 ± 3.7
SI	1.20	**3.49**		0.86	1.75		0.79	**2.06**	
Doxorubicin (μg/mL)	0.339 ± 1.2	1.268 ± 0.2	1.364 ± 0.15	0.258 ± 0.1	0.189 ± 0.1	0.224 ± 0.1	0.050 ± 0.0	0.005 ± 0.01	0.018 ± 0.1
SI	**4.02**	1.07		0.86	1.183		0.36	**3.6**	

2.3. Selectivity Index

In terms of the selectivity of the compounds, the *n*-butanol extract and the compounds were selective for the THP-1 cell line, mainly at 24 h, since the selectivity indices are between two and three, whereas for the Jurkat cell line, the SI was lower than one (Table 1). The differences in cytotoxicity between Jurkat and the THP-1 cells can be explained by the presence of intracellular signaling proteins, such as caveolin 1, that can affect membrane transport and the cell cycle. Some studies report an increase in the expression of this protein in cells of myeloid origin, increasing the sensitivity of these cells to molecules with antiproliferative potential [38,39]. In the literature, extracts or molecules with SI values of two or more are considered to be selective for tumor cells; this means that the evaluated compound is twice as cytotoxic for the tumor cell line as it is for normal cells [40]. Peripheral blood mononuclear cells (PBMCs) were used as normal cells. Considering the results obtained, apoptosis assays were performed in the THP-1 cell line.

2.4. Nuclear Morphology of Cells Treated with an n-Butanol Extract from the Inner Bark of Tabebuia rosea and Pretreated with Apicidin

THP-1 cells were exposed to high, medium, or low concentrations of the extract for 24 h (Figure 2). Compared with the control, the *n*-butanol extract increased the number of cells with nuclear fragmentation, suggesting that the *n*-butanol extract has an apoptotic effect on THP-1 cells. Similarly, studies with oral carcinoma cells revealed increased internucleosomal DNA fragmentation after treatment with β-lapachone and its 3-iodine derivatives isolated from *T. avellanedae* extract [28]. In this study, pretreatment with APC increased apoptosis in cells treated with the lowest concentration of the extract (25 μg/mL). HDAC inhibitors such as apicidin have been shown to modify the expression of different genes related to cell cycle regulation, growth inhibition, and apoptosis induction [41].

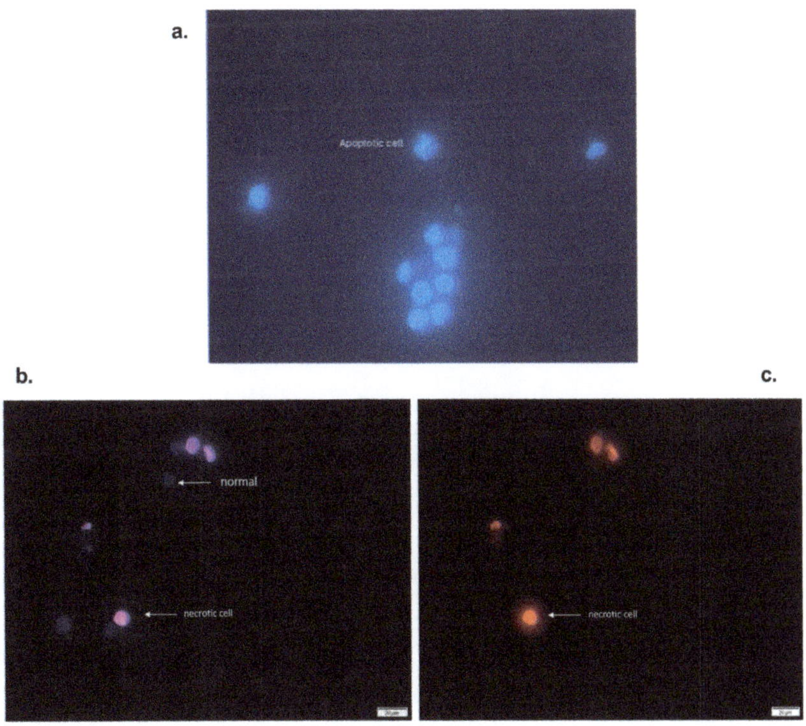

Figure 2. Viable and apoptotic THP-1 cells (with fragmented nuclei) were exposed to different concentrations of the *n*-butanol extract obtained from the inner bark of *T. rosea* for 24 h. (**a**) Viable (normal) THP-1 cells marked with Hoechst 33342. (**b**) THP-1 cells stained with propidium iodide were observed, and necrotic cells were detected. In contrast, viable cells are not observed because propidium iodide is not permeable (**c**).

These results are similar to those reported by Kwon et al., who reported that APC induces nuclear fragmentation and decreases nuclear size in HL-60 cells [42]. Another study revealed that in addition to nuclear fragmentation, APC induces apoptosis through the intrinsic pathway because it increases the level of cytochrome c and the regulation of caspase 3, 7, and 9 [43]. Moreover, a change in the membrane morphology of Ishikawa cells, from a polygonal or elongated shape to a filamentous shape, was observed after 24 h of APC treatment [44]. In this study, no changes were observed in the shape of the cell membrane, and only characteristic changes in apoptotic processes, such as nuclear fragmentation, were observed.

2.5. *Effects of Extract, Specioside, and Catalposide on Cell Apoptosis*

Apoptosis can prevent carcinogenic processes, eliminating or inhibiting the development of abnormal cells. Therefore, the induction of cancer cell apoptosis is necessary to determine the antiproliferative properties of various agents and compounds with anticancer activity [45]. The concentrations of the *n*-butanol extract evaluated in THP-1 cells at 24 h resulted in a greater percentage of early apoptotic cells. Similarly, the molecule naphthofurandione, which is present in the inner bark of *Tabebuia*, has been shown to have apoptotic effects on breast cancer cells by increasing the expression of proapoptotic proteins such as Bax [46]. Compared with catalposide or specioside treatment, apicidin pretreatment increased the percentage of apoptotic cells (Figure 3), which, at the same exposure time, increased the percentage of late apoptotic cells. Notably, only plant extracts contain bioactive molecules such as sugars, fatty acids, and antioxidants that can affect the activation of cell death pathways. In contrast, isolated compounds can directly affect late apoptosis [47].

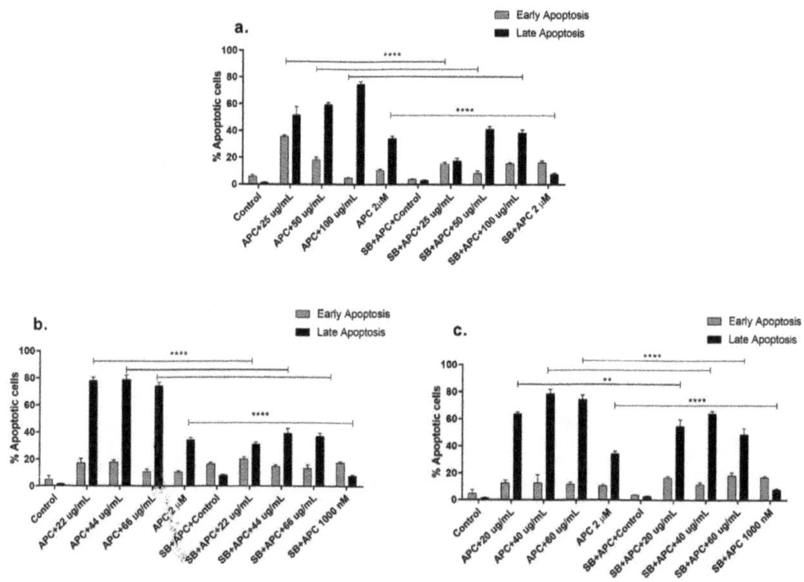

Figure 3. Apoptosis of THP-1 cells stained with annexin V-CF647 and 7-AAD at different concentrations of (**a**) *n*-butanol extract, (**b**) catalposide, (**c**) and specioside for 24 h and pretreated with APC and the p38 inhibitor SB202190 (SB) at 5 μM. ** $p \leq 0.05$ **** $p \leq 0.0001$. ANOVA, Bonferroni post hoc correction.

In addition to having a more significant effect on early apoptosis, the *n*-butanol extract also significantly increased ($p < 0.05$) the depolarization of the mitochondrial membrane (Figure 4) and the expression of *Bax* and *MAPK14* mRNAs at a concentration of 25 μg/mL

(Figures 5 and 6). However, no significant change in the protein expression of Bax or Bcl-2 was observed compared with those in the control group. In addition, *Bcl-2* mRNA expression was significantly decreased at several concentrations tested, except for 50 µg/mL, 100 µg/mL, and 25 µg/mL with APC pretreatment. It is essential to highlight that new transcripts of the *Bax* gene have been found in different tissues, where the encoded proteins undergo post-translational modifications that could reduce the detection of the protein with the Western blot technique [48].

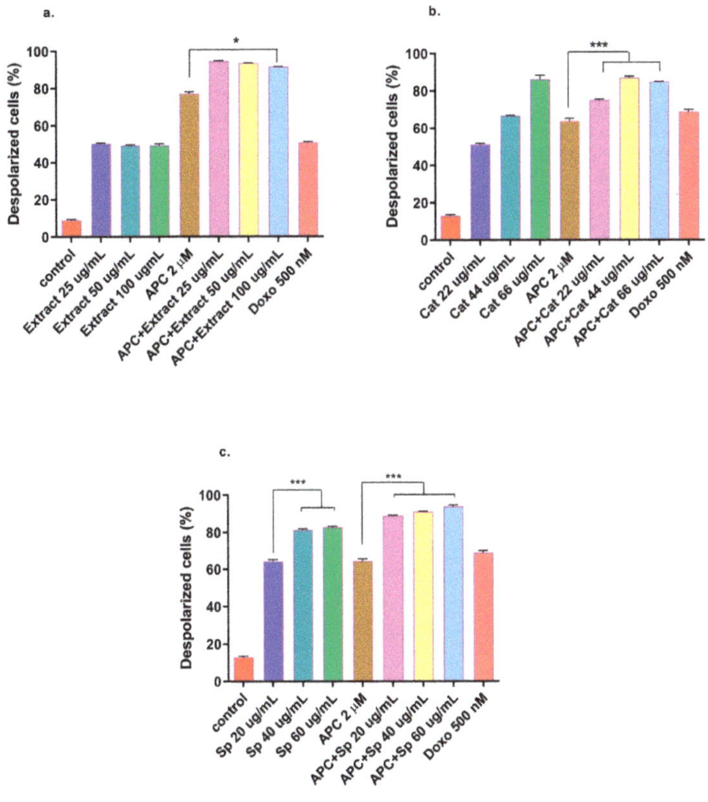

Figure 4. THP-1 cells with mitochondrial membrane depolarization were labeled with JC-1 and exposed to (**a**) the *n*-butanol extract obtained from the inner bark of *T. rosea* or (**b**) catalposide (Cat). (**c**) Specioside (Sp.) treatment for 24 h and pretreatment with APC for 24 h. * $p \leq 0.05$ *** $p \leq 0.001$. ANOVA, Tukey's post hoc test.

In this study, compared with the control, THP-1 cells treated with catalposide or specioside presented increased apoptosis (Supplementary Materials, Figure S5). However, Saracoglu and Harpuin reported that in Hep-G2 cells, catalposide only had cytotoxic and cytostatic effects [49]. Therefore, iridoid glucosides such as catalposide may have different effects depending on the type of cancer cell.

Therefore, pretreatment with catalposide and specioside (44 and 40 µg/mL) in combination with APC induced apoptosis through the intrinsic pathway because of decreased Bcl-2 protein expression and mitochondrial membrane polarization and consequently increased expression of the Bax protein at all concentrations of the compounds and the extract used. Additionally, the conserved binding domains of Bax heterodimerize with those of Bcl-2 to decrease its antiapoptotic capacity [50]. Under normal conditions, the Bax protein is located in the cytoplasm and, in the presence of apoptotic stimuli, it migrates to the outer membrane of the mitochondria, generating the opening of the mitochondrial pores and the subsequent release of cytochrome-c into the cytoplasm [48].

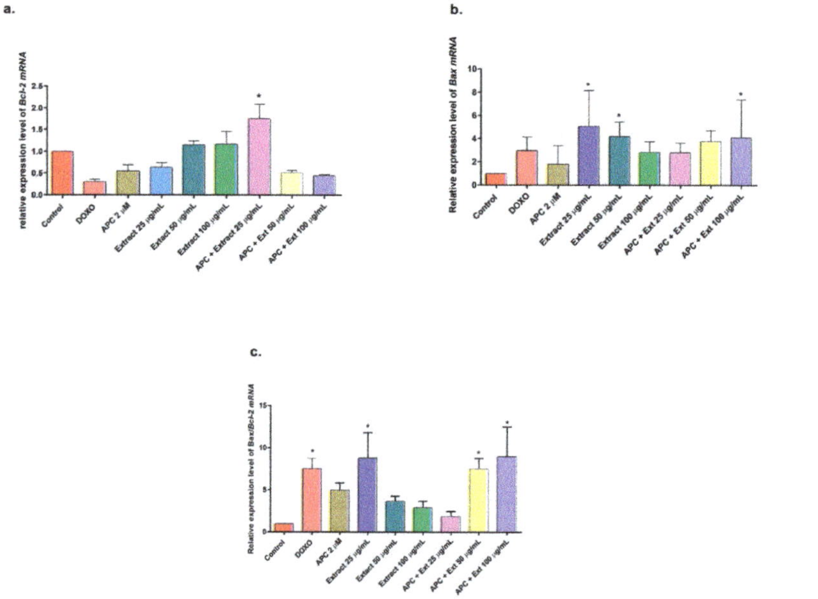

Figure 5. Gene expression: BCL2 and BAX genes in THP-1 cells treated with the *n*-butanol extract at different concentrations and pretreated with APC for 24 h. (**a**) BCL2 expression. (**b**) BAX expression. (**c**) Relative expression of the BAX/BCL2 genes. * $p \leq 0.05$. Kruskal–Wallis, Dunn's post hoc test.

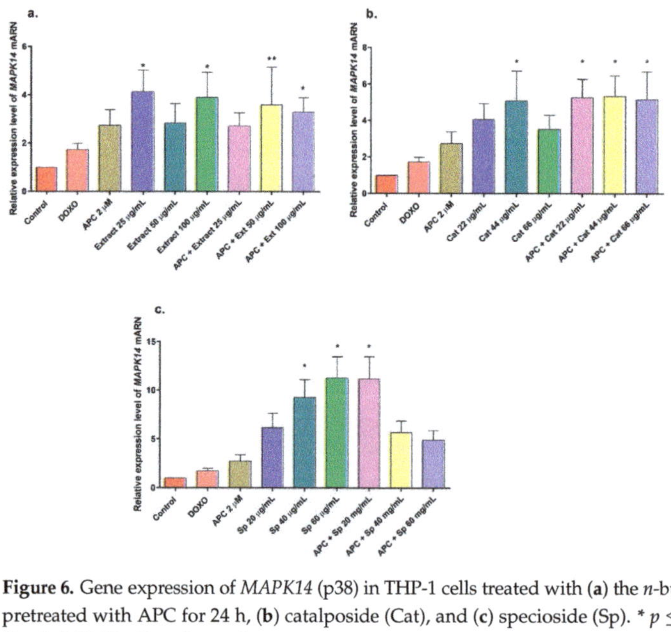

Figure 6. Gene expression of *MAPK14* (p38) in THP-1 cells treated with (**a**) the *n*-butanol extract and pretreated with APC for 24 h, (**b**) catalposide (Cat), and (**c**) specioside (Sp). * $p \leq 0.05$, ** $p \leq 0.01$. Kruskal–Wallis, Dunn's post hoc test.

In this study, APC decreased mitochondrial membrane polarization, and some studies reported that APC induced the accumulation of reactive oxygen species and the loss of the mitochondrial membrane potential in neuroblastoma cells [51]. Catalposide at concentrations of 44 μg/mL and 66 μg/mL, specioside at concentrations of 20 μg/mL, 40 μg/mL, and 60 μg/mL, and pretreatment with APC increased the expression of *Bax* mRNA and protein (Figures 7 and 8).

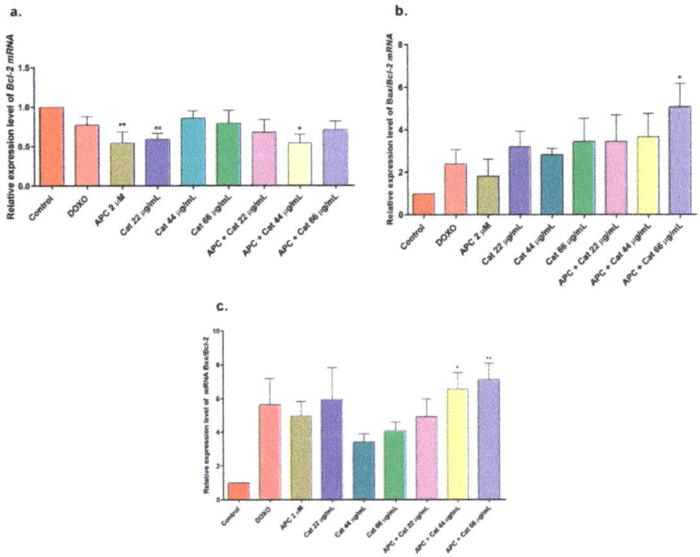

Figure 7. Gene expression: BCL2 and BAX in THP-1 cells treated with catalposide (Cat) and pretreated with APC for 24 h. (**a**) BCL2 expression; (**b**) BAX expression; (**c**) relative expression of the BAX/BCL2 genes. * $p \leq 0.05$, ** $p \leq 0.01$. Kruskal–Wallis, Dunn's post hoc test.

When the concentration of catalposide was 44 μg/mL and that of specioside was 40 μg/mL, APC decreased the expression of *Bcl-2* mRNA. Therefore, the mean concentrations of catalposide and specioside, 44 μg/mL and 40 μg/mL, respectively, promoted apoptosis through the intrinsic pathway because of a decrease in the antiapoptotic protein Bcl-2 and an increase in the proapoptotic protein Bax (Figure 9). Additionally, a decrease in mitochondrial membrane polarization was observed at all concentrations of the compounds and the extract. The conserved binding domains of Bax heterodimerize with those of Bcl-2 to decrease its antiapoptotic capacity [50]. Under normal conditions, the Bax protein is located in the cytoplasm and, in the presence of apoptotic stimuli, migrates to the outer membrane of the mitochondria, generating the opening of the mitochondrial pores and the subsequent release of cytochrome c into the cytoplasm [48].

Some studies have reported the antiproliferative effects of the inner bark of *Tabebuia avellanedae* in MCF-7AROM cells and the extract of *Tabebuia pallida* leaves in the cancerous cells of Erlich's ascites, which resulted in the overexpression of the *BAX* gene and decreased the expression of *BCL2* [36,46]. The evaluation of the apoptotic effect of the inner bark extract of *T. avellanedae* and some isolated compounds, such as lapacol and furanonaptoquinones, revealed that the intrinsic pathway mediates the apoptotic effect in A549 cells and canine osteosarcoma cells and that the proapoptotic proteins Bax, p53, and caspase 3 are activated [52,53]. These data demonstrate that various *Tabebuia* extracts have an apoptotic effect on cancer cells through the intrinsic pathway. Some iridoids, such as geniposidic acid, are the main compounds of *Genipa americana*; they have an apoptotic effect on synoviocytes through the intrinsic pathway, overexpressing the Bax protein and decreasing the Bcl-2 protein [54].

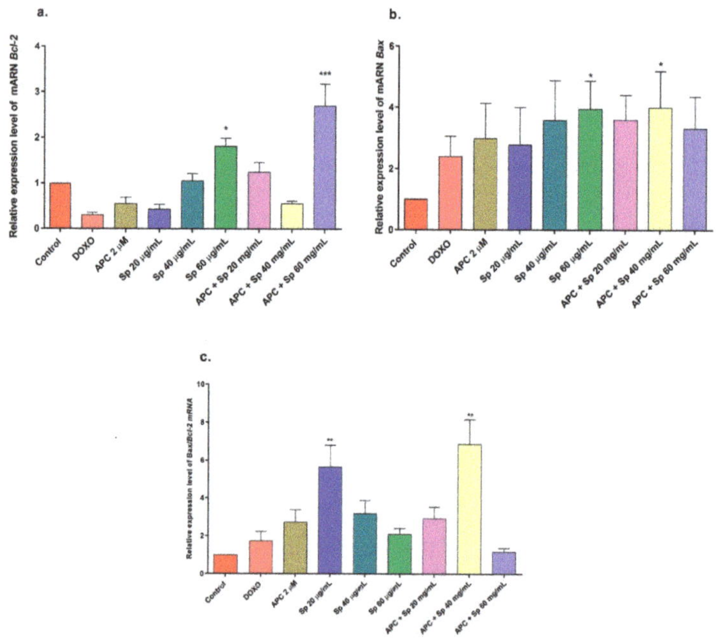

Figure 8. Gene expression of *BCL2* and *BAX* in THP-1 cells treated with specioside (Sp) and pretreated with APC for 24 h. (**a**) *BCL2* expression; (**b**) *BAX* expression; (**c**) relative expression of the *BAX*/*BCL2* genes. * $p \leq 0.05$, ** $p \leq 0.01$, *** $p \leq 0.001$ Kruskal–Wallis, Dunn's post hoc test.

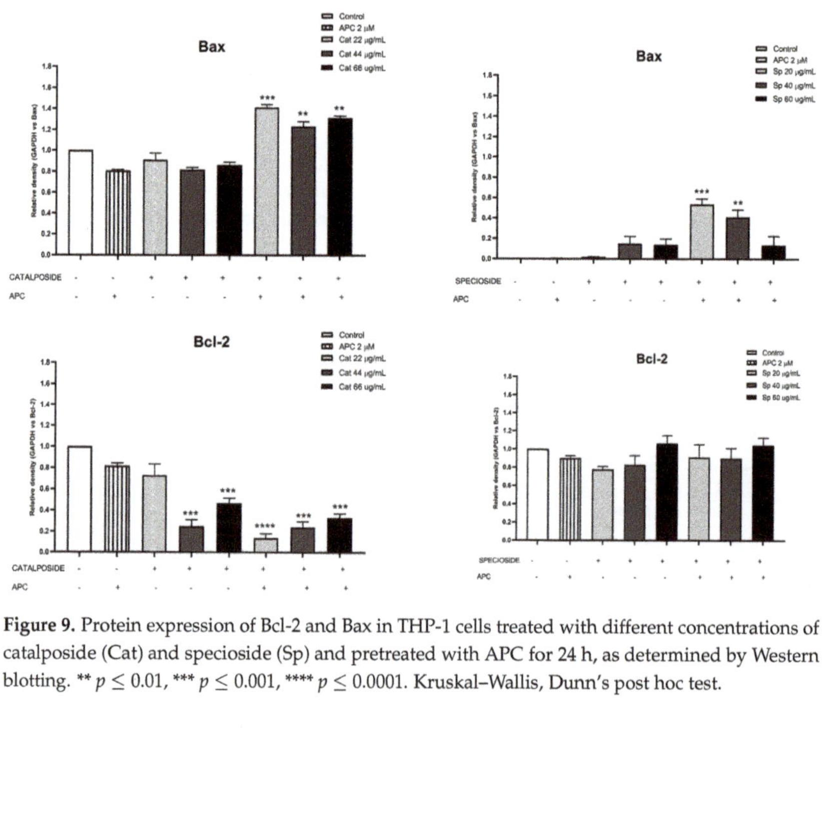

Figure 9. Protein expression of Bcl-2 and Bax in THP-1 cells treated with different concentrations of catalposide (Cat) and specioside (Sp) and pretreated with APC for 24 h, as determined by Western blotting. ** $p \leq 0.01$, *** $p \leq 0.001$, **** $p \leq 0.0001$. Kruskal–Wallis, Dunn's post hoc test.

In this study, the *n*-butanol extract increased the mRNA expression of the *MAPK14* gene, which encodes p38, in THP-1 cells, mainly at concentrations of 25 and 100 μg/mL and in combination with APC at 50 μg/mL (Figure 6); a slight increase in the phosphorylation of the p38 protein was observed at all the concentrations evaluated compared with that in the control (Figure 10a,b). The JNK protein was significantly phosphorylated at all the concentrations of the *n*-butanol extract evaluated; pretreatment with APC and 25 μg/mL had the greatest effect on the level of the protein (Figure 10c,d), whereas catalposide did not significantly change the level of JNK compared with that of the control. Specioside significantly phosphorylated the JNK protein at all concentrations tested, except at 60 μg/mL, in the presence of APC. Compared with the control, the *n*-butanol extract and specioside did not significantly change the phosphorylation of the ERK protein (Figure 10e,f). In contrast, compared with the control, catalposide decreased protein phosphorylation but not significantly. Some secoiridoids, such as oleuropein, have been shown to induce apoptosis through the JNK pathway in A549 cells and decrease the mitochondrial membrane potential [55,56].

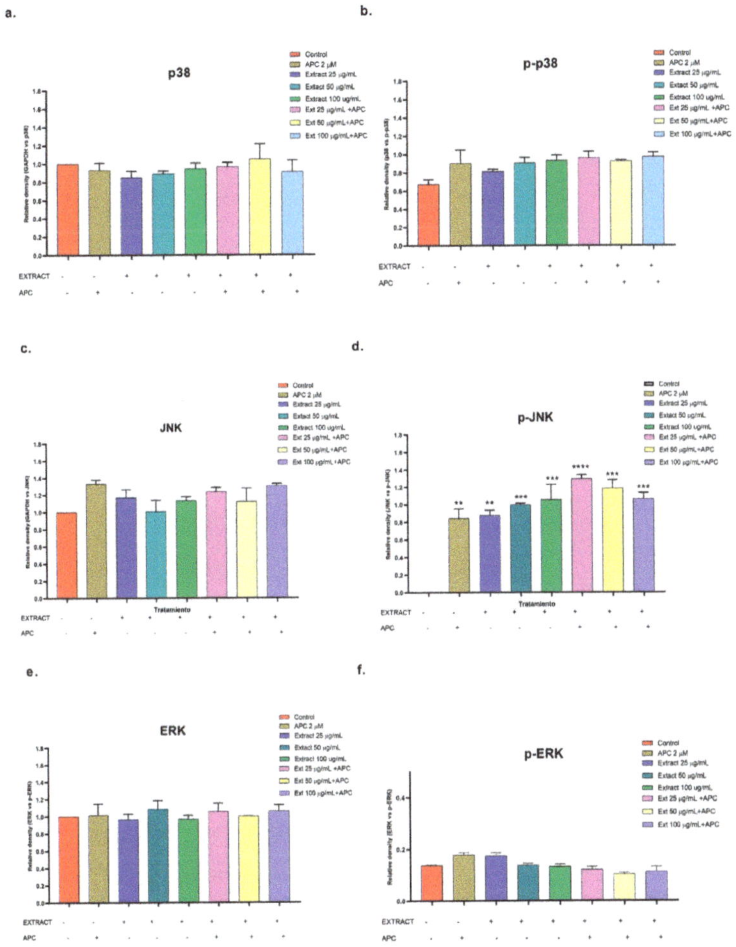

Figure 10. Relative protein expression density of (**a**) p38 protein, (**b**) p-p38, (**c**) JNK, (**d**) p-JNK, (**e**) ERK, (**f**) p-ERK in their basal and phosphorylated forms in THP-1 cells treated with the *n*-butanol extract and pretreated with APC for 24 h. ** $p \leq 0.01$, *** $p \leq 0.001$, **** $p \leq 0.0001$. Kruskal–Wallis, Tukey post hoc test.

Catalposide and specioside significantly increased the phosphorylation of p38 in the cells pretreated with APC compared with the control ($p < 0.001$) (Figures 11 and 12). These data are related to the increase in the expression of *MAPK14* mRNA. It has been reported that the phosphorylation of MAPK kinases such as p38 can be inhibited by some molecules that are present in plant extracts, such as flavonoids that inhibit the kinases MKK3 and MKK6, proteins that participate in the phosphorylation of the conserved Thr-Gly-Tyr (TGY) motif of p38 [57].

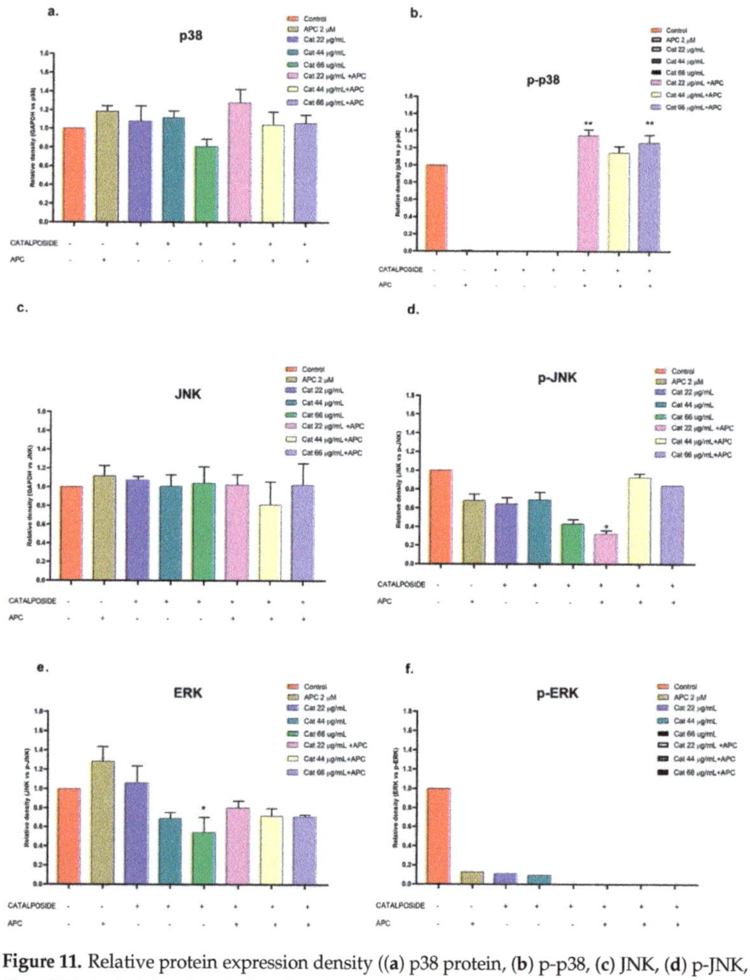

Figure 11. Relative protein expression density ((**a**) p38 protein, (**b**) p-p38, (**c**) JNK, (**d**) p-JNK, (**e**) ERK, (**f**) p-ERK) in their basal and phosphorylated forms in THP-1 cells treated with catalposide (Cat) and pretreated with APC for 24 h. * $p \leq 0.05$, ** $p \leq 0.01$. Kruskal–Wallis, Dunn's post hoc test.

Cell cycle alteration is an essential feature in the transformation of normal cells into tumor cells and, therefore, has therapeutic potential for several regulatory molecules because it controls cell proliferation. The cell cycle distribution was analyzed to identify the mechanism of action of the *n*-butanol extract, and the compounds were evaluated for their ability to decrease the activity of THP-1 cells. The results with the *n*-butanol extract revealed a slight increase in the percentage of cells in the G0/G1 phase (Supplementary Materials, Figure S6a), whereas for catalposide and specioside, the increase was significant compared with that of the control (Supplementary Materials, Figure S6b,c). In addition,

APC pretreatment increased G0/G1 phase arrest. The cell cycle regulates cell growth and proliferation; when it is arrested, it can inhibit proliferation and induce apoptosis in cancer cells [58]. In this study, compared with control cells, cells treated with catalposide, specioside, or APC presented significant phosphorylation of the p38 protein; these findings suggest that this protein is involved in cell cycle arrest in the G0/G1 phase. However, identifying the activity of other proteins, such as cyclin D1, related to this cell cycle phase is necessary. In one study, the extract obtained from *Galium aparine*, a plant that contains large amounts of iridoids, arrested the cell cycle at 72 h in G0/G1 and increased the fraction of cells in the subG1 phase, generating an apoptotic effect in MCF-7 cells [59,60]. It has also been reported that some flavonoids, such as apigenin and monoterpenes (1,8 cineol), are able to arrest the cell cycle in the G0/G1 phase and phosphorylate the p38 protein after 24 h of exposure. Additionally, they induce the expression of the p21 protein, which acts upstream of the p38 MAPK pathway [61,62].

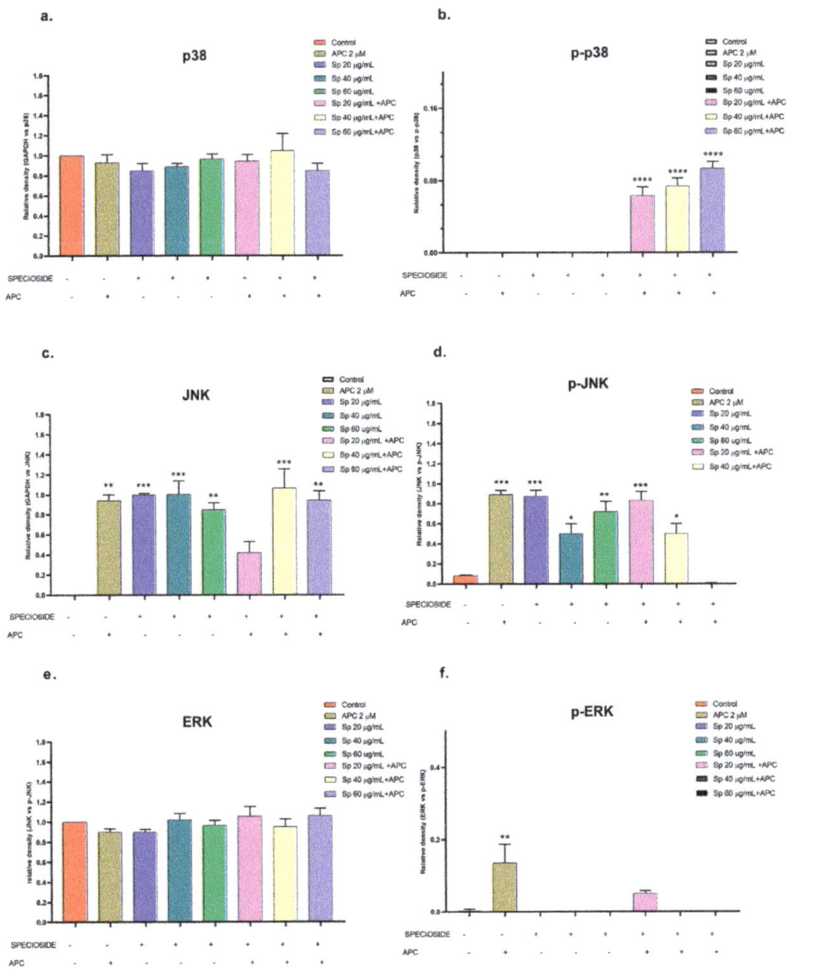

Figure 12. Relative protein expression density (**a**). p38 protein, (**b**). p-p38, (**c**). JNK, (**d**). p-JNK, (**e**). ERK, (**f**). p-ERK) in their basal and phosphorylated forms in THP-1 cells treated with specioside (Sp) and pretreated with APC for 24 h. * $p \leq 0.05$, ** $p \leq 0.01$, *** $p \leq 0.001$, **** $p \leq 0.0001$. Kruskal–Wallis, Dunn's post hoc test.

The findings of this study highlight the potential of natural products in the search for plant extracts and new molecules with antineoplastic activity. The *n*-butanol extract obtained from the inner bark of *Tabebuia rosea* (Bertol.) DC and the iridoids catalposide and specioside, in the presence of apicidin, induces apoptosis in leukemia cells. This work also has ethnopharmacological importance, since several indigenous groups in Central and South America use *Tabebuia* bark as an herbal or medicinal tea to treat diseases such as cancer and infectious diseases [23,63,64]. However, the cell signaling pathways involved in the antiproliferative and anticancer activities of *T. rosea* inner bark need further study.

3. Materials and Methods

3.1. Plant Material and Preparation of Extract

The inner bark of *T. rosea* (Bertol.) DC was collected at the Universidad Tecnológica de Pereira Campus. The plants were identified at the Colombian National Herbarium (Voucher No. COL 582577 for *T. rosea*). The collection and processing of the material were covered by collection permission number 1133/2014, which was issued by the Autoridad Nacional de Licencias Ambientales (ANLA) de Colombia.

All the chemicals used in this study were of analytical grade. The extract was obtained by the Polifenoles Research Group, as described by Jimenez et al. in 2018 [23]. Briefly, the plant material from the inner bark of *T. rosea* (2 kg) was dried and macerated in analytical-grade methanol (14 L) for 48 h. To obtain the crude extract, it was necessary to homogenize, filter, and concentrate it under vacuum using a rotary evaporator (Heidolph, Laborota model, Wood Dale, IL, USA) at 40 °C. This procedure was repeated three times. The crude extract was dissolved in 400 mL of distilled water and subjected to liquid—liquid extraction with n-butanol; the extract was vacuum dried by a vacuum rotary evaporator, and a mass of 12.5 g was obtained. Endotoxin levels in the extract were assayed using the Limulus Amebocyte Lysate Test, E-Toxate Kit (Sigma Chemical Co., Saint Louis, MO, USA; Cat No. ET0200-1KT). The sample was negative for the presence of endotoxins (detection limit 0.05–0.1 EU/mL). The extract was refrigerated at −20 °C in an amber tube protected from light, heat, air, and moisture. For each of the biological assays, the extracts were dissolved in DMSO (dimethyl sulfoxide, Merck, Darmstadt, Germany; Cat No. 1029521000).

3.2. Preliminary Phytochemical Analysis

Preliminary phytochemical analysis was performed by selective derivatization reactions to characterize the secondary metabolites present in the *n*-butanol extract obtained from the inner bark of *T. rosea*. The characterization was carried out using thin-layer chromatography (TLC) in the normal phase (silica) and reversed-phase (RP-18) with hexane-ethyl acetate (7:3) and water-isopropanol (7:3) elution systems, respectively. The chromatographic plates were developed with aluminum chloride ($AlCl_3$, Sigma Chemical Co., Saint Louis, MO, USA), ferric chloride ($FeCl_3$, Sigma Chemical Co., Saint Louis, MO, USA), and a mixture of vanillin-phosphoric acid (H_3PO_4) for the detection of flavonoids, phenols, and lignans. Potassium hydroxide (KOH, Merck, Darmstadt, Germany) in analytical-grade ethanol was used for the detection of anthrones, quinones, and coumarins; a mixture of anisaldehyde–acetic acid–sulfuric acid (H_2SO_4) with vanillin-phosphoric acid (H_3PO_4) was used for the detection of iridoids; a mixture of anisaldehyde–acetic acid–sulfuric acid (H_2SO_4) with antimony chloride ($SbCl_3$) was used for the detection of saponins and triterpenes; oleum (Sigma Chemical Co., Saint Louis, MO, USA) was used for the detection of sesquiterpene lactones; 2,4-dinitrophenylhydrazine was used for the determination of aldehydes and ketones; and the Liebermann–Burchard reagent was used for the detection of terpenes and steroids. The extract showed a specific color when reacted with the developing reagents for each test. The absence or presence of this color was taken as a negative (−) or positive (+) result for the presence of these phytochemical components.

3.3. Fractionation and Isolation of Specioside

The isolation and structural identification of specioside (the principal constituent of the *n*-butanol extract from *T. rosea*) was previously reported [22]. The *n*-butanol extract was concentrated via rotary evaporation under reduced pressure, and a dark brown extract (12.5 g, yield 4.25%) was obtained. The *n*-butanol extract (8.0 g) was subjected to separation by column chromatography (CC) on a Diaion® HP-20 (Mitsubishi Chemical Corp., Tokyo, Japan), with a water—isopropanol elution gradient (90:10 to 10:90), obtaining subfractions A–J. Tr-1 (Specioside, 25.9 mg) was isolated from subfraction D with a semipreparative HPLC–DAD system (Hitachi-Merck, Tokyo, Japan) in reverse phase (LiChrocart 250-10; LiChrospher 100; 10 μm, Merck, Darmstadt, Germany) by isocratic elution with H_2O–ACN (70:30% *v*/*v*) containing 1% *v*/*v* CH_3COOH. Specioside (Figure S7) was obtained as a dark brown amorphous solid (m.p. 142–162 °C). The FTIR spectrum displayed absorption bands attributable to carbonyl groups ($\nu_{C=O}$ 1698 cm^{-1}), hydroxyl groups ($\nu_{O\text{-}H}$ 3383 cm^{-1}), and aromatic rings ($\nu_{C=C}$ 1605 cm^{-1}).

Full assignments from the ^1H and ^{13}C NMR spectra were made through the use of ^1H-^1H COSY, HSQC, and HMBC experiments. All the experiments were performed on a 400 MHz Agilent spectrometer (Agilent, Santa Clara, CA, USA) using deuterated methanol as the solvent. The ^1H NMR spectrum showed two olefinic protons at δ H 6.37 (H-3, dd) and δ H 4.98 (H-4, dd), characteristic of the iridoid nucleus. This structure was confirmed by correlations shown in the HMBC spectrum with carbons at δ C 140.95 (C-3) and δ C 101.50 (C-4). In addition, two olefinic protons at δ H 7.67 (1H, d, *J* = 16.0 Hz, H-7″) and δ H 6.38 (1H, d, *J* = 15.9 Hz, H-8″) suggested the presence of an E configuration, which is characteristic of a p-coumaroyl skeleton. The p-coumaroyl structure was confirmed by the observation of two signals at δ H 7.48 (2H, d, *J* = 8.7 Hz, H-2″, H-6″) and δ H 6.81 (2H, d, *J* = 8.7 Hz, H-3″, H-5″), characteristic of an AA′XX′ system; these data were confirmed by the ^{13}C NMR spectrum, which exhibited eight carbon signals, including the carbonyl carbon at δ C 164.49 (C-9″), which was attributed to the p-coumaroyl ester. The presence of anomeric protons at δ H 4.79 (1H, d, *J* = 7.9 Hz, H-1′) and methine signals at δ H 3.42–3.23 (4H, m) are characteristic of a sugar moiety. Analysis of the 1D and 2D NMR spectra, in addition to comparisons with the literature data for glucoside analogs, suggested that the saccharide portion was a glucose moiety. Characteristic ^1H NMR, ^{13}C NMR, COSY, HSQC, and HMBC spectra are provided in the Supplementary Materials (Figures S7–S13).

The molecule catalposide, an iridoid glycoside also isolated from the plants of the genus *Tabebuia* [65], was purchased from Sigma Chemical Company (SMB00094).

3.4. Cell Culture

Jurkat and THP-1 cell lines were purchased from the American Type Culture Collection (ATCC, Rockville, MD, USA); Jurkat is a human lymphocytic cell line representing acute T-cell leukemia, and THP-1 is a monocytic cell line that represents acute myelogenous leukemia (AML). Jurkat and THP-1 cells were maintained in RPMI 1640 medium (Sigma) supplemented with 10% heat-inactivated fetal bovine serum (FBS) (Gibco Cat No. 16140071, Waltham, MA USA), 200 μg/mL penicillin, 200 μg/mL streptomycin, 400 μg/mL neomycin (GIBCO, Cat No. 15640-055), 5 μg/mL amphotericin, and 1 mM sodium pyruvate (all from Sigma Chemical Co., Saint Louis, MO, USA; Cat Nos. A9528-50 MG, M7522-100ML, and S8636-100ML, respectively). The cells were maintained at 37 °C in a humidified atmosphere with 5% CO_2. The culture medium was exchanged with fresh medium every 2–3 days. Peripheral blood mononuclear cells (PBMCs) were isolated from normal human venous blood. Further, 10 milliliters of human blood was mixed with 10 mL of RPMI-1640 containing 50 μL of heparin and gradually poured over 1 mL of HISTOPAQUE®-1119 (Sigma). The plasma was removed by centrifugation at 3000 rpm for 30 min. The peripheral blood mononuclear cell-containing layer was collected with a pipette and diluted in 4 mL of PBS. PBMCs were harvested by centrifugation at 1500 rpm for 10 min at room temperature, resuspended in RPMI-1640 with 10% FBS, and incubated at 37 °C in 5% CO_2 humidified air.

3.5. Cell Viability Assay (MTT)

Cell viability was determined by measuring the mitochondrial activity of live cells via the metabolism of the tetrazolium substrate 3-(4,5-dimethylthiazol-2-yl)-2,5-diphenyl tetrazolium bromide (MTT) and converting it to purple formazan crystals [66]. Briefly, the cells (2×10^4 cells/well) were treated with 25, 50, 100, 200, or 400 μg/mL extract diluted in DMSO (at a final concentration of 0.5%) and incubated for 12, 24, or 48 h. Catalposide and specioside were tested at concentrations of 20, 50, and 100 μg/mL for 12, 24, and 48 h. For apicidin, 0.5, 1, and 2 μM apicidin were tested for 24 and 48 h. Doxorubicin was used as a reference standard drug (positive control). After treatment, the medium was discarded; 200 μL of RPMI 1640 medium without phenol red containing 0.5 mg/mL MTT (Sigma Chemical Co., Saint Louis, MO, USA; Cat. No. M2128-500MG) was then added to each well. The plates were incubated for four hours at 37 °C with 5% CO_2 in a humidified atmosphere. The medium was discarded, and 100 μL of DMSO was added to solubilize the formazan crystals. The absorbance was measured with an ELISA microplate reader at 492 nm (ELx800; BioTek Instruments Inc., Winooski, VT, USA). The percentage of viable cells was calculated on the basis of the nontreated control (taken as 100%). The IC_{50} (concentration causing a 50% reduction in cellular viability) values for all the tested compounds were evaluated in Excel using the nonlinear regression curve method. Three independent assays were performed, each in triplicate.

3.6. Estimation of the Selectivity Index (SI)

The selectivity index corresponds to the ratio of the IC_{50} value calculated for the activity of synthesized compounds on a regular cell line (PBMCs) to that of the IC_{50} calculated for cancer cell lines (Jurkat and THP-1) [67]. Values greater than two were optimal for an efficient selectivity index.

Selectivity index:

$$SI = \frac{IC_{50}\ \text{normal cells}}{IC_{50}\ \text{cancer cells}} \quad (1)$$

3.7. Fluorescence Microscopic Analysis of Cell Death (Propidium Iodide and Hoechst Staining)

Fluorescence microscopy was used to observe cell nuclear morphology, followed by propidium iodide (50 μg/mL) and Hoechst 333342 (1 mg/mL) staining. THP-1 cells (1×10^5 cells/well) were treated with fresh media (control) and with 25, 50, or 100 μg/mL extract for 24 h; 400 μM doxorubicin was used as a positive control. Further, 10 microliters of the cell suspension was mixed with 90 μL of the dye, incubated in a water bath for 5 min at 37 °C, and wrapped in aluminum foil. The cells were examined under an Olympus IX53 fluorescence microscope (Olympus Corporation, Tokyo, Japan). The following formula was used to calculate the percentage of apoptotic cells [68].

3.8. Flow Cytometric Analysis of Apoptosis via the ANNEXIN V-CF647/7-AAD Double-Staining Assay

In 96-well plates, 8×10^4 cells were treated with 25, 50, and 100 μg/mL extract and 400 μM doxorubicin (positive control) for 24 and 48 h. The cells were washed with 1X PBS, and apoptotic cells were detected by staining with 100 μL of Annexin V-CF647 and 5 μL of the 7-AAD Apoptosis Annexin Red Kit (FCCH100108 FlowCellect, Millipore, Darmstadt, Germany). The cells were incubated at room temperature for 15 min in the dark and analyzed on a Guava Millipore flow cytometer (Merck Millipore, Bedford, MA, USA) using InCyte software (version 3.1, Merck Millipore). The percentage of annexin V-positive cells was evaluated.

3.9. Determination of Mitochondrial Membrane Potential ($\Delta\Psi m$)

The $\Lambda\psi$m was measured using a Guava Mitochondrial Depolarization Kit (4500-0250 Millipore, Darmstadt, Germany). After pretreatment with 1 μM apicidin for 24 h, the cells were exposed to various concentrations of the extract (25, 50, and 100 μg/mL) for 24 h.

The cells were collected and suspended in 100 μL of PBS containing JC-1 and 7-AAD after incubation at 37 °C for 15 min. The fluorescence intensity of the cells was analyzed in a Guava Millipore flow cytometer (Merck Millipore, Bedford, MA, USA) using InCyte software (version 3.1, Merck Millipore).

3.10. Cell Cycle Analysis

After treatment with the extract, 7×10^4 cells were harvested, washed with PBS, fixed with 200 μL of ice-cold 70% ethanol, and maintained at 4 °C for 4 h before staining. The cell pellet was washed in 1X PBS, resuspended in 200 μL of Guava Cell Cycle reagent (#4500-0220, Millipore), and incubated in the dark at 37 °C for 30 min before analysis with a Guava flow cytometer (Merck Millipore, Bedford, MA, USA) using InCyte software (version 3.1, Merck Millipore).. Centrifugation was performed at 1200 rpm for 5 min at room temperature for each step.

3.11. Western Blot Analysis

THP-1 cells were seeded in 24-well plates (5×10^5 cells/well), and after 24 h of incubation, they were pretreated with 1 μM apicidin for 24 h and then treated with different concentrations of the *n*-butanol extract, catalposide, and specioside for 24 h. After treatment, the cells were lysed with an Abcam protein extraction kit (ab270054), and a phosphatase inhibitor cocktail (ab201115) was added. The supernatants of the cell extracts were quantified with a BCA protein assay (Thermo Scientific Pierce #23227, Waltham, MA, USA). Equivalent amounts of protein were electrophoresed on 10% SDS polyacrylamide gels and then electroblotted onto 0.45 μm polyvinylidene difluoride (PVDF) membranes (GE Healthcare, Chicago, IL, USA). After blocking with 5% nonfat milk in TBS/0.5% Tween 20 (TBST) for 1 h at room temperature, the membranes were incubated with p-p38 MAPK (1:1000 dilution, cat 701057), p38 MAPK (1:2000 dilution, cat PA5-17713), p-ERK1/2 (1:100 dilution, 44680G), ERK1/2 (1:2000 dilution, 44654G), p-JNK1/2 (1:1000 dilution, PA5-37698), JNK1/2 (1:2000 dilution, cat 44690G), bcl-2 (1:2000 dilution, PA1-28275), Bax (1:2000 dilution, PA5-70418), and GAPDH (1:10,000 dilution, PA1-16777) antibodies overnight at 4 °C. All the antibodies were purchased from Invitrogen-Thermo Fisher Scientific (Waltham, MA, USA). Afterward, the membranes were washed with TBST three times and incubated with horseradish peroxidase (HRP)-conjugated secondary antibody for 1 h at room temperature. The signals were detected using SuperSignal™ West Pico PLUS Chemiluminescent Substrate (Thermo Scientific Pierce cat 34577) and analyzed with a ChemiDoc XRS+ system (Bio-Rad, Hercules, CA, USA). The density of each band was measured using ImageJ software V. 1.53n, 7 November 2021 (NIH, Bethesda, MD, USA), and the protein levels were normalized to the GAPDH levels. The data are expressed as the means of three independent experiments. The Western blot images are presented in the Supplementary Materials (Figures S1–S4).

3.12. RT–qPCR

THP-1 cells (3×10^5 cells/well) were pretreated with 1 μM apicidin for 24 h and then treated with different concentrations of the extract, catalposide, and specioside (25, 50, 100 μg/mL) for 24 h. After treatment, mRNA extraction was performed using the RNeasy Plus Mini Kit (Qiagen, Germantown, MD, USA; Cat No. 74134). The mRNA was quantified with a NanoDrop 2000c (Thermo Fisher Scientific, Waltham, MA, USA). The expression of the *MAPK14* (gene encoding p38), *BCL2*, and *BAX* genes was evaluated by qRT–PCR and quantified with the $2^{-\Delta\Delta Ct}$ method in the Applied Biosystems StepOnePlus Real-Time PCR System (Applied Biosystems, Foster City, CA, USA), which uses predesigned TaqMan Gene Expression Assays (codes Hs00608023_m1, Hs00608023_m1, and Hs00180269_m1, respectively) (Applied Biosystems, Foster City, CA, USA) and the TaqMan® RNA-to-CT TM 1-Step Kit (Applied Biosystems, Foster City, CA, USA, Cat No. 4392653). The reaction mixture was incubated at 48 °C for 15 min and 95 °C for 10 min and then cycled (40 cycles) at 95 °C for 15 s and 60 °C for 1 min. GAPDH was used as an endogenous control.

3.13. Statistical Analysis

Each experiment was performed at least in duplicate. The results are expressed as the means ± SDs of at least three independent experiments. Statistical analysis was performed using ANOVA and the Kruskal–Wallis test. Values were considered significantly different at $p < 0.05$. The statistical tests were performed using GraphPad Prism, version 8.01 (GraphPad Software, San Diego, CA, USA).

4. Conclusions

Pretreatment with APC, the *n*-butanol extract obtained from the inner bark of *Tabebuia rosea*, and the evaluated compounds (catalposide and specioside) activated the MAPK pathway, specifically p38, which affected the G0/G1 phase of the cell cycle and subsequent cell death; although the JNK and ERK proteins were expressed in the cells treated with the catalposide and specioside compounds, the phosphorylation of these proteins was not significant. In addition, there was depolarization of the mitochondrial membrane, an effect that was related to the participation of the proapoptotic protein Bax.

Supplementary Materials: The following supporting information can be downloaded at https://www.mdpi.com/article/10.3390/molecules29173986/s1, Supplementary information Guerrero-Pepinosa et al. Table S1. Preliminary phytochemical analysis of extracts prepared from the inner bark of *T. rosea*. Figure S1. Blotting of MAPK proteins (p38 protein, p.p38, JNK, p-JNK, ERK, p-ERK). in their basal and phosphorylated forms in THP-1 cells treated with the n-butanol extract and pretreated with APC for 24 h. Figure S2. Protein expression of Bcl-2 and Bax in THP-1 cells treated with different concentrations of catalposide (Cat) (a) and specioside (Sp) (b) and pretreated with APC for 24 h, as determined by western blotting. Figure S3. Relative protein expression density (p38 protein, p-p38, JNK, p-JNK, ERK, p-ERK). in their basal and phosphorylated forms in THP-1 cells treated with catalposide (Cat) and pretreated with APC for 24 h. Figure S4. Relative protein expression density (p38 protein, p-p38, JNK, p-JNK, ERK, p-ERK). in their basal and phosphorylated forms in THP-1 cells treated with specioside (Sp) and pretreated with APC for 24 h. Figure S5. THP-1 cells labeled with Annexin V-CF647 and 7-AAD in early and late apoptosis and treated with different concentrations of Catalposide (a) and Specioside (b) for 24 hours. ** $p \leq 0.01$,**** $p \leq 0.0001$. ANOVA, Bonferroni post hoc. Figure S6. (a) THP-1 cells in each phase of the cell cycle were exposed to the n-butanol extract obtained from the inner bark of *T. rosea*. (b) Pretreatment with the catalposide (Cat) and (c) specioside (Sp) and pretreatment with APC for 24 h. * $p \leq 0.05$, *** $p \leq 0.001$. Kruskal–Wallis, Dunn's post hoc test. Figure S7. Specioside structure. Figure S8. The ^{1}H NMR spectrum of Specioside in CD3OD, 400 MHz. Figure S9. The ^{13}C NMR spectrum of Specioside in CD3OD, 125.6 MHz. Figure S10. The COSY spectrum of Specioside in CD3OD, 400 MHz. Figure S11. The HSQC spectrum of Specioside in CD3OD, 400 MHz. Figure S12. The HMBC spectrum of Specioside in CD3OD, 400 MHz. Figure S13. The HMBC expanded spectrum of Specioside (δ 6.4–3.2). Figure S14. The HMBC expanded spectrum of Specioside (δ 7.8–6.2).

Author Contributions: Conceptualization, N.Y.G.-P., L.A.V. and J.C.S.-A.; methodology, N.Y.G.-P. and L.A.V.; investigation, N.Y.G.-P., L.A.V. and J.C.S.-A.; formal analysis, N.Y.G.-P., L.A.V., and J.C.S.-A.; resources, L.A.V. and J.C.S.-A.; writing—original draft preparation, N.Y.G.-P. and J.C.S.-A.; writing—review and editing, N.Y.G.-P., L.A.V. and J.C.S.-A.; supervision, L.A.V. and J.C.S.-A.; project administration, J.C.S.-A.; funding acquisition, L.A.V. and J.C.S.-A. All authors have read and agreed to the published version of the manuscript.

Funding: This study was supported by Universidad Tecnológica de Pereira (Grants 5-21-8, 5-24-2 and 5-23-1) and Sistema General de Regalías de Colombia (Código BPIN 2012000100050 and BPIN 2020000100077).

Institutional Review Board Statement: Not applicable.

Informed Consent Statement: Not applicable.

Data Availability Statement: The original contributions presented in the study are included in the article, and further inquiries can be directed to the corresponding author.

Acknowledgments: The authors wish to thank all the members of the Infección e Inmunidad and Polifenoles Research Groups for their support. Nancy Guerrero-Pepinosa acknowledges Minciencias for a PhD fellowship (Convocatoria 647-2014), Colombia.

Conflicts of Interest: The authors declare no conflict of interest. The funders had no role in the design of the study, the collection, analysis, or interpretation of data, the writing of the manuscript, or the decision to publish the results.

References

1. Bray, F.; Ferlay, J.; Soerjomataram, I.; Siegel, R.L.; Torre, L.A.; Jemal, A. Global cancer statistics 2018: GLOBOCAN estimates of incidence and mortality worldwide for 36 cancers in 185 countries. *CA Cancer J. Clin.* **2018**, *68*, 394–424. [CrossRef]
2. Stacy, C.P.; Brown, A. Treatment of Pediatric Acute Lymphoblastic Leukemia. *Pediatr. Clin. N. Am.* **2015**, *62*, 13.
3. Miller, K.D.; Nogueira, L.; Mariotto, A.B.; Rowland, J.H.; Yabroff, K.R.; Alfano, C.M.; Jemal, A.; Kramer, J.L.; Siegel, R.L. Cancer treatment and survivorship statistics, 2019. *CA Cancer J. Clin.* **2016**, *69*, 363–385. [CrossRef] [PubMed]
4. Cragg, G.M.; Newman, D.J. Natural products: A continuing source of novel drug leads. *Biochim. Biophys. Acta Gen. Subj.* **2013**, *1830*, 3670–3695. [CrossRef]
5. Newman, D.J.; Cragg, G.M. Natural Products as Sources of New Drugs over the Nearly Four Decades from 01/1981 to 09/2019. *J. Nat. Prod.* **2020**, *83*, 770–803. [CrossRef] [PubMed]
6. Abotaleb, M.; Samuel, S.M.; Varghese, E.; Varghese, S.; Kubatka, P.; Liskova, A.; Büsselberg, D. Flavonoids in Cancer and Apoptosis. *Cancers* **2019**, *11*, 28. [CrossRef]
7. Murray, V.; Shaw, D. WHO Monographs on Selected Medicinal Plants, Volume 1. *Health Hyg.* **2000**, *21*, 129.
8. Vogl, S.; Picker, P.; Mihaly Bison, J.; Fakhrudin, N.; Atanasov, A.G.; Heiss, E.H.; Wawrosch, C.; Reznicek, G.; Dirsch, V.M.; Saukel, J. Ethnopharmacological in vitro studies on Austria's folk medicine—An unexplored lore in vitro anti-inflammatory activities of 71 Austrian traditional herbal drugs. *J. Ethnopharmacol.* **2013**, *149*, 750–771. [CrossRef] [PubMed]
9. Gentry, A.H. A Synopsis of Bignoniaceae Ethnobotany and Economic Botany. *Ann. Mo. Bot. Gard.* **1992**, *79*, 53–64. [CrossRef]
10. Hamed, A.N.E.; Mahmoud, B.K.; Samy, M.N.; Kamel, M.S. An extensive review on genus "Tabebuia", family bignoniaceae: Phytochemistry and biological activities (1967 to 2018). *J. Herb. Med.* **2020**, *24*, 100410. [CrossRef]
11. Olmstead, R.G.; Zjhra, M.L.; Lohmann, L.G.; Grose, S.O.; Eckert, A.J. A molecular phylogeny and classification of Bignoniaceae. *Am. J. Bot.* **2009**, *96*, 1731–1743. [CrossRef]
12. Michel, A.F.R.M.; Melo, M.M.; Campos, P.P.; Oliveira, M.S.; Oliveira, F.A.S.; Cassali, G.D.; Ferraz, V.P.; Cota, B.B.; Andrade, S.P.; Souza-Fagundes, E.M. Evaluation of anti-inflammatory, antiangiogenic and antiproliferative activities of *Arrabidaea chica* crude extracts. *J. Ethnopharmacol.* **2015**, *165*, 29–38. [CrossRef] [PubMed]
13. Lorenzi, H.; Matos, F. *Medicinal Plants in Brazil: Native and Exotic*; Instituto Plantarum de Estudosda Flora, Editora Plantarum: Nova Odessa, Brazil, 2008; p. 576.
14. Mafioleti, L.; da Silva Junior, I.F.; Colodel, E.M.; Flach, A.; de Oliveira Martins, D.T. Evaluation of the toxicity and antimicrobial activity of hydroethanolic extract of *Arrabidaea chica* (Humb. & Bonpl.) B. *Verl. J. Ethnopharmacol.* **2013**, *150*, 576–582. [PubMed]
15. Moya, E.; Brea, M. First Pleistocene record of fossil wood of Bignoniaceae in the Americas and a comparison with the extant Tabebuia alliance and Tecomeae. *Bot. J. Linn. Soc.* **2018**, *187*, 303–318. [CrossRef]
16. Gómez-Estrada, H.; Díaz-Castillo, F.; Franco-Ospina, L.; Mercado-Camargo, J.; Guzmán-Ledezma, J.; Medina, J.D.; Gaitán-Ibarra, R. Folk medicine in the northern coast of Colombia: An overview. *J. Ethnobiol. Ethnomed* **2011**, *7*, 27. [CrossRef]
17. Hajdu, Z.; Hohmann, J. An ethnopharmacological survey of the traditional medicine utilized in the community of Porvenir, Bajo Paraguá Indian Reservation, Bolivia. *J. Ethnopharmacol.* **2012**, *139*, 838–857. [CrossRef]
18. Lima Bezerra, J.J.; Johanes, I.; Vieira Pinheiro, A.A. Anticancer potential and toxicity of the genus *Handroanthus* Mattos (Bignoniaceae): A systematic review. *Toxicon* **2022**, *217*, 131–142. [CrossRef]
19. Garzón-Castaño, S.C.; Lopera-Castrillón, I.A.; Jiménez-González, F.J.; Siller-López, F.; Veloza, L.A.; Sepúlveda-Arias, J.C. Nrf2-Mediated Antioxidant Activity of the inner bark extracts obtained from *Tabebuia rosea* (Bertol) DC and *Tabebuia chrysantha* (JACQ) G. *Nicholson. F1000Research* **2018**, *7*, 1937. [CrossRef]
20. Queiroz, M.L.; Valadares, M.C.; Torello, C.O.; Ramos, A.L.; Oliveira, A.B.; Rocha, F.D.; Arruda, V.A.; Accorci, W.R. Comparative studies of the effects of *Tabebuia avellanedae* bark extract and β-lapachone on the hematopoietic response of tumor-bearing mice. *J. Ethnopharmacol.* **2008**, *117*, 228–235. [CrossRef]
21. Cardona-Trujillo, M.C.; Jiménez-González, F.J.; Veloza, L.A.; Sepúlveda-Arias, J.C. In Vitro Anti-Toxoplasma Activity of Extracts Obtained from *Tabebuia rosea* and *Tabebuia chrysantha*: The Role of β-Amyrin. *Molecules* **2024**, *29*, 920. [CrossRef]
22. Garzón-Castaño, S.C.; Jiménez-González, F.J.; Veloza, L.A.; Sepúlveda-Arias, J.C. Activation of the Keap1-Nrf2 pathway by specioside and the *n*-butanol extract from the inner bark of *Tabebuia rosea* (Bertol) DC. *F1000Research* **2020**, *9*, 1262. [CrossRef] [PubMed]
23. Jimenez-Gonzalez, F.J.; Vélez-Gómez, J.M.; Melchor-Moncada, J.J.; Veloza, L.A.; Sepúlveda-Arias, J.C. Antioxidant, anti-inflammatory, and antiproliferative activity of extracts obtained from *Tabebuia rosea* (Bertol.) DC. *Pharmacogn. Mag.* **2018**, *14*, 25.
24. Compadre, C.; Jáuregui, J.; Nathan, P.J.; Enríquez, R. Isolation of 6-O-(p-Coumaroyl)-Catalpol from *Tabebuia rosea*. *Planta Medica* **1982**, *46*, 42–44. [CrossRef]

25. Inagaki, R.; Ninomiya, M.; Tanaka, K.; Watanabe, K.; Koketsu, M. Synthesis and cytotoxicity on human leukemia cells of furonaphthoquinones isolated from *Tabebuia* plants. *Chem. Pharm. Bull.* **2013**, *61*, 670–673. [CrossRef]
26. Khandelwal, P.; Singh, P. Tabebuin and tecomaquinone-III-dimeric quinones from *Tabebuia rosea*. *J. Indian Chem. Soc.* **2008**, *85*, 310–312.
27. Kang, N.; Wang, M.-M.; Wang, Y.-H.; Zhang, Z.-N.; Cao, H.-R.; Lv, Y.-H.; Yang, Y.; Fan, P.-H.; Qiu, F.; Gao, X.-M. Tetrahydrocurcumin induces G2/M cell cycle arrest and apoptosis involving p38 MAPK activation in human breast cancer cells. *Food Chem. Toxicol.* **2014**, *67*, 193–200. [CrossRef]
28. Dias, R.B.; de Araújo, T.B.S.; de Freitas, R.D.; da Cruz Rodrigues, A.C.B.; Sousa, L.P.; Sales, C.B.S.; de Faro Valverde, L.; Soares, M.B.P.; Dos Reis, M.G.; Della Coletta, R. β-Lapachone and its iodine derivatives cause cell cycle arrest at G2/M phase and reactive oxygen species-mediated apoptosis in human oral squamous cell carcinoma cells. *Free Radic. Biol. Med.* **2018**, *126*, 87–100. [CrossRef] [PubMed]
29. Lee, J.K.; Kim, N.-J. Recent advances in the inhibition of p38 MAPK as a potential strategy for the treatment of Alzheimer's disease. *Molecules* **2017**, *22*, 1287. [CrossRef] [PubMed]
30. Chinembiri, T.N.; Du Plessis, L.H.; Gerber, M.; Hamman, J.H.; Du Plessis, J. Review of natural compounds for potential skin cancer treatment. *Molecules* **2014**, *19*, 11679–11721. [CrossRef]
31. Bauden, M.; Tassidis, H.; Ansari, D. In vitro cytotoxicity evaluation of HDAC inhibitor Apicidin in pancreatic carcinoma cells subsequent time and dose dependent treatment. *Toxicol. Lett.* **2015**, *236*, 8–15. [CrossRef]
32. Kumar, S.; Chaudhary, A.K.; Kumar, R.; O'Malley, J.; Dubrovska, A.; Wang, X.; Yadav, N.; Goodrich, D.W.; Chandra, D. Combination therapy induces unfolded protein response and cytoskeletal rearrangement leading to mitochondrial apoptosis in prostate cancer. *Mol. Oncol.* **2016**, *10*, 949–965. [CrossRef] [PubMed]
33. Al-Lazikani, B.; Banerji, U.; Workman, P. Combinatorial drug therapy for cancer in the postgenomic era. *Nat. Biotechnol.* **2012**, *30*, 679. [CrossRef]
34. Newman, D.J.; Cragg, G.M. Natural products as sources of new drugs over the last 25 years. *J. Nat. Prod.* **2007**, *70*, 461–477. [CrossRef]
35. Singh, J.; Hatcher, S.; Ku, A.; Ding, Z.; Feng, F.; Sharma, R.; Pfister, S. Model selection for the preclinical development of new drug–radiotherapy combinations. *Clin. Oncol.* **2021**, *33*, 694–704. [CrossRef] [PubMed]
36. Rahman, M.M.; Reza, A.S.M.A.; Khan, M.A.; Sujon, K.M.; Sharmin, R.; Rashid, M.; Sadik, M.G.; Reza, M.A.; Tsukahara, T.; Capasso, R.; et al. Unfolding the apoptotic mechanism of antioxidant enriched-leaves of *Tabebuia pallida* (lindl.) Miers in EAC cells and mouse model. *J. Ethnopharmacol.* **2021**, *278*, 114297. [CrossRef] [PubMed]
37. Kuete, V.; Efferth, T. African flora has the potential to fight multidrug resistance of cancer. *BioMed Res. Int.* **2015**, *2015*, 914813. [CrossRef]
38. Huertas-Martínez, J.; Rello-Varona, S.; Herrero-Martín, D.; Barrau, I.; García-Monclús, S.; Sáinz-Jaspeado, M.; Lagares-Tena, L.; Núñez-Álvarez, Y.; Mateo-Lozano, S.; Mora, J.; et al. Caveolin-1 is downregulated in alveolar rhabdomyosarcomas and negatively regulates tumor growth. *Oncotarget* **2014**, *5*, 9744. [CrossRef]
39. Feldman, R.; Martinez, J.D. Growth suppression by ursodeoxycholic acid involves caveolin-1 enhanced degradation of EGFR. *Biochim. Et Biophys. Acta (BBA)—Mol. Cell Res.* **2009**, *1793*, 1387–1394. [CrossRef]
40. Oliveira, P.F.d.; Alves, J.M.; Damasceno, J.L.; Oliveira, R.A.M.; Dias, H.; Crotti, A.E.M.; Tavares, D.C. Cytotoxicity screening of essential oils in cancer cell lines. *Rev. Bras. Farmacogn.* **2015**, *25*, 183–188. [CrossRef]
41. Feinberg, A.P.; Ohlsson, R.; Henikoff, S. The epigenetic progenitor origin of human cancer. *Nat. Rev. Genet.* **2006**, *7*, 21–33. [CrossRef]
42. Kwon, S.H.; Ahn, S.H.; Kim, Y.K.; Bae, G.-U.; Yoon, J.W.; Hong, S.; Lee, H.Y.; Lee, Y.-W.; Lee, H.-W.; Han, J.-W. Apicidin, a Histone Deacetylase Inhibitor, Induces Apoptosis and Fas/Fas Ligand Expression in Human Acute Promyelocytic Leukemia Cells. *J. Biol. Chem.* **2002**, *277*, 2073–2080. [CrossRef] [PubMed]
43. Ahn, M.-Y.; Ahn, S.-G.; Yoon, J.-H. Apicidin, a histone deaceylase inhibitor, induces both apoptosis and autophagy in human oral squamous carcinoma cells. *Oral. Oncol.* **2011**, *47*, 1032–1038. [CrossRef]
44. Ahn, M.Y.; Lee, J.; Na, Y.J.; Choi, W.S.; Lee, B.M.; Kang, K.W.; Kim, H.S. Mechanism of apicidin-induced cell cycle arrest and apoptosis in Ishikawa human endometrial cancer cells. *Chem. Biol. Interact.* **2009**, *179*, 169–177. [CrossRef]
45. Cai, X.; Guo, L.; Pei, F.; Chang, X.; Zhang, R. Polyphyllin G exhibits antimicrobial activity and exerts anticancer effects on human oral cancer OECM-1 cells by triggering G2/M cell cycle arrest by inactivating cdc25C-cdc2. *Arch. Biochem. Biophys.* **2018**, *644*, 93–99. [CrossRef]
46. Telang, N.; Nair, H.B.; Wong, G.Y.C. Growth inhibitory efficacy and anti-aromatase activity of *Tabebuia avellanedae* in a model for postmenopausal luminal a breast cancer. *Biomed. Rep.* **2019**, *11*, 222–229. [PubMed]
47. Nobili, S.; Lippi, D.; Witort, E.; Donnini, M.; Bausi, L.; Mini, E.; Capaccioli, S. Natural compounds for cancer treatment and prevention. *Pharmacol. Res.* **2009**, *59*, 365–378. [CrossRef] [PubMed]
48. Husain, M.A.; Ishqi, H.M.; Sarwar, T.; Rehman, S.U.; Tabish, M. Identification and expression analysis of alternatively spliced new transcript isoform of Bax gene in mouse. *Gene* **2017**, *621*, 21–31. [CrossRef]
49. Saracoglu, I.; Harput, U.S. In vitro cytotoxic activity and structure-activity relationships of iridoid glucosides derived from Veronica species. *Phytother. Res.* **2012**, *26*, 148–152. [CrossRef] [PubMed]

50. Kale, J.; Osterlund, E.J.; Andrews, D.W. BCL-2 family proteins: Changing partners in the dance toward death. *Cell Death Differ.* **2018**, *25*, 65–80. [CrossRef]
51. Gupta, R.; Ambasta, R.K.; Kumar, P. Pharmacological intervention of histone deacetylase enzymes in the neurodegenerative disorders. *Life Sci.* **2020**, *243*, 1–26. [CrossRef]
52. Zhang, L.; Tatsuno, T.; Hasegawa, I.; Tadano, T.; Ohta, T. Furanonaphthoquinones from Tabebuia avellanedae induce cell cycle arrest and apoptosis in the human non-small cell lung cancer cell line A549. *Phytochem. Lett.* **2015**, *11*, 9–17. [CrossRef]
53. Cruz, V.S.; Rodrigues, F.A.; Braga, K.; Machado, P.A.; Bianchi Filho, C.; Prado, Y.C.; Araújo, E.G. β Lapachone blocks the cell cycle and induces apoptosis in canine osteosarcoma cells. *Pesqui. Veter Bras.* **2018**, *38*, 2224–2232. [CrossRef]
54. Dinda, B. Pharmacology of Iridoids. In *Pharmacology and Applications of Naturally, Occurring Iridoids*; Dinda, B., Ed.; Springer International Publishing: Cham, Switzerland, 2019; pp. 145–254.
55. Cao, S.; Zhu, X.; Du, L. P38 MAP kinase is involved in oleuropein-induced apoptosis in A549 cells by a mitochondrial apoptotic cascade. *Biomed. Pharmacother.* **2017**, *95*, 1425–1435. [CrossRef]
56. Xu, J.; Wang, Z.; Huang, Y.; Wang, Y.; Xiang, L.; He, X. A spirostanol saponin isolated from *Tupistra chinensis* Baker simultaneously induces apoptosis and autophagy by regulating the JNK pathway in human gastric cancer cells. *Steroids* **2017**, *164*, 108737. [CrossRef] [PubMed]
57. Xie, X.; Liu, K.; Liu, F.; Chen, H.; Wang, X.; Zu, X.; Ma, X.; Wang, T.; Wu, Q.; Zheng, Y.; et al. Gossypetin is a novel MKK3 and MKK6 inhibitor that suppresses esophageal cancer growth in vitro and in vivo. *Cancer Lett.* **2019**, *442*, 126–136. [CrossRef] [PubMed]
58. Yang, B.; Zhu, R.; Tian, S.; Wang, Y.; Lou, S.; Zhao, H. Jatamanvaltrate P induces cell cycle arrest, apoptosis and autophagy in human breast cancer cells in vitro and in vivo. *Biomed. Pharmacother.* **2017**, *89*, 1027–1036. [CrossRef]
59. Atmaca, H.; Bozkurt, E.; Cittan, M.; Dilek Tepe, H. Effects of Gallium aparine extract on the cell viability, cell cycle and cell death in breast cancer cell lines. *J. Ethnopharmacol.* **2016**, *186*, 305–310. [CrossRef]
60. Bokhari, J.; Khan, M.R.; Shabbir, M.; Rashid, U.; Jan, S.; Zai, J.A. Evaluation of diverse antioxidant activities of Gallium aparine. *Spectrochim. Acta Part A Mol. Biomol. Spectrosc.* **2013**, *102*, 24–29. [CrossRef]
61. Li, Y.; Cheng, X.; Chen, C.; Huijuan, W.; Zhao, H.; Liu, W.; Xiang, Z.; Wang, Q. Apigenin, a flavonoid constituent derived from P. villosa, inhibits hepatocellular carcinoma cell growth by CyclinD1/CDK4 regulation via p38 MAPK-p21 signaling. *Pathol. Res. Pract.* **2020**, *216*, 152701. [CrossRef]
62. Rodenak-Kladniew, B.; Castro, A.; Stärkel, P.; Galle, M.; Crespo, R. 1,8-Cineole promotes G0/G1 cell cycle arrest and oxidative stress-induced senescence in HepG2 cells and sensitizes cells to anti-senescence drugs. *Life Sci.* **2020**, *243*, 117271. [CrossRef]
63. Jiménez-González, F.J.; Veloza, L.A.; Sepúlveda-Arias, J.C. Anti-infectious activity in plants of the genus *Tabebuia*. *Univ. Sci.* **2013**, *18*, 257–267. [CrossRef]
64. Melchor Moncada, J.J.; Socarrás Cárdenas, A.; Mantilla Muriel, L.E.; Sepúlveda Arias, J.C.; Mancilla Estacio, L.I.; Felipe Villalba, M.F.; Caballero, L.C. Actividad Biológica de Plantas de la Familia Bignoniaceae. In *Biotecnología y sus Aplicaciones en el Sector Salud*; Editorial Universidad Tecnológica de Pereira: Pereira, Colombia, 2020; pp. 358–386.
65. Dal Piaz, F.; Vassallo, A.; Temraz, A.; Cotugno, R.; Belisario, M.A.; Bifulco, G.; Chini, M.G.; Pisano, C.; De Tommasi, N.; Braca, A. A chemical-biological study reveals C9-type iridoids as novel heat shock protein 90 (Hsp90) inhibitors. *J. Med. Chem.* **2013**, *56*, 1583–1595. [CrossRef] [PubMed]
66. Mosmann, T. Rapid colorimetric assay for cellular growth and survival: Application to proliferation and cytotoxicity assays. *J. Immunol. Methods* **1983**, *65*, 55–63. [CrossRef] [PubMed]
67. Badisa, R.B.; Darling-Reed, S.F.; Joseph, P.; Cooperwood, J.S.; Latinwo, L.M.; Goodman, C.B. Selective cytotoxic activities of two novel synthetic drugs on human breast carcinoma MCF-7 cells. *Anticancer. Res.* **2009**, *29*, 2993–2996. [PubMed]
68. Khanam, R.; Ahmad, K.; Hejazi, I.I.; Siddique, I.A.; Kumar, V.; Bhat, A.R.; Azam, A.; Athar, F. Inhibitory growth evaluation and apoptosis induction in MCF-7 cancer cells by new 5-aryl-2-butylthio-1,3,4-oxadiazole derivatives. *Cancer Chemother. Pharmacol.* **2017**, *80*, 1027–1042. [CrossRef]

molecules

MDPI

Article

Comparative Analysis of Estragole, Methyleugenol, Myristicin, and Elemicin Regarding Micronucleus Formation in V79 Cells

Andreas Eisenreich *, Lucas Wittek, Marlies Sagmeister, Mia Kruse, Josephine Krüger, Benjamin Sachse, Jakob Menz, Mario E. Götz and Bernd Schäfer

Department of Food Safety, German Federal Institute for Risk Assessment, Max-Dohrn-Straße 8-10, 10589 Berlin, Germany

* Correspondence: andreas.eisenreich@bfr.bund.de; Tel.: +49-30-18412-25202

Abstract: Alkenylbenzenes occur as natural constituents in a variety of edible plants, in particular those herbs and spices used to give a distinctive flavor to a range of food and feed items. Some alkenylbenzenes with relevance for food, such as estragole and methyleugenol, are known to be genotoxic and carcinogenic in rodents. However, the genotoxic and carcinogenic potential of other structurally related alkenylbenzenes, such as myristicin and elemicin, is still under scientific discussion. Here, we investigated the potential of myristicin and elemicin to induce micronuclei (MN) in V79 cells in comparison to that of estragole and methyleugenol. In addition, we determined the impact of these alkenylbenzenes on cell viability and on the induction of apoptosis and necrosis. All tested alkenylbenzenes affected cell viability in a concentration-dependent manner, albeit to varying degrees. Regarding MN formation, elemicin induced a weak but statistically significant response at 100 μM and 500 μM in the absence of an exogenous metabolizing system (S9 mix). Negative results were obtained for estragole and myristicin at the highest tested non-cytotoxic concentration of 10 μM and 100 μM, respectively. For methyleugenol, the MN assay results were considered equivocal, since the observed change in MN induction was rather small and not supported by a concentration-related trend. These findings indicate that traditional in vitro test systems utilizing exogenous metabolizing systems have limited explanatory power with regard to the genotoxic potential of alkenylbenzenes.

Keywords: alkenylbenzenes; genotoxicity; micronucleus assay; viability; apoptosis; necrosis

1. Introduction

Alkenylbenzenes are secondary plant metabolites, occurring as characteristic flavor constituents of various herbs and spices, such as nutmeg, fennel, and basil [1]. As they are components of essential oils [2], particularly high concentrations can be found in food products made from aromatic parts of different herbs and spices, such as basil-based oily condiments (e.g., "pesto"), non-alcoholic or alcoholic beverages (e.g., fennel tea or anis-based liqueurs), or plant-based food supplements [3].

For many alkenylbenzenes occurring in food, the toxicological data required for a conclusive risk assessment are sparse [1,2]. However, some alkenylbenzenes, such as estragole (EST), methyleugenol (ME), and safrole (SAF), are well studied and known to be genotoxic and carcinogenic in rodents [4–6]. Tumors, observed mainly in the liver but also in other organs, seem to be induced by reactive metabolites. These are formed via cytochrome P450 (CYP)-mediated 1′-hydroxylation followed by sulfotransferase (SULT)-catalyzed sulfonation [3]. The resulting allylic sulfate esters spontaneously form electrophilic carbocation intermediates [3]. They are expected to react with cellular nucleophiles, including DNA and proteins, and are therefore likely to act as ultimate carcinogens [4–7]. Due to their genotoxic potential, the addition of the above-mentioned alkenylbenzenes as such to food has already been prohibited and maximum levels of these substances, when naturally present in flavorings and food ingredients with flavoring properties as well as in certain compound foods, have been defined in the European Union (EU) via Regulation (EC) No 1334/2008.

Based on structural similarities to EST, ME, and SAF, it is reasonable to assume that other allylic alkenylbenzenes, like myristicin (MYR) and elemicin (ELE), may also exhibit a genotoxic and carcinogenic potential [1]. However, as is also true for other structurally related substances, the toxicological profiles of MYR and ELE, including genotoxicity, have not yet been comprehensively studied. Those data, together with reliable data on exposure (which are still lacking), are required for a conclusive risk assessment which could support regulation in the EU [3].

In this study, we asked whether a high-throughput micronucleus assay (MNT) with V79 cells can provide relevant comparative insights into the genotoxic potential of yet less characterized alkenylbenzenes. As examples, we analyzed MYR and ELE in comparison to the structurally related and well-studied alkenylbenzenes EST and ME (Figure 1). Moreover, we characterized the differential composition of the cytotoxic effects of these alkenylbenzenes and analyzed the mRNA expression of different exemplary metabolic factors in Chinese hamster (ch) V79 cells. This information may help to ameliorate—at least in part—the insufficient data situation regarding alkenylbenzenes in food.

estragole (EST) (CAS# 140-67-0) | methyleugenol (ME) (CAS# 93-15-2) | myristicin (MYR) (CAS# 607-91-0) | elemicin (ELE) (CAS# 487-11-6)

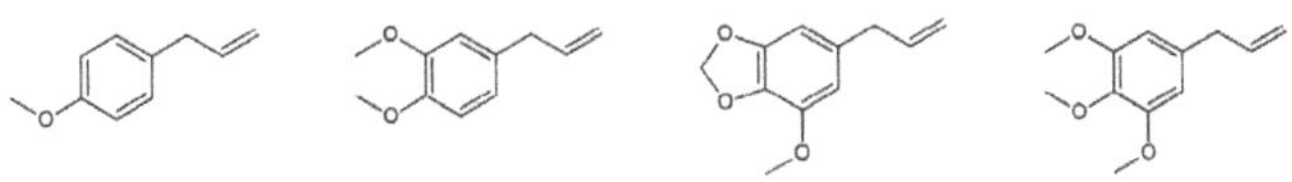

Figure 1. Structural formulas of estragole (EST), methyleugenol (ME), myristicin (MYR), and elemicin (ELE). CAS# = Chemical Abstracts Service number.

2. Results

2.1. *Impact of EST, ME, MYR, and ELE on Micronucleus Formation in V79 Cells*

The influence of EST, ME, MYR, and ELE (1–500 μM each) on micronucleus (MN) formation, the percentage of dead (ethidium monoazide positive; EMA+) cells, and cytotoxicity based on relative nuclei counts was analyzed in V79 cells sampled after 24 h including 4 h exposure in absence (Figure 2A–J), as well as in the presence (Figure 2K–T) of an exogenous metabolizing system (S9).

Positive Controls (−S9): Treatment of V79 cells with 30 μM mitomycin C (MC, used as positive control for an alkylating agent in the absence of S9) significantly increased the frequency of MN. In contrast to MC, 20 μM cyclophosphamide (CP, used as positive control in the presence of S9) had no notable influence on MN generation in the absence of exogenous metabolization (Figure 2A), as expected. Changes in EMA+ cells and relative nuclei counts were considered to fall in an acceptable range (Figure 2F).

EST (−S9): EST did not induce a significant increase in MN frequency up to the highest tested concentration of 10 μM, at which no critical cytotoxicity was observed (Figure 2B). At 100 μM and 500 μM, excessive cytotoxicity was evident in a high percentage of EMA+ cells, as was a sharp decrease in relative nuclei counts (Figure 2G). Therefore, the reliable measurement of MN induction was not possible in this concentration range.

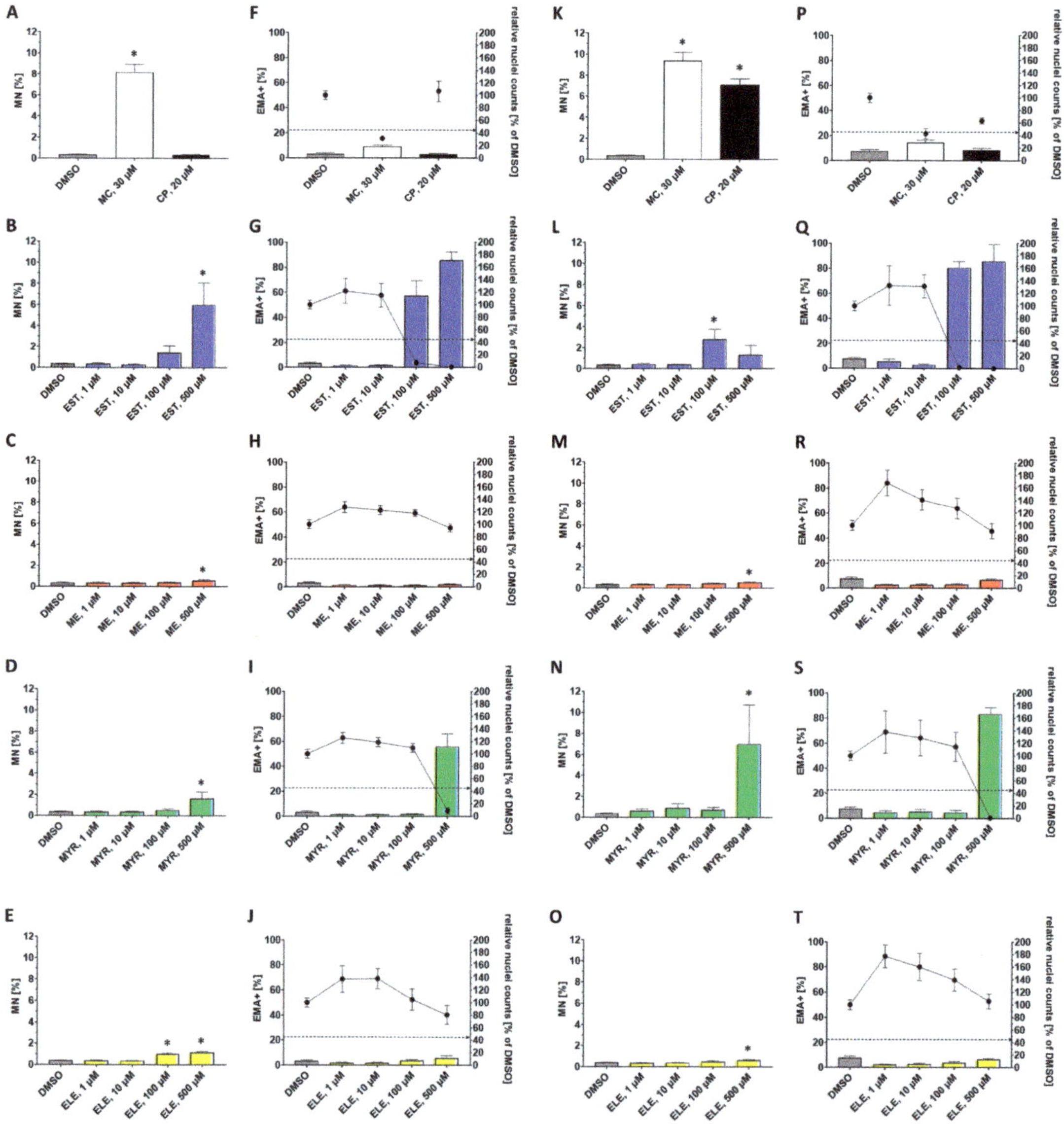

Figure 2. Effect of the studied alkenylbenzenes on micronucleus (MN) formation and viability in V79 cells exposed for 4 h and sampled after 24 h. Shown is the percentage of MN events in the absence (**A–E**) or in the presence (**K–O**) of exogenous metabolization (S9) as well as the percentage of EMA-positive (EMA+) cells and relative nuclei counts (used as cytotoxicity marker and as indicator of cell viability) related to 1% DMSO (negative control) in the absence (**F–J**) or in the presence (**P–T**) of S9, respectively. Cells were treated with 1–500 µM estragole (EST), methyleugenol (ME), myristicin (MYR), or elemicin (ELE), respectively. The positive controls were 30 µM mitomycin C (MC; −S9) and 20 µM cyclophosphamide (CP; +S9). In (**F–J**,**P–T**), the interlinked or single dots represent the relative nuclei counts (% of DMSO) and the dashed line indicates a cytotoxicity limit of 55%. The mean ± SEM of at least 3 independent experiments is shown. (*) = $p < 0.05$.

ME (−S9): Treatment of cells with 1–100 µM ME had no effect on MN induction, whereas 500 µM ME induced a small but significant ($p < 0.05$) increase in MN formation

(Figure 2C). ME treatments at 1–500 μM had no impact on the percentage of EMA+ cells or relative nuclei counts (Figure 2H). However, since the increase in MN induction at 500 μM was minor and not supported by a concentration-related trend, this result was considered equivocal.

MYR (−S9): Similar to EST, MYR produced excessive cytotoxicity at 500 μM, characterized by an increased rate of EMA+ cells and a sharp decrease in relative nuclei counts. At 1–100 μM, the concentration range at which cytotoxicity did not interfere with MN measurements, no significant difference in MN formation was found (Figure 2I).

ELE (−S9): Treatment of V79 cells with ELE significantly increased the MN formation rate at 100 μM and 500 μM (Figure 2E). At 1–500 μM ELE, no excessive cytotoxicity based on the EMA+ cell rate or relative nuclei counts was observed. However, at 500 μM ELE, a slightly increased amount of EMA+ cells and moderately reduced relative nuclei count, compared to the lower concentrations of ELE, was found (Figure 2J). As the increase in MN was rather small but concentration-related and no excessive cytotoxicity occurred, this was interpreted as a weakly positive result.

Positive Controls (+S9): Both 30 μM MC as well as 20 μM CP significantly increased the occurrence of MN after 24 h (Figure 2K), the latter demonstrating sufficient effectiveness of the exogenous metabolic activation system. Changes in EMA+ cells and relative nuclei counts were considered to fall in an acceptable range (Figure 2P).

EST (+S9): Treatment with 1–10 μM EST had no effect on MN formation, EMA+ cells, and relative nuclei counts (Figure 2L,Q), whereas treatment with 100–500 μM EST produced excessive cytotoxicity. Therefore, also in the presence of S9, a reliable measurement of MN induction was not possible at the two highest concentrations.

ME (+S9): Similar to the results obtained in the absence of S9, 1–100 μM ME had no influence on MN formation, whereas 500 μM ME led to a slight but significant increase of the MN induction rate after 24 h (Figure 2M). There was a slight increase in the EMA+ cell rate at 500 μM and a trend towards a decrease in the relative nuclei count compared to lower concentrations of ME but not to the control (Figure 2R). Since the observed change in MN induction was rather small and not supported by a concentration-related trend, this result was considered equivocal.

MYR (+S9): Treatment of V79 cells with 500 μM MYR was accompanied by excessive cytotoxicity, indicated by a strong increase in EMA+ cells and a sharp decrease in relative nuclei counts, compared to the negative control (Figure 2S). In the concentration range of 1–100 μM (Figure 2S), at which no critical cytotoxicity occurred, no significant increase in MN frequency was observed (Figure 2N).

ELE (+S9): Treatment of cells with ELE slightly but significantly induced the formation of MN at 500 μM (Figure 2O). Similar to ME, there was a slight trend towards an increase in EMA+ cell rate and a decrease in relative nuclei counts compared to lower concentrations of ME but not to the control in this setting (Figure 2T). Since the increase in MN induction at 500 μM was minor and not supported by a concentration-related trend, this result was considered equivocal.

In conclusion, ELE induced a weak increase in MN formation at 100 μM and 500 μM in absence of an exogenous metabolizing system (S9 mix). Negative results were obtained for EST and MYR up to the highest tested concentration of 10 μM and 100 μM, respectively, at which no critical cytotoxicity occurred. For ME, the results of the MN assay were considered equivocal.

2.2. Impact of EST, ME, MYR, and ELE on Apoptosis and Necrosis in V79 Cells

The influence of EST, ME, MYR, and ELE exposure on the proportions of V79 cells in viable, early apoptotic, and late apoptotic/necrotic states were assessed after 24 h including 4 h exposure in the absence or in the presence of an exogenous metabolizing system, respectively.

In the absence of metabolic activation (−S9), 10 µM of the positive control camptothecin (CPT) reduced cell viability and increased early- and late-stage apoptosis and necrosis compared to DMSO (Figure 3). The same applied for 500 µM tert-butylhydroperoxide (tBHP), a positive control for peroxide-induced apoptosis and necrosis. Treatment of V79 with 10 µM or 100 µM EST had no notable effect on cell viability or induction of apoptosis and necrosis. However, 500 µM EST obviously lowered cell viability and increased apoptosis and necrosis. Compared to the negative control, 10–500 µM ME, MYR, and ELE led to a dose-dependent and moderate reduction of cell viability and to an increase of early- and late-stage apoptosis and necrosis (Figure 3).

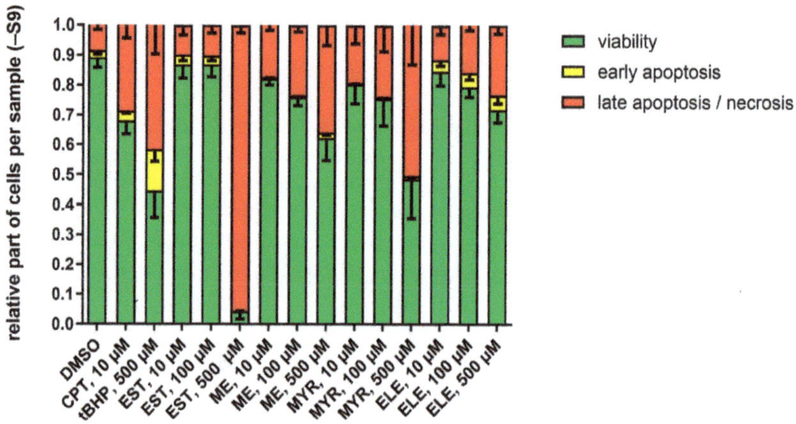

Figure 3. Effect of alkenylbenzenes on the proportions of viable, early apoptotic, and late apoptotic/necrotic cells in the absence of exogenous metabolization (S9). V79 cells were exposed for 4 h and sampled after 24 h. Treatment was performed with 10–500 µM estragole (EST), methyleugenol (ME), myristicin (MYR), or elemicin (ELE), respectively, 10 µM camptothecin (CPT) or 500 µM tert-butylhydroperoxide (tBHP) were used as positive controls, and 1% DMSO was used as negative control. The mean ± SEM of at least 3 independent experiments is shown.

In the presence of metabolic activation (+S9), the DMSO control exhibited a lower rate of viable cells and a higher rate of cells in early- and late-stage apoptosis and necrosis, compared to the absence of S9 (Figure 3). Treatment of cells with 10 µM CPT as well as with 500 µM tBHP (positive controls) in the presence of S9 reduced cell viability and increased apoptosis/necrosis, compared to DMSO (Figure 4). Treatment of V79 cells with 10–500 µM EST, ME, MYR, or ELE led to a concentration-dependent decrease of cell viability and to an increase of cells in early- and late-stage apoptosis and necrosis. The intensity of these effects was comparable between the tested alkenylbenzenes in the presence of S9 (Figure 4).

2.3. Expression of Selected Genes Encoding Cytochrome P450 and Sulfotransferase Enzymes on mRNA Level in V79 Cells

Based on results on functional analyses in V79 cells published in 1990, it is assumed that these cells exhibit negligible endogenous metabolic capacity [8]. However, it is unknown whether these cells express metabolic factors, such as CYPs or SULTs. Therefore, we performed a database search and identified exemplarily representatives of CYPs or SULTs expressed in Chinese hamster (ch) cells. The expression of selected genes encoding chCYP1A1, 1A2, and 2E1, as well as those encoding chSULT1A1 and 2B1, was studied at the mRNA level (Figure 5). In V79 cells, chCYP1A1 and chSULT2B1 mRNA was only detectable at low levels. Compared to chCYP1A1 and chSULT2B1, the expression of chCYP2E1 and chSULT1A1 was much higher, whereas chCYP1A2 was not detectable at the mRNA level (Figure 5).

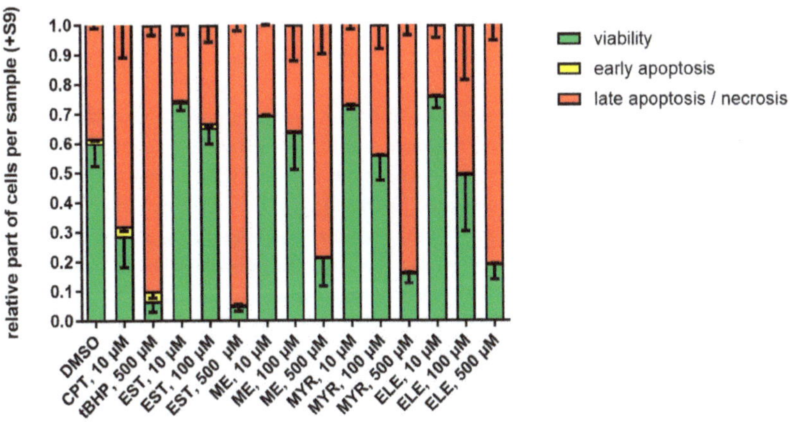

Figure 4. Effect of alkenylbenzenes on the proportions of viable, early apoptotic, and late apoptotic/necrotic cells in the presence of exogenous metabolization (S9). V79 cells were exposed for 4 h and sampled after 24 h. Treatment was performed with 10–500 µM estragole (EST), methyleugenol (ME), myristicin (MYR), and elemicin (ELE), respectively, 1% DMSO was used as negative control, and 10 µM camptothecin (CPT) or 500 µM tert-butylhydroperoxide (tBHP) were used as positive controls. The mean ± SEM of at least 3 independent experiments is shown.

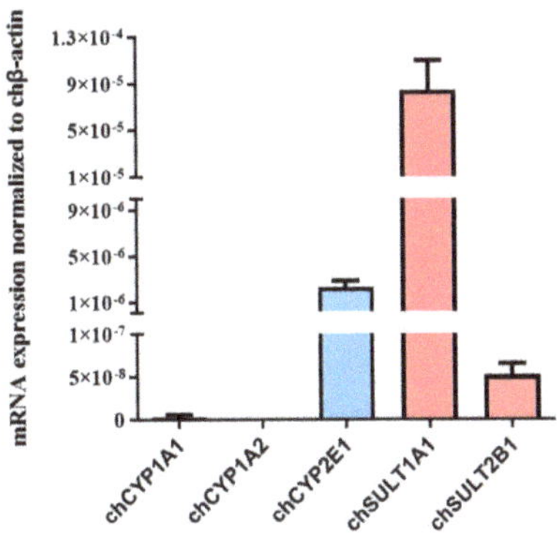

Figure 5. Expression of selected genes encoding cytochrome P450 and sulfotransferase in the V79 cell line. Shown is the mRNA abundance of Chinese hamster cytochrome P450 1A1 (chCYP1A1), 1A2 (chCYP1A2), 2E1 (chCYP2E1), sulfotransferase 1A1 (chSULT1A1), and 2B1 (chSULT2B1) in V79 cells. The abundance of the mRNAs was normalized to that of Chinese hamster beta-actin (chβ-actin) mRNA.

3. Discussion

In recent years, several relevant data gaps were identified regarding alkenylbenzenes in foods, highlighting genotoxicity as one of the most important toxicological aspects [1,9]. To evaluate whether a high-throughput MNT using V79 cells could shed more light on the potential genotoxic effects of less characterized alkenylbenzenes, we performed a comparative analysis using EST, ME, MYR, and ELE as examples.

For the assessment of MN testing results, it is usually recommended to interpret results obtained at cytotoxicity > 55 ± 5% with caution [10]. This is based on the observation that higher levels of cytotoxicity can induce chromosome damage as a secondary effect [11,12].

In this context, Meintieres et al. showed in 2004 that increased apoptosis may also lead to the generation of micronucleated cells, which can potentially affect the outcome of the in vitro MNT, e.g., when performed under extreme conditions [13]. Therefore, in the case of a treatment resulting in excessive cytotoxicity, as observed for higher concentrations of EST and MYR in the present study, increases in MN percentage cannot be interpreted as positive findings.

In the present study, negative MN assay results were obtained for EST at the highest tested concentration of 10 μM, without critical cytotoxicity, while higher concentrations of EST caused excessive cytotoxicity. In line with our findings, EST was also found to be negative in chromosomal aberration tests at 10–1000 μM performed with V79 cells [14,15]. Additionally, predominantly negative in vitro findings regarding the mutagenic potential of EST in the bacterial reverse mutation assay have been published [16,17]. However, this does not exclude that EST induces genotoxicity per se. For example, Martins et al. showed in 2012 that EST induces DNA strand breaks at 250–1000 μM (assessed via an alkaline comet assay) and sister chromatid exchanges (SCE) at 100–750 μM in V79 cells in the absence of S9 [15]. They also found 500–1000 μM EST to induce the formation of DNA adducts in absence of S9 in V79 cells in a dose-dependent manner. Based on their results and the assumption that V79 cells exhibit negligible endogenous metabolic capacity [8], the authors suggested that EST is a weak food-borne genotoxin [15]. Beside this, as comprehensively reviewed elsewhere [18], there is strong evidence of the genotoxic and carcinogenic potential of EST and its metabolites from in vivo studies. Consequently, EST was evaluated as genotoxic and carcinogenic [1,5].

ME is also known to be genotoxic and carcinogenic in rodents [1,4,9]. In our study, however, the in vitro MN assay produced equivocal results for ME. In previous studies, testing of its genotoxic potential in vitro let to negative and positive results, depending on the utilized experimental setting [1,4]. On the one hand, ME was found to be negative in different bacterial test systems, such as the bacterial reverse mutation assay (+/−S9) at 30–300 μg/plate or 0–666 μg/plate and the *Bacillus subtilis* DNA repair test (+/−S9) at 1 mg/disk, as well as in an in vitro chromosome aberration test at 50–500 μg/mL with Chinese hamster ovary (CHO) cells (+/−S9) [17,18]. Moreover, Groh et al. found no significant impact of 10–100 μM ME on the MN frequency in V79 or human colon carcinoma cells (HT29) in the absence of S9 [19,20]. On the other hand, 50–100 μM ME were positive in an unscheduled DNA synthesis (UDS) test in primary cultures of freshly isolated rat hepatocytes [21]. Further, 167 μg/mL ME induced SCE in CHO cells with but not without S9 [18]. ME was also positive in a Comet assay at 10–100 μM with V79 and at 50–100 μM with HT29 cells in absence of S9. Moreover, ME metabolites (methyleugenol-2′,3′-epoxide and 3′-oxomethylisoeugenol) were positive at 10–100 μM in MNT in V79 and at 25–100 μM with HT29 cells in the absence of S9, substantiating the important role of adequate metabolic competence in this context [19,20].

In this study, negative MN assay results were obtained for MYR at the highest tested concentration of 100 μM, at which no critical cytotoxicity occurred, while 500 μM MYR caused excessive cytotoxicity. However, this does not rule out genotoxicity of MYR in other experimental settings, as also discussed for EST. So far, limited data are available on the potential genotoxic effects of MYR. According to a report published by the National Toxicology Program (NTP) in 2019 [22], MYR was assessed to be negative in the bacterial reverse mutation assay at 0–833 μg/plate with or without S9. Moreover, in three-month in vivo studies, no increase in micronucleated polychromatic erythrocytes (PCEs) was found in B6C3F1/N mice. However, 600 mg/kg MYR induced a small but statistically significant increase in micronucleated PCEs in Fisher (F344) rats. MYR was also shown to induce genotoxic effects by Kobets et al. in 2016. They demonstrated in an in vivo avian egg model that 50 mg/egg MYR induced DNA stand breaks in a Comet assay as well as the formation of DNA adducts [23]. Even if our MNT in V79 cells produced negative results, the abovementioned findings of others, especially those obtained in vivo, suggest that MYR exhibits genotoxic potential.

In our experiments, ELE tested positive for MN induction in the absence of S9, whereas an equivocal result was obtained in the presence of S9. This adds to the growing evidence suggesting that ELE has genotoxic potential (reviewed in [1,3]). For example, Hasheminejad et al. [24] showed in 1994 that ELE was positive in an UDS assay (maximum response at 500 µM) performed with rat hepatocytes isolated from male Fischer (F344) rats. Genotoxic effects of ELE were also observed in two in vivo models. In 2016, Kobets and colleagues showed that ELE induced DNA stand breaks in a Comet assay at 20 and 50 mg/egg as well as DNA adduct formation at 50 mg/egg in an avian egg model, indicating genotoxic potential in this setting [23]. More recently, Ishii et al. demonstrated that 400 mg/kg ELE induced genotoxicity in a transgenic rodent model (*gpt* delta rats), as determined by significantly increased *gpt* mutant frequencies [25]. Moreover, they found that 400 mg/kg ELE increased the number and area of glutathione S-transferase placental form-positive foci, which was interpreted as a preneoplastic effect pointing to hepatocarcinogenic potential. Taken together, the aforementioned findings increasingly indicate that ELE exhibits genotoxic potential.

The data obtained from the MNT in V79 cells exposed for 4 h and sampled after 24 h indicate that EST, ME, MYR, and ELE differentially affected relative nuclei counts (as an indicator of cytotoxicity) and rates of dead (EMA+) cells (Figure 2). Therefore, we performed additional experiments to further characterize the impact of EST, ME, MYR, and ELE on cell viability as well as on rates of early- and late-stage apoptosis and necrosis (Figures 3 and 4). Our data show that in V79 cells exposed for 4 h and sampled after 24 h, the fraction of cells in the early phase of apoptosis is in all samples much smaller than that of cells in the late apoptosis/necrosis phase after 24 h. At this relatively late sampling timepoint, the early phase of apoptosis is already over and most of the remaining cells are either viable or in the late apoptosis phase or in necrosis, respectively.

We further found that treatment of V79 cells with 10–500 µM EST, ME, MYR, or ELE, respectively, led to a concentration-dependent decrease of cell viability and increased rate of apoptosis/necrosis after 24 h. As also found in the MNT (Figure 2), the cytotoxic effects of EST and MYR, especially at high concentrations (500 µM), were much more intensive than those of ME and ELE (Figures 3 and 4). In line with our findings, other groups also showed that alkenylbenzenes, such es EST, MYR, eugenol, and *trans*-anethole, reduced cell viability and induced apoptosis in a concentration-dependent manner in different experimental settings [26–29]. For example, Martins et al. demonstrated in 2011 MYR to reduce cell viability and to induce apoptotic processes in DNA-repair-deficient EM9 Chinese hamster ovary cells, especially at higher doses > 500 µM [27]. In another study published in 2015, Andrade and colleagues showed that 25 µg/mL EST induced cytotoxic effects in human MCF-7 and NCIH292 cells after 24 h [26].

Moreover, we found that the effects of EST, ME, MYR, or ELE, as well as the positive controls (CPT and tBHP), on viability and apoptosis/necrosis were much higher in the presence of S9, compared to experiments performed in the absence of S9. This is in line with findings of others also showing increased cytotoxic effects of different metabolically activated substances, such as eugenol or benzo[a]pyrene, in V79 cells in the presence of S9 [30,31]. Further substantiating the cytotoxic effects of S9, Cox et al. demonstrated in 2015 that higher concentrations of human S9 also led to higher cytotoxicity in different settings and cell lines, including Chinese hamster cells [32].

Overall, the results of our study, as well as data reported in the literature, clearly show that alkenylbenzenes often give inconclusive or conflicting results in in vitro genotoxicity studies, whereas many derivatives have been shown to be genotoxic in vivo. These conflicting results are probably due to the complex bioactivation of alkenylbenzenes leading to genotoxic metabolites. The main pathway leading to the bioactivation of alkenylbenzenes is thought to be side-chain hydroxylation followed by sulfo conjugation to give reactive sulfate esters [1]. However, when external metabolizing systems such as S9 are used, these molecules are formed outside the cells. As the sulfate esters are charged, these metabolites are often unable to penetrate the cell sufficiently. As a consequence, such an approach may lead to cytotoxicity rather than genotoxicity, as has been demonstrated in the Ames test for some furan derivatives that are also activated via the SULT pathway [33]. This may also explain, in part, the higher cytotoxicity that has been observed in our study in the presence of S9. Thus, equivocal or weakly positive in vitro results, as observed in our study for ME and ELE and in some other studies reported in the literature for these and other alkenylbenzenes, may be a result of different factors, e.g., the cell line exhibiting residual metabolic activity (such as indicated by mRNA expression of different CYPs and SULTS in the present study), the formation of other genotoxic metabolites, or artefacts, e.g., those caused by cytotoxicity. However, these results may not appropriately reflect the SULT-mediated bioactivation of alkenylbenzenes that is thought to be of high toxicological relevance.

Thus, at this time, standard in vitro genotoxicity tests, including the MNT applied in our study, are currently not suitable models to investigate the genotoxic potency of alkenylbenzenes. The same is probably true for other compounds that are bioactivated to charged metabolites. In this context, mutagenicity analyses in vitro, e.g., via the *hypoxanthine phosphoribosyl transferase* (*HPRT*) gene test could—at least in part—help to approach this issue.

However, in vitro assays to investigate the mutagenic and genotoxic potency of alkenylbenzenes need to be performed with cell lines that express functional phase I (activation) and phase II (conjugation) metabolic enzymes [34,35]. In the case of alkenylbenzenes, at least functional CYPs, SULTs, and glutathione transferases as can be found in the liver would be needed to mimic in vivo metabolism by in vitro test systems [1,36]. This may be reached by using cell lines able or induced to proliferate and to express these enzymes (e.g., cell division as well as metabolically competent liver cells or artificial genetically modified V79 cells expressing specific CYPs and SULTs) in the in vitro MNT or HPRT gene mutation test [34,37–40]. In addition, the presence of sufficient amounts of co-factors required for the metabolic activation of alkenylbenzenes must be ensured [3]. As for now, in vivo models, in particular the transgenic rodent assay, appear to be the most appropriate test systems to address the mutagenic and genotoxic potential of this class of compounds. Results obtained from in vivo tests could also be used to get an impression of the relative potency of individual alkenylbenzenes [41].

On the other hand, animal testing is increasingly being avoided due to ethical obligations and high costs. In fact, the genotoxicity testing strategy of the European Food Safety Authority (EFSA) only recommends a battery of Ames tests and MNT as a first step. If the results of this battery are negative, no in vivo follow-up is recommended [42]. In turn, the genotoxic activity of alkenylbenzenes would not be detected by the standard procedure.

4. Materials and Methods

4.1. Cell Culture

In this study, we used V79 cells (Chinese hamster lung fibroblasts) for assessment of genotoxic effects induced by EST, ME, MYR, and ELE. These cells offer different features useful for adequate performance of the MNT. V79 have a doubling time of about

12 h, which is helpful, since cell division is essential for the formation and detection of MN [34,43]. Moreover, these cells exhibit a high sensitivity for genotoxins, due to a reduced DNA repair capacity [44]. V79 cells were cultured in Dulbecco's Modified Eagle Medium (DMEM; Pan-Biotech, Aidenbach, Germany) containing 10% fetal bovine serum (FBS; Pan-Biotech, Aidenbach, Germany) and 1% penicillin/streptomycin (Capricorn Scientific, Ebsdorfergrund, Germany) at 37 °C in a humidified incubator (5% CO_2, 95% air).

For experimental testing, V79 cells were treated with 1, 10, 100, and 500 µM EST (Chemical Abstracts Service number (CAS#) 140-67-0, purity = 98%), ME (CAS# 93-15-2, purity > 98%), MYR (CAS# 607-91-0, purity ≥ 85%), and ELE (CAS# 487-11-6, purity = 98%), each provided by Sigma-Aldrich, Taufkirchen, Germany. The selection of the dose range used for alkenylbenzene treatment was based on results of preliminary apoptosis/necrosis tests performed as described below. Treatment was performed for 4 h in the presence (+) or the absence (−) of a 10% S9 mix consisting of 2.85 mL liver S9 (supernatant fraction from homogenized liver after centrifugation at 9000× *g*) from 5- to 6-week-old male Sprague Dawley rats induced with phenobarbital and 5,6-benzoflavone (Trinova Biochem GmbH, Gießen, Germany), 4.65 mL sterile water, and 15 mL co-factor solution (8.0 mM $MgCl_2/6H_2O$ (Supelco, St. Louis, MO, USA), 33.0 mM KCl (Merck, Darmstadt, Germany), 67.2 mM $Na_2HPO_4/2H_2O$ (Merck), 15.8 mM $NaH_2PO_4/2H_2O$ (Merck), 5.62 mM glucose-6-phosphate (Carl Roth, Karlsruhe, Germany), 4.1 mM NADPH (Carl Roth), and 4.3 mM NADH (Carl Roth)). This was done in a volume of 500 µL/well (+S9: 350 µL DMEM + 100 µL S9 mix + 50 µL DMEM with substance or control; −S9: 450 µL DMEM + 50 µL DMEM with substance). After that, the medium was replaced by fresh medium for a further 20 h (recovery phase). As controls for genotoxicity, cells were treated with 20 µM cyclophosphamide (CP, positive control in the presence of S9; Sigma-Aldrich) or with 30 µM mitomycin C (Mito, positive control in the absence of S9; Sigma-Aldrich). All test substances and positive controls were solved in dimethyl sulfoxide (DMSO; Merck) and 1% DMSO was used as negative control.

4.2. Micronucleus Test

For the treatment phase, 8000 V79 cells/well were seeded in 48-well plates for 24 h in 500 µL DMEM. After that, medium was changed and cells were treated as described above. After 24 h, medium was removed and the percentages of MN and dead (EMA+) cells, as well as cytotoxicity based on relative nuclei counts (as % of DMSO control) were determined via flow cytometry using the MicroFlow In Vitro-250/50 Kit (NC1938779, Litron Laboratories, Rochester, NY, USA) following the manufacturer's protocol. Flow cytometric analyses were done using the BD Accuri™ C6 Plus (Biosciences Products, Becton, NJ, USA) device.

4.3. Apoptosis/Necrosis Assay

At 24 h prior to treatment, 8000 V79 cells/well were seeded in DMEM in 48-well plates. Next, the medium was changed and V79 cells were treated with 10, 100, and 500 µM EST, ME, MYR, ELE, 1% DMSO (negative control), and 10 µM CPT (Sigma-Aldrich) or 500 µM tBHP (Sigma-Aldrich), respectively, as positive controls (+/−S9). Treatment was done as described above. Post 24 h, the supernatant was transferred to a 2 mL tube and kept on ice. Then, cells were washed with 500 µL PBS/well which was then conveyed to a 2 mL tube. Next, V79 cells were detached with 100 µL trypsin/well for 2–3 min and 500 µL DMEM/well as the stop reagent. Then, cells solved in 600 µL trypsin/DMEM were pooled with the treatment medium and PBS in the corresponding 2 mL tube. All samples were centrifugated for 10 min at 300× *g* and 4 °C (Multifuge 3SR+, Thermo Fisher Scientific, Waltham, MA, USA) and the supernatant was discarded. Cells were washed with 100 µL calcium buffer (0.1 M HEPES, pH 7.4; 1.4 M NaCl; 25 mM $CaCl_2$; each provided by Carl Roth), centrifugated (10 min at 300× *g* and 4 °C), and the supernatant was discarded. Then, cells were dyed with 80 µL of 5% 7-amino-actinomycin D (7-AAD; BioGems, Via Colinas, CA, USA)/5% Annexin-V-phycoerythrin (AV-PE; Biosciences Products)/90% calcium buffer mix per sample for 20 min in the dark on ice. The measurement was done via flow cytometry using the BD Accuri™ C6 Plus (Biosciences Products) device and following the manufacturer's protocol. Characterizations of the cell populations were done as follows: PE^-/7-AAD^-: viable; PE^+/7-AAD^-: early-apoptotic; and $PE^{-/+}$/7-AAD^+: late-apoptotic and necrotic.

4.4. Quantitative Real-Time Polymerase Chain Reaction

Prior to the performance of quantitative real-time polymerase chain reaction (qRT-PCR), total RNA was isolated from V79 cell using the RNeasy mini Kit (Qiagen, Hilden, Germany) following the manufacturer's instructions, 1 µg of total RNA was reverse transcribed using the High-Capacity cDNA Reverse Transcription Kit (Thermo Fisher Scientific), And 1 µL complementary (c)DNA and 9 µL master mix (2,8 µL water; 5 µL Absolute qPCR SYBR Green ROX mix and 1.2 µL primer (5 µM), respectively) were mixed per well. For qRT-PCR, an AriaDX (Agilent technologies, Waldbronn, Germany) was used. Conditions were 95 °C, 15 s; 40 cycles: 95 °C, 15 s; and 60 °C, 1 min; followed by (each 1x) 60 °C, 10 min; 95 °C, 15 min; 60 °C, 20 min; and 95 °C, 15 min). Determined was the expression of Chinese hamster *(ch)CYP1A1* (all 5′->3′; forward: AGCTTCTGCATCCTCTTGCT; reverse: AAGGGTCAAAGTGGCCAACC), *chCYP1A2* (forward: TAGCCTCAGACCCAACCTCA; reverse: TCTGCCGTTAGCTTCTGCAA), *chCYP2E1* (forward: CGGGATGTGACGGACTGTTT; reverse: AGTCCGCCAAAGTCACAGAA), *chSULT1A1* (forward: GGGTGCCCTTCCTTGAGTTT; reverse: GCAAGGACAGAGGCAGATGT), chSULT2B1 (forward: GGGTTCATGCACACTCTGGA; reverse: CACGTGGTACCTGACTTGGG), normalized against the expression of actin (*chActin:* forward: CACCACAGCTGAGAGGGAAA; reverse: GGAGGAAGAGGATGCAGCAG) in V79.

4.5. Statistical Analysis

All data were expressed as mean ± SEM. Data were analyzed by Student's *t*-test or one-way ANOVA as appropriate. A probability value (p) < 0.05 was regarded as significant. Statistical analyses were done using GraphPad Prism, version 10.1.2 (GraphPad Software, Boston, MA, USA).

5. Conclusions

In summary, the findings reported and discussed in this manuscript emphasize the need to further develop existing in vitro genotoxicity testing systems that do not rely on exogenous metabolizing systems in order to increase the sensitivity to genotoxins that are bioactivated to highly reactive but charged compounds.

Author Contributions: Conceptualization, A.E., M.E.G., and B.S. (Bernd Schäfer); investigation, L.W., M.S., J.K., and M.K.; data curation, A.E., L.W., J.K., M.K., and J.M.; writing—original draft preparation, A.E., L.W., M.E.G., J.K., M.S., M.K., B.S. (Benjamin Sachse), and J.M.; writing—review and editing, A.E., M.E.G., J.M., B.S. (Benjamin Sachse), and B.S. (Bernd Schäfer); supervision, A.E., B.S. (Bernd Schäfer), and M.S.; project administration, A.E., M.E.G., and B.S. (Bernd Schäfer). All authors have read and agreed to the published version of the manuscript.

Funding: This research received no external funding.

Institutional Review Board Statement: Not applicable.

Informed Consent Statement: Not applicable.

Data Availability Statement: The data presented in this study are available on request from the corresponding author (the data are not publicly available due to privacy).

Acknowledgments: We thank Anja Köllner for technical support and Matthias Peiser for methodological and administrative support.

Conflicts of Interest: The authors declare no conflicts of interest.

References

1. Eisenreich, A.; Götz, M.E.; Sachse, B.; Monien, B.H.; Herrmann, K.; Schäfer, B. Alkenylbenzenes in foods: Aspects impeding the evaluation of adverse health effects. *Foods* **2021**, *10*, 2139. [CrossRef] [PubMed]
2. Götz, M.E.; Eisenreich, A.; Frenzel, J.; Sachse, B.; Schafer, B. Occurrence of Alkenylbenzenes in Plants: Flavours and Possibly Toxic Plant Metabolites. *Plants* **2023**, *12*, 2075. [CrossRef] [PubMed]
3. Götz, M.E.; Sachse, B.; Schäfer, B.; Eisenreich, A. Myristicin and Elemicin: Potentially Toxic Alkenylbenzenes in Food. *Foods* **2022**, *11*, 1988. [CrossRef] [PubMed]
4. Scientific Committee on Food; European Commision. Opinion of the Scientific Committee on Food on Methyleugenol (4-Allyl-1,2-dimethoxybenzene). In *SCF/CS/FLAV/FLAVOUR/4 ADD1 FINAL*; European Commision: Luxembourg, 2001; pp. 1–10.
5. Scientific Committee on Food; European Commision. Opinion of the Scientific Committee on Food on Estragole (1-Allyl-4-methoxybenzene). In *SCF/CS/FLAV/FLAVOUR/6 ADD2 FINAL*; European Commision: Luxembourg, 2001; pp. 1–10.
6. Scientific Committee on Food; European Commision. Opinion of the Scientific Committee on Food on the safety of the presence of safrole (1-allyl-3,4-methylene dioxy benzene) in flavourings and other food ingredients with flavouring properties. In *SCF/CS/FLAV/FLAVOUR/6 ADD3 Final*; European Commision: Luxembourg, 2002; pp. 1–15.
7. Burkey, J.L.; Sauer, J.M.; McQueen, C.A.; Sipes, I.G. Cytotoxicity and genotoxicity of methyleugenol and related congeners-- a mechanism of activation for methyleugenol. *Mutat. Res.* **2000**, *453*, 25–33. [CrossRef] [PubMed]
8. Glatt, H.; Gemperlein, I.; Setiabudi, F.; Platt, K.L.; Oesch, F. Expression of xenobiotic-metabolizing enzymes in propagatable cell cultures and induction of micronuclei by 13 compounds. *Mutagenesis* **1990**, *5*, 241–249. [CrossRef] [PubMed]
9. Martins, C.; Rueff, J.; Rodrigues, A.S. Genotoxic alkenylbenzene flavourings, a contribution to risk assessment. *Food Chem. Toxicol.* **2018**, *118*, 861–879. [CrossRef]
10. Honma, M. Cytotoxicity measurement in in vitro chromosome aberration test and micronucleus test. *Mutat. Res.* **2011**, *724*, 86–87. [CrossRef]
11. Aimonen, K.; Suhonen, S.; Hartikainen, M.; Lopes, V.R.; Norppa, H.; Ferraz, N.; Catalan, J. Role of Surface Chemistry in the In Vitro Lung Response to Nanofibrillated Cellulose. *Nanomaterials* **2021**, *11*, 389. [CrossRef]
12. Hilliard, C.A.; Armstrong, M.J.; Bradt, C.I.; Hill, R.B.; Greenwood, S.K.; Galloway, S.M. Chromosome aberrations in vitro related to cytotoxicity of nonmutagenic chemicals and metabolic poisons. *Environ. Mol. Mutagen.* **1998**, *31*, 316–326. [CrossRef]
13. Meintieres, S.; Marzin, D. Apoptosis may contribute to false-positive results in the in vitro micronucleus test performed in extreme osmolality, ionic strength and pH conditions. *Mutat. Res.* **2004**, *560*, 101–118. [CrossRef]
14. Muller, L.; Kasper, P.; Muller-Tegethoff, K.; Petr, T. The genotoxic potential in vitro and in vivo of the allyl benzene etheric oils estragole, basil oil and trans-anethole. *Mutat. Res.* **1994**, *325*, 129–136. [CrossRef]
15. Martins, C.; Cacao, R.; Cole, K.J.; Phillips, D.H.; Laires, A.; Rueff, J.; Rodrigues, A.S. Estragole: A weak direct-acting food-borne genotoxin and potential carcinogen. *Mutat. Res.* **2012**, *747*, 86–92. [CrossRef]
16. Zeiger, E.; Anderson, B.; Haworth, S.; Lawlor, T.; Mortelmans, K.; Speck, W. Salmonella mutagenicity tests: III. Results from the testing of 255 chemicals. *Environ. Mutagen.* **1987**, *9* (Suppl. 9), 1–109. [CrossRef]
17. Sekizawa, J.; Shibamoto, T. Genotoxicity of safrole-related chemicals in microbial test systems. *Mutat. Res. Genet. Toxicol.* **1982**, *101*, 127–140. [CrossRef]
18. National Toxicology Program. *NTP Technical Report on the Toxicology and Carcinogenesis Studies of Methyleugenol (CAS NO. 93-15-2) in F344/N Rats and B6C3F1 Mice (Gavage Studies)*; NTP Toxicity Report Series; NTP TR 491 (NIH Publication No. 00-3950); National Toxicology Program: Triangle Park, NC, USA, 2000; pp. 1–412.
19. Groh, I.A.M.; Cartus, A.T.; Vallicotti, S.; Kajzar, J.; Merz, K.H.; Schrenk, D.; Esselen, M. Genotoxic potential of methyleugenol and selected methyleugenol metabolites in cultured Chinese hamster V79 cells. *Food. Funct.* **2012**, *3*, 428–436. [CrossRef]
20. Groh, I.A.M.; Rudakovski, O.; Gründken, M.; Schroeter, A.; Marko, D.; Esselen, M. Methyleugenol and oxidative metabolites induce DNA damage and interact with human topoisomerases. *Arch. Toxicol.* **2016**, *90*, 2809–2823. [CrossRef]
21. Chan, V.S.W.; Caldwell, J. Comparative induction of unscheduled DNA synthesis in cultured rat hepatocytes by allylbenzenes and their 1′-hydroxy metabolites. *Food Chem. Toxicol.* **1992**, *30*, 831–836. [CrossRef]
22. National Toxicology Program. *NTP Technical Report on the Toxicity Studies of Myristicin (CASRN 607-91-0) Administered by Gavage to F344/NTac Rats and B6C3F1/N Mice*; National Toxicology Program Technical Report Series; National Toxicology Program: Triangle Park, NC, USA, 2019; Volume 95, pp. 1–65.

23. Kobets, T.; Duan, J.D.; Brunnemann, K.D.; Etter, S.; Smith, B.; Williams, G.M. Structure-activity relationships for DNA damage by alkenylbenzenes in Turkey egg fetal liver. *Toxicol. Sci.* **2016**, *150*, 301–311. [CrossRef]
24. Hasheminejad, G.; Caldwell, J. Genotoxicity of the alkenylbenzenes alpha- and beta-asarone, myristicin and elimicin as determined by the UDS assay in cultured rat hepatocytes. *Food Chem. Toxicol.* **1994**, *32*, 223–231. [CrossRef] [PubMed]
25. Ishii, Y.; Shi, L.; Takasu, S.; Ogawa, K.; Umemura, T. A 13-week comprehensive toxicity study with adductome analysis demonstrates the toxicity, genotoxicity, and carcinogenicity of the natural flavoring agent elemicin. *Food. Chem. Toxicol.* **2023**, *179*, 113965. [CrossRef]
26. Andrade, T.C.B.; Lima, S.G.D.; Freitas, R.M.; Rocha, M.S.; Islam, T.; Silva, T.G.D.; Militão, G.C.G. Isolation, characterization and evaluation of antimicrobial and cytotoxic activity of estragole, obtained from the essential oil of croton zehntneri (euphorbiaceae). *Anais Acad. Bras. Cienc.* **2015**, *87*, 173–182. [CrossRef]
27. Martins, C.; Doran, C.; Laires, A.; Rueff, J.; Rodrigues, A.S. Genotoxic and apoptotic activities of the food flavourings myristicin and eugenol in AA8 and XRCC1 deficient EM9 cells. *Food Chem. Toxicol.* **2011**, *49*, 385–392. [CrossRef] [PubMed]
28. Harakeh, S.; Al-Raddadi, R.; Alamri, T.; Al-Jaouni, S.; Qari, M.; Qari, Y.; Kumar, A.; Tashkandi, H.M.; Moulay, M.; Aldahlawi, A.M.; et al. Apoptosis induction in human hepatoma cell line HepG2 cells by trans- Anethole via activation of mitochondria-mediated apoptotic pathways. *Biomed. Pharmacother.* **2023**, *165*, 115236. [CrossRef] [PubMed]
29. Martins, C.; Doran, C.; Silva, I.C.; Miranda, C.; Rueff, J.; Rodrigues, A.S. Myristicin from nutmeg induces apoptosis via the mitochondrial pathway and down regulates genes of the DNA damage response pathways in human leukaemia K562 cells. *Chem.-Biol. Interact.* **2014**, *218*, 1–9. [CrossRef]
30. Maralhas, A.; Monteiro, A.; Martins, C.; Kranendonk, M.; Laires, A.; Rueff, J.; Rodrigues, A.S. Genotoxicity and endoreduplication inducing activity of the food flavouring eugenol. *Mutagenesis* **2006**, *21*, 199–204. [CrossRef]
31. O'Donovan, M.R. Mutation assays of ethyl methanesulphonate, benzidine and benzo[a]pyrene using Chinese hamster V79 cells. *Mutagenesis* **1990**, *5*, 9–13.
32. Cox, J.A.; Fellows, M.D.; Hashizume, T.; White, P.A. The utility of metabolic activation mixtures containing human hepatic post-mitochondrial supernatant (S9) for in vitro genetic toxicity assessment. *Mutagenesis* **2016**, *31*, 117–130. [CrossRef]
33. Glatt, H.; Schneider, H.; Murkovic, M.; Monien, B.H.; Meinl, W. Hydroxymethyl-substituted furans: Mutagenicity in Salmonella typhimurium strains engineered for expression of various human and rodent sulphotransferases. *Mutagenesis* **2012**, *27*, 41–48. [CrossRef] [PubMed]
34. Xie, J.; Tu, H.; Chen, Y.; Chen, Z.; Yang, Z.; Liu, Y. Triphenyl phosphate induces clastogenic effects potently in mammalian cells, human CYP1A2 and 2E1 being major activating enzymes. *Chem. Biol. Interact.* **2023**, *369*, 110259. [CrossRef]
35. Zhu, N.; Hu, K.; Li, Z.; Chen, Y.; Liu, Y. Micronuclei Formation by Promutagens in Metabolism-Incompetent V79 Cells Interacting with Activation-Proficient Cells in Various Experimental Settings. *Environ. Mol. Mutagen.* **2020**, *61*, 224–234. [CrossRef]
36. Yao, H.; Peng, Y.; Zheng, J. Identification of glutathione and related cysteine conjugates derived from reactive metabolites of methyleugenol in rats. *Chem. Biol. Interact.* **2016**, *253*, 143–152. [CrossRef] [PubMed]
37. Rutz, L.; Gao, L.; Kupper, J.H.; Schrenk, D. Structure-dependent genotoxic potencies of selected pyrrolizidine alkaloids in metabolically competent HepG2 cells. *Arch. Toxicol.* **2020**, *94*, 4159–4172. [CrossRef] [PubMed]
38. Jiang, H.; Lai, Y.; Hu, K.; Chen, D.; Liu, B.; Liu, Y. Genotoxicity of 1-methylpyrene and 1-hydroxymethylpyrene in Chinese hamster V79-derived cells expressing both human CYP2E1 and SULT1A1. *Environ. Mol. Mutagen.* **2015**, *56*, 404–411. [CrossRef]
39. Haas, M.; Wirachowski, K.; Thibol, L.; Kupper, J.H.; Schrenk, D.; Fahrer, J. Potency ranking of pyrrolizidine alkaloids in metabolically competent human liver cancer cells and primary human hepatocytes using a genotoxicity test battery. *Arch. Toxicol.* **2023**, *97*, 1413–1428. [CrossRef]
40. Josse, R.; Rogue, A.; Lorge, E.; Guillouzo, A. An adaptation of the human HepaRG cells to the in vitro micronucleus assay. *Mutagenesis* **2012**, *27*, 295–304. [CrossRef]
41. Nohmi, T.; Masumura, K.; Toyoda-Hokaiwado, N. Transgenic rat models for mutagenesis and carcinogenesis. *Genes Environ.* **2017**, *39*, 11. [CrossRef]
42. EFSA Scientific Committee. Scientific opinion on genotoxicity testing strategies applicable to food and feed safety assessment. *EFSA J.* **2011**, *9*, 2379. [CrossRef]
43. Sommer, S.; Buraczewska, I.; Kruszewski, M. Micronucleus Assay: The State of Art, and Future Directions. *Int. J. Mol. Sci.* **2020**, *21*, 1534. [CrossRef]
44. Elkind, M.M.; Sutton, H. Radiation response of mammalian cells grown in culture. 1. Repair of X-ray damage in surviving Chinese hamster cells. *Radiat. Res.* **1960**, *13*, 556–593. [CrossRef]

molecules

MDPI

Article

In Situ Antimicrobial Properties of Sabinene Hydrate, a Secondary Plant Metabolite

Asta Judžentienė *, Dalė Pečiulytė and Irena Nedveckytė

Institute of Biosciences, Life Sciences Center, Vilnius University, Saulėtekio Avenue 7, LT-10257 Vilnius, Lithuania; irena.nedveckyte@gf.vu.lt (I.N.)
* Correspondence: asta.judzentiene@gmc.vu.lt

Abstract: The objective of this research was to investigate natural products for their potential against pathogenic microorganisms. Sabinene hydrate (SH), a monoterpenoid, is synthesised by numerous different plants as a secondary metabolite. At present, there is a lack of definite investigations regarding the antimicrobial activity of SH itself and its different isomers. The antimicrobial effects of commercially available SH (composed mainly of *trans*-isomer) were evaluated within a range of concentrations in three types of contact tests: solid and vapor diffusion and the macro-broth dilution method. Moreover, the effects of SH on the rate of linear growth and spore germination were also examined. Ethanolic SH solutions were tested against an array of microorganisms, including blue-stain fungi (*Ceratocystis polonica, Ophiostoma bicolor, O. penicillatum*), frequently originating from bark beetle galleries; three fungal strains (*Musicillium theobromae, Plectosphaerella cucumerina*, and *Trichoderma* sp.) isolated from a sapwood underneath bark beetle galleries (*Ips typographus*) on spruce (*Picea abies*) stems; *Verticillium fungicola*, isolated from diseased *I. typographus* larvae; two Gram-positive bacteria (*Bacillus subtilis* and *Staphylococcus aureus*), two Gram-negative bacteria (*Escherichia coli* and *Pseudomonas aeruginosa*); five yeasts (*Candida albicans, C. krusei, C. parapsilosis, Saccharomyces cerevisiae*, and *Rhodotorula muscilaginosa*), and two saprophytic fungi (*Aspergillus niger* and *Penicillium notatum*). In solid agar disc diffusion tests, Gram-positive bacteria exhibited greater susceptibility to SH than Gram-negative bacteria, followed by yeasts and fungi. The most resistant to SH in both the disc diffusion and broth macro-dilution methods were *P. aeruginosa, A. niger*, and *Trichoderma* sp. strains. Blue-stain fungi and fungi isolated from the *Picea* sapwood were the most resistant among the fungal strains tested. The minimum inhibition concentrations (MICs) generated by SH and determined using a disc volatilization method were dependent on the fungal species and played an important role in the development of microorganism inhibition. The two Gram-positive bacteria, *B. subtilis* and *S. aureus* (whose MICs were 0.0312 and 0.0625 mg/mL, respectively), were the organisms most susceptible to SH, followed by the Gram-negative bacterium, *E. coli* (MIC = 0.125 mg/mL) and two yeasts, *C. albicans* and *C. kruei* (MIC was 0.125 mg/mL and 0.25 mg/mL, respectively). *C. parapsilosis* (MIC = 0.75 mg/mL) was the yeast most resistant to SH. The investigation of antimicrobial properties of plant secondary metabolites is important for the development of a new generation of fungicides.

Keywords: sabinene hydrate; fungi associated with *Ips typographus*; Gram-positive and Gram-negative bacteria; fungi; yeasts; inhibition

1. Introduction

Sabinene hydrate (SH, also known as 4-thujanol) is a volatile organic compound and belongs to the class of bicyclic monoterpene alcohols. Biosynthesis of monoterpenes occurs mainly by the 2-methyl-erythritol-4-phosphate pathway in plant cell plastids, and geranyl/neryl diphosphate is a key intermediary in the formation of cyclic monoterpenoids [1]. It is important to note that in many cases, the enzymatic synthesis of SH isomers occurs without the formation of free intermediates, e.g., via sabinene or α-thujene [2]. The role of metal ions (such as Mn^{2+} or Mg^{2+}) as catalysts is very important for the biosynthesis of SH in plants [2,3]. SH could be in *cis* or *trans* form, it has optical isomers [2,4], and different enzymes are responsible for the biosynthesis of (1*S*,2*R*,4*S*)-(*Z*)-sabinene hydrate and (1*S*,2*S*,4*R*)-(*E*)-sabinene hydrate [4]. This secondary metabolite occurs naturally in a large number of plants and their essential oils (EOs), including *Citrus* [5,6], *Salvia* [7], *Myristica* [8–10], *Origanum* [11–22], *Thymus* [3,23–28], *Mentha* [22,29], *Juniperus* [30,31] and other species. It has been observed that the presence of terpinen-4-ol in the mature leaves and in the steam distillates of *Melaleuca argentea*, *M. dissitiflora*, and *M. linariifolia* is related to high levels of *cis*- and *trans*-sabinene hydrate in the young leaves. Isomers of SH serve as the precursors of terpinen-4-ol, which is formed through non-enzymatic chemical conversion [32]. A significant number of EOs containing appreciable quantities of SH isomers have demonstrated bioactive properties, including strong antifungal and antibacterial activities [12,18,20,28,29,33–40]. A valuable study was conducted to investigate the cultivable bacterial communities of *Origanum* species, from which EOs containing high amounts of SH were obtained [41]. EOs were found to be rich in *trans*-sabinene hydrate (24.0% and 30.8% for *O. vulgare* ssp. *vulgare* and *O. vulgare* ssp. *hirtum*, respectively), and a high degree of biodiversity was found in the bacterial endophytic microbiome. A hypothesis has been proposed that the composition of the EOs may be involved in the formation of microbial communities and that bacteria may be able to colonize the plants by resisting the antimicrobial activity exhibited by the EOs themselves and/or by using some compounds as carbon and energy sources. The composition of microbial communities of plants can impact or modify the EOs' composition [41].

Plants produce volatile organic compounds for many reasons, and one of them is as a defensive activity against pests and their associated fungi. Terpenoids can be involved in the systemic resistance mechanisms of plants [42–44]. It has been reported how the profile of main terpenoids and enantiomeric ratio of major monoterpenes changed in the stem bark of Norway spruce (*Picea abies*) trees inoculated with blue-stain fungus *Ceratocystis polonica* [45]. However, it has also been found that various fungal strains can degrade tree defence metabolites (phenolic compounds) and use them as a carbon source [46–48]. Furthermore, the different strains of *Endoconidiophora*, *Ophiostoma* or *Grosmannia* associated with the bark beetle *Ips typographus* Linnaeus (Coleoptera, Curculionidae: Scolytinae) can metabolize monoterpenes in Norway spruce resin, producing volatiles with attractant properties [49]. Bornyl acetate can be metabolized into camphor and α- and β-pinene to *trans*-4-thujanol (SH); both monoterpenoids at specific doses attracted the *I. typographus* beetles in the above study. Additionally, it has been discussed how the volatile emissions of conifers may provide clues regarding tree vitality and suitability for *I. typographus* attacks, i.e., to find suitable host trees for the beetles [50]. On other hand, the repellent effects of SH on both sexes of bark beetle *I. typographus* have been evaluated [51–53]. *I. typographus* is a common pest of conifers that attacks Norway spruce, a dominant tree species in the European boreal, montane, and sub-alpine forests, as well as Yezo spruce (*Picea jezoensis*) and Sakhalin spruce (*Picea glehnii* (Fr. Schm.) Masters), dominant trees in eastern Asia [54–58]. During periods when the beetles are not active, they breed in felled, fallen, or windthrown trees, i.e., stumps and logs. During outbreaks, they kill healthy trees, which can have a considerable impact on the forest ecosystem and global environment [59,60].

The interaction between plants and herbivores is often not a simple two-way process; rather, it is mediated by microorganisms, resulting in a complex three-way interaction between plants, herbivores, and microorganisms [55]. The bark beetle *I. typographus* carries spores of several phytopathogenic fungi, including *Ceratocystiopsis minuta*, *Ceratocystis polonica* (Siem.) C. Moreau, *Ophiostoma bicolor* Davidson & Wells, *O. penicillatum* (Grosmann.) Siemaszko (syn., *Grosmannia penicillata*), *O. piceae* and *O. japonicum* [55–58]. A well-studied example of a three-way, plant–herbivore–microbe interaction is that observed between conifer trees and tree-killing bark beetles, in which fungal pathogens, developed in the phloem and cambium, are thought to facilitate the beetles' ability to kill trees [57,58,61].

The main objectives of the investigation were to evaluate the activity of SH (composed mainly of *trans-isomer*), a volatile secondary metabolite of plants against pests' associated microorganisms:

(i) blue-stain fungi: *Ceratocystis polonica*, *Ophiostoma bicolor* and *O. penicillatum* (syn. *Grosmannia penicillata*)), frequently originating from bark beetle galleries;
(ii) other fungi associated with *Ips. typographus*, i.e., three fungal strains: *Musicillium theobromae, Plectosphaerella cucumerina and Trichoderma* sp., isolated from sapwood underneath bark beetle galleries (*Ips typographus*) on spruce (*Picea abies*) stems;
(iii) *Verticillium fungicola*, isolated from diseased *I. typographus* larvae;
(iv) and to compare SH activity against:
(v) two Gram-positive bacteria (*Bacillus subtilis* and *Staphylococcus aureus*),
(vi) two Gram-negative bacteria (*Escherichia coli* and *Pseudomonas aeruginosa*);
(vii) five yeasts (*Candida albicans, C. krusei, C. parapsilosis, Saccharomyces cerevisiae*, and *Rhodotorula muscilaginosa*),
(viii) two saprophytic fungi (*Aspergillus niger* and *Penicillium notatum*).

As we mentioned above, a significant number of studies have been conducted on the antimicrobial activity of plant EOs containing appreciable amounts of SH. However, to the best of our knowledge, at present there is a definite lack of publications on the antimicrobial properties of SH itself and its different isomers [12].

It must be emphasised that there are no previous reports related to SH's effects on most of the microorganisms tested in the present research.

2. Results

2.1. Agar Disc Diffusion Method

The diameters of inhibition zones (IZs), including paper disc diameter (6 mm), are presented in Table 1.

Microbial strains belonging to different groups (bacteria, yeasts, blue-stain, and other fungi) were differently susceptible to SH in the disc diffusion method. SH was more active against Gram-positive bacteria, followed by Gram-negative bacteria and yeasts. Fungi were more resistant than yeasts and bacteria. Blue-stain fungi as well as other fungi showed low susceptibility to SH in the disc diffusion method. The most resistant blue-stain fungus was *O. penicillatum*, with an IZ of only 13.1 ± 0.7 mm even at the highest SH concentration (1000 µg/disc corresponding 100 mg/mL SH concentration). At the lowest SH concentrations (25 µg/disc and 250 µg/disc), *O. penicillatum* (syn. *Grosmannia penicillata*) showed the full resistance to this monoterpene alcohol. Moreover, a stimulation of melanin synthesis by SH was noticeable in fungus cultures. A similar SH resistance level was detected for *C. polonica*. *O. bicolor* was the most sensitive to SH among the blue-stain fungi as well as among all tested fungi. Very low, albeit detectable, growth inhibition was detected even at the lowest SH concentration (125 µg/disc); IZ diameter increased with SH concentration on the paper disc and exceeded 17.2 ± 3.8 mm at 1000 µg/disc SH concentration.

Surprisingly, in this investigation, the saprotrophic fungi and fungi used (whose trophic attribution is not yet determined), isolated from bark beetle galleries, were more resistant to SH than blue-stain fungi were (Table 1). *A. niger* was chosen for our treatments due to its versatility and ability to grow well in a variety of media with different parameters. None of the SH concentrations inhibited *A. niger* or *Trichoderma sp.* strains. All these strains were developed on the paper discs impregnated with 125–250 µg/disc SH content. *A. niger* tolerated also at 500 µg/disc SH concentration. Additionally, *A. niger* was found as a fungus whose sporulation and colony pigmentation were stimulated by SH. *P. notatum* was inhibited only at an SH concentration of 1000 µg/disc, and its IZ was very low (7.9 ± 0.6 mm). *P. notatum* was selected for our studies as a fungus that is ubiquitous in its environment and is able to produce biologically active secondary metabolites. *M. theobromae* showed the largest IZ (average 15.4 mm) as well as *P. cucumerina*, which was susceptible to the lower SH concentration (750 µg/disc).

Table 1. Mean diameters of inhibition zones (mm) of microorganisms using sabinene hydrate in an agar disc diffusion test *.

Microorganisms	Samples						
	Sabinene Hydrate, mg/mL (μg/disc)					ETA [1]	Reference [2]
	12.5 (125)	25.0 (250)	50.0 (500)	75.0 (750)	100 (1000)		
Mycelial fungi							
Ceratocystis polonica	0.0 [3]	0.0 ^{a}	6.0 ± 0.2 ^{a}	13.4 ± 0.5 ^{b,c}	15.5 ± 0.5 ^{b}	11.5 ± 1.5 ^{c}	30.0 ± 3.4
Ophiostoma bicolor	7.2 ± 0.3 ^{a,b,e}	7.6 ± 0.6 ^{a,f}	9.2 ± 0.8 ^{b,c,d,g}	12.3 ± 2.1 ^{c}	17.2 ± 3.8 ^{d}	9.0 ± 0.9 ^{e,f,g}	41.9 ± 2.7
Ophiostoma penicillatum [4]	0.0 ^{a}	0.0 ^{a}	6.0 ± 0.1	7.8 ± 0.6 ^{b}	13.1 ± 0.7	10.5 ± 1.5 ^{b}	30.5 ± 3.1
Musicillium theobromae	0.0	6.0 ± 0.1 ^{a,b,d}	6.0 ± 0.1 ^{a,c,e}	6.0 ± 0.3 ^{b,c,f}	15.4 ± 0.2	6.8 ± 1.3 ^{d,e,f}	36.8 ± 2.9
Plectosphaerella cucumerina	0.0 ^{a}	0.0 ^{a}	6.0 ± 0.0	7.4 ± 0.5 ^{b}	11.8 ± 0.6 ^{c}	7.0 ± 0.3 ^{b}	12.6 ± 1.8 ^{c}
Aspergillus niger	0.0 ^{a,b}	0.0 ^{a,c}	0.0 ± 0.0 ^{b,c}	6.0 ± 0.1 ^{d,e}	6.0 ± 0.0 ^{d,f}	6.0 ± 0.0 ^{e,f}	30.0 ± 1.0
Penicillium notatum	0.0 ^{a}	0.0 ^{a}	6.0 ± 0.0 ^{b,c}	6.0 ± 0.0 ^{b,d}	7.9 ± 0.6	6.0 ± 0.2 ^{c,d}	28.2 ± 2.3
Trichoderma sp.	0.0 ^{a}	0.0 ^{a}	6.0 ± 0.1 ^{b,c,e}	6.0 ± 0.0 ^{b,d,f}	6.0 ± 0.2 ^{c,d,g}	6.5 ± 0.3 ^{e,f,g}	30.3 ± 3.5
Yeasts							
Candida albicans	6.0 ± 0.1 ^{a}	8.2 ± 0.3 ^{a}	11.7 ± 1.5	16.1 ± 0.4 ^{b}	21.4 ± 0.8 c	10.2 ± 0.9	26.4 ± 6.1 ^{b,c}
Candida krueii	6.0 ± 0.2 ^{a,b,e}	6.0 ± 0.1 ^{a,c,f}	8.5 ± 1.8 ^{b,d,g}	8.6 ± 0.9 ^{d,h}	15.5 ± 0.7	7.1 ± 0.8 ^{e,f,g,h}	29.0 ± 2.3
Candida parapsilosis	6.0 ± 0.1 ^{a,b,c,d}	6.0 ± 0.2 ^{a,e}	6.0 ± 0.3 ^{b,c,d,f}	7.0 ± 0.0 ^{d}	18.4 ± 0.9 ^{g}	6.6 ± 0.0 ^{d,e,f}	16.8 ± 1.8 ^{g}
Saccharomyces cerevisiae [5]	6.0 ± 0.2 ^{a,d}	6.0 ± 0.1 ^{a,b,c,e}	6.0 ± 0.1 ^{b,c,f}	8.1 ± 0.3	18.3 ± 0.6	6.5 ± 0.2 ^{d,e,f}	36.9 ± 4.2
Rhodotorula muscilaginae [4]	6.0 ± 0.1 ^{a,d}	6.0 ± 0.1 ^{a,b,e}	7.0 ± 0.2 ^{b,c,f}	9.2 ± 1.3 ^{c}	14.4 ± 0.6	8.2 ± 0.4 ^{d,e,f}	33.7 ± 3.2
Bacteria							
Bacillus subtilis	7.0 ± 0.4 ^{a,b}	7.9 ± 0.8 ^{a}	14.8 ± 2.3 ^{c}	18.9 ± 2.1 ^{d}	33.5 ± 2.7 ^{e}	6.0 ± 0.3 ^{b}	22.4 ± 6.1 ^{c,d,e}
Staphylococcus aureus	6.0 ± 0.1 ^{b}	8.0 ± 0.3 ^{a}	9.1 ± 0.7 ^{a}	13.4 ± 0.4	28.8 ± 1.6 ^{c}	6.0 ± 0.2 ^{b}	36.5 ± 4.8 ^{c}
Escherichia coli	6.0 ± 0.0 ^{a}	7.8 ± 0.5 ^{a,b,d,e,f}	7.6 ± 0.2 ^{c}	8.4 ± 0.9 ^{b,c}	23.8 ± 1.2	7.2 ± 0.4 ^{d,e,f}	31.7 ± 1.6
Pseudomonas aeruginosa	6.0 ± 0.1 ^{a,b,d,k}	6.0 ± 0.1 ^{a,e,f,g,l}	6.0 ± 0.2 ^{b,e,h,i,m}	6.0 ± 0.3 ^{c,f,h,j}	6.0 ± 0.4 ^{d,g,i,j,n}	7.5 ± 0.7 ^{k,l,m,n}	45.7 ± 8.6

* Inhibition zone diameter of 6 mm value is equal to disc diameter, implying no activity. The results are presented as means ± SD (standard deviation) of three replicate tests from three experiments (n = 9); paper of disc diameter is included. [1] Solvent ethanol as negative control is presented only at the highest concentration (10 μL/disc). [2] Reference compounds are chloramphenicol (30 μg/disc) for bacteria and nystatin-dihydrate (30 μg/disc) for fungi. [3] Fungus growth on the paper disc. [4] Strains whose cultures are stimulated by vapor phase. [5] Strains whose cultures are negatively influenced by the vapor phase. Unmarked values are significantly different ($p < 0.05$). For each individual microorganism, obtained values (at different SH concentrations and references) with no significant difference are marked by the same letters (^{a,b,c,d,e,f,g,h,i,j,k,l,m,n}) ($p > 0.05$).

Gram-positive *B. subtilis* was the most sensitive to SH; its average IZ ranged from 7.0 to 33.5 mm with increased SH concentration, followed by *S. aureus* (Gram-positive), whose average IZ values were 28.8 mm at the highest SH concentration (100 mg/mL) (Table 1). None of the SH concentrations tested inhibited Gram-negative bacterium *P. aeruginosa*. This strain as well as the saprotrophic fungi *A. niger* and *Trichoderma* sp. strains were the microorganisms most resistant to SH in the agar disc diffusion test.

2.2. Broth Macro-Dilution Method

The minimum inhibitory concentrations (MICs) of SH were determined against four bacterial and five yeast strains (Table 2).

Gram-positive bacteria, *B. subtilis* and *S. aureus*, with MIC values of 0.0312 and 0.0625 mg/mL, respectively, were the organisms most susceptible to SH, followed by the Gram-negative bacterium *E. coli* (MIC = 0.125 mg/mL) and two yeasts, *C. albicans* and *C. kruei* (MIC values were determined to be 0.125 mg/mL and 0.25 mg/mL, respectively). *C. parapsilosis* was the yeast most resistant to SH (MIC = 0.75 mg/mL), while *S. cerevisiae* and *R. muscilaginosa* showed a medium resistance to this monoterpenoid. None of the concentrations of SH inhibited *P. aeruginosa* (Gram-negative) in this investigation.

Table 2. Minimum inhibition concentrations (mg/mL) of SH for microbial strains by the macro-broth dilution method.

Organisms	Sabinene Hydrate, mg/mL (μg/mL)	Nystatin-Dihydrate, μg/mL	Chloramphenicol, μg/mL
Yeasts			
Candida albicans	0.125 (125)	9.375	–
Candida kruei	0.25 (250)	37.5	–
Candida parapsilosis	0.75 (750)	150.0	–
Saccharomyces cerevisiae	0.5 (500)	18.75	–
Rhodotorula muscilaginosa	0.5 (500)	9.375	–
Gram-positive bacteria			
Bacillus subtilis	0.0312 (30)	–	62.50
Staphylococcus aureus	0.0625 (62.5)	–	<15.625
Gram-negative bacteria			
Escherichia coli	0.125 (125)	–	31.25
Pseudomonas aeruginosa	>1.0 mg/mL *	–	62.50

* *P. aeruginosa* was revealed to be resistant to all tested SH concentrations.

The MICs induced in the microbial cultures by SH were from 10 to 100 times lower than those induced by the standard antibiotics (Table 2). Strains of *B. subtilis* and *P. aeruginosa* were the most resistant to chloramphenicol (MICs = 62.50 μg/mL). *E. coli* (MIC = 31.25 μg/mL) was less sensitive, followed by *S. aureus*, as the most susceptible to chloramphenicol.

All filamentous fungi tested were more resistant to SH than yeasts and bacteria; however, none of the SH concentrations induced 100% inhibition of the fungi in their early development stages (germination or germ-tube formation rate). The most susceptible blue-stain fungus was *O. bicolour* (Table 3).

Table 3. Germination effects (%) of sabinene hydrate on fungi development with the macro-broth dilution method *.

Fungi	Sabinene Hydrate Concentration, mg/mL (μg/mL)					
	0.0625 (62.5)	0.125 (125)	0.25 (2500)	0.5 (500)	0.75 (750)	1.0 (1000)
Ceratocystis polonica	0.0 ± 0.0 [a]	0.0 ± 0.0 [a]	8.62 ± 4.80 [b]	17.11 ± 4.35 [b, c]	31.19 ± 5.17	29.64 ± 7.07 [c]
Ophiostoma bicolor	0.52 ± 0.21 [a]	1.59 ± 1.43 [a]	21.21 ± 9.01	47.98 ± 10.09 [b, c, d]	59.93 ± 19.08 [b, c, d]	67.35 ± 9.93 [d]
O. penicillatum	0.0 ± 0.0 [a]	0.0 ± 0.01 [a]	18.93 ± 7.17	32.14 ± 5.74	49.46 ± 12.38 [b]	49.21 ± 3.67 [b]
Plectosphaerella cucumerina	0.0 ± 0.0 [a, b]	0.0 ± 0.01 [a]	0.0 ± 0.01 [b]	7.35 ± 2.51 [c]	7.68 ± 5.22 [c]	19.89 ± 6.47
Aspergillus niger	0.0 ± 0.0 [a, b]	0.0 ± 0.00 [a, c]	0.0 ± 0.01 [b]	0.0 ± 0.00 [c]	0.82 ± 0.31 [d]	1.45 ± 0.82 [d]
Musicillium theobromae	0.0 ± 0.0 [a]	0.0 ± 0.00 [a]	6.73 ± 2.98 [b]	13.25 ± 4.91 [c, d]	8.97 ± 6.14 [b, c]	24.00 ± 9.45 [d]
	Nystatin-Dihydrate (N-D) Concentration, mg/mL (μg/mL)					
	0.009375 (9.375)	0.01875 (18.75)	0.0375 (37.5)	0.075 (75)	0.15 (150)	0.3 (300)
C. polonica	0.0 ± 0.0 [a]	0.0 ± 0.0 [a]	26.71 ± 11.14	63.28 ± 24.41	98.55 ± 1.23 [a]	100 [a]
O. bicolor	0.92 ± 0.55	13.07 ± 4.46	48.92 ± 20.02	80.27 ± 19.22 [a]	100 [a, b]	100 [b]
O. penicillatum	0.08 ± 0.03	0.88 ± 0.22	37.52 ± 11.55	96.27 ± 3.71 [a, b]	100 [a, b, c]	100 [c]
P. cucumerina	0.19 ± 0.08	14.38 ± 9.71 [a]	33.61 ± 22.04 [a]	87.23 ± 10.71 [b]	99.01 ± 0.04 [b, c]	100 [c]
A. niger	0.04 ± 0.01	3.56 ± 1.88	22.83 ± 6.47	86.87 ± 5.23 [a]	86.17 ± 13.64 [a, b]	100 [b]
M. theobromae	0.62 ± 0.17	31.05 ± 27.91 [a]	66.37 ± 33.06 [a, b, c, d]	90.87 ± 6.61 [b, c, d]	96.14 ± 2.87 [b, c, d]	100 [b, c, d]

* Results are presented as an inhibition of spore (or conidium) germination by SH percentages as compared to control. The results are expressed as a mean ± SD (standard deviation) of three agar plates (with emerged colonies) for each of three wells/each SH dilution. Unmarked values are significantly different ($p < 0.05$). For each individual microorganism, values (at different SH and N-D concentrations) with no significant difference are marked with the same letters ([a, b, c, d]) ($p > 0.05$)

Inhibition of spores started from the lowest tested SH concentration (0.0625 mg/mL) and gradually increased with the increased concentration of the monoterpenoid. Spore germination and inhibition of the ophiostomatoid fungi *C. polonica* and *O. penicillatum* also started from the same SH concentration (2.25 μg/mL). However, *O. penicillatum* showed higher susceptibility (higher inhibition percentages) than *C. polonica* at all SH concentrations tested. Conidia of *A. niger* germinated and were resistant even to very high SH concentrations. An average 0.82% and 1.45% inhibition were caused at 7.5 and 10.0 μg/mL SH concentrations, respectively. Surprisingly, very high resistance to SH was shown by the *M. theobromae* and *P. cucumerina* strains isolated from partially decomposed spruce sapwood underneath *I. typographus* galleries.

As in the case of the broth macro-dilution method used for bacteria and yeasts, nystatin-dihydrate (N-D) activity against the fungi tested was significantly higher than SH activity (Table 3). In the broth macro-dilution method, all fungal strains were fully inhibited by N-D at a concentration of 300 μg/mL, and only a small portion of the propagules of four fungi, including *C. polonica* and fungi associated with beetle galleries (*P. cucumerina*, *A. niger*, and *M. theobromae*) survived at an N-D concentration of 150 μg/mL. *C. polonica* was the strain most resistant to N-D among the all fungi tested. The lowest concentration of N-D, causing 26.71 ± 11.14% inhibition, was 37.5 μg/mL. The lowest N-D concentration inhibited spore germination of both *Ophiostoma* species, and the conidium germination of other fungi was 9.375 μg/mL. However, inhibition percentages were low and insignificant due to the high dispersal of the data.

2.3. *Sabinene Hydrate Volatilization from Paper Disc (Vapour Phase Activity Test)*

In Petri dishes, the atmosphere created from paper discs containing 1 mg, 2 mg, or 3 mg of SH induced inhibition of the radial growth rate, which was fungus species-dependent (Figure 1). Inhibition of the radial growth (%) of the blue-stain fungi by SH supplied during the vapor phase was contradictory. Rate of radial growth of *C. polonica* and other fungi tested were inhibited by SH vapor, while *O. penicillatum* was stimulated up to 47.57% compared to the control by the vapor phase obtained from 1 mg SH in the 9 cm^3 Petri dish. Less stimulation was detected with increasing SH content. *C. polonica* was the least susceptible to SH supplied in the vapor phase, followed by *O. bicolor*.

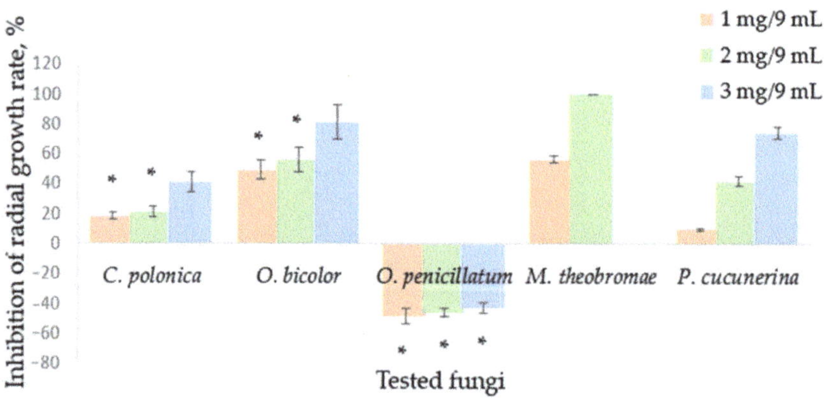

Figure 1. Inhibition of the radial growth rate of fungi by sabinene hydrate supplied in the vapor phase: *Ceratocystis polonica*, *Ophiostoma bicolour*, *Ophiostoma penicillatum* (syn. *Grosmannia penicillata*), *Musicillium theobromae*, and *Plectosphaerella cucunerina*. Mean values represent data from three replicate experiments, bar—SD (standard deviation). Unmarked values are significantly different ($p < 0.05$). A lack of statistically significant difference between the experimental data is marked with asterisks (*).

Two yeasts investigated were also affected by SH supplied in the vapor phase. Neither of the two strains was stimulated by SH in the disc volatilization method (Figure 2). Yeast cell budding as well as pseudo-mycelium formation rate was influenced in the atmosphere containing SH vapor evaporated from 3 mg SH (Figure 2). Greater damage from SH vapor, evaluated as cell budding inhibition percentage (Figure 2), and determined for *C. albicans*. *C. parapsilosis* was more resistant in both cell budding (Figure 2) and pseudo-hypha development (Figure 3).

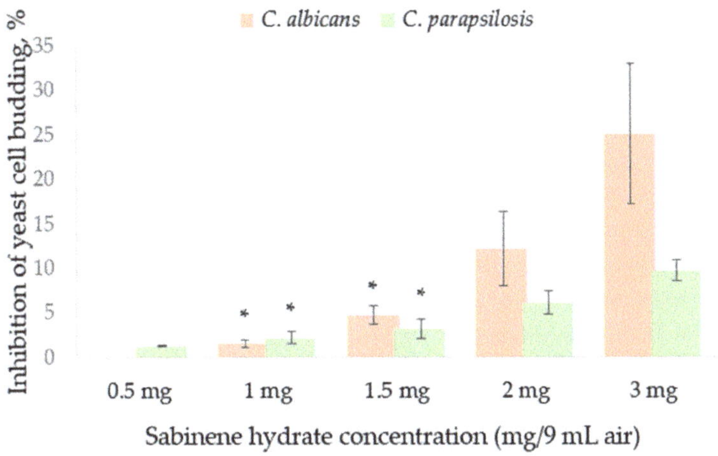

Figure 2. Inhibition of yeast cell budding by the sabinene hydrate supplied in the vapor phase in the disc volatilization method. Mean from three experiments ($n = 3$), bar—SD (standard deviation). Unmarked values are significantly different ($p < 0.05$). A lack of statistically significant difference between the experimental data is marked with asterisks (*).

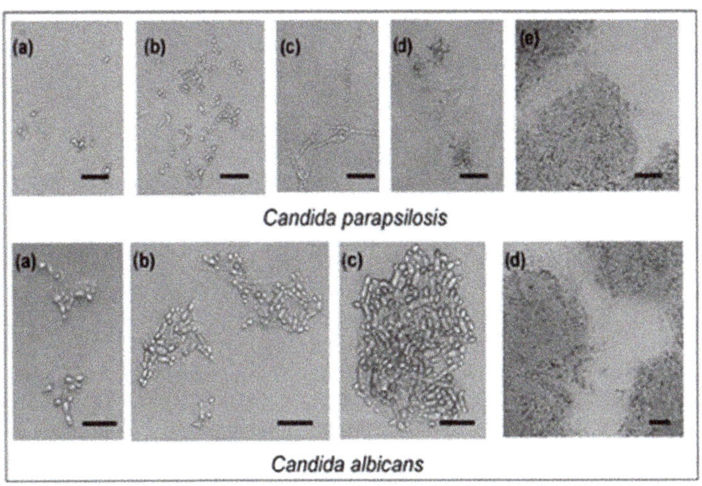

Figure 3. Effect of sabinene hydrate supplied in the vapor phase (volatile fraction evaporating into 9 cm^3 Petri dish atmosphere from paper disc impregnated with 1 g of this compound) on yeast cell budding and pseudo-mycelium formation. Scale is 10 µm; (**a**–**c**) conidia and conidiophores; (**d**,**e**) conidiophores and conidial masses in preparations. The most representative images were selected from each of the three replicates ($n = 3$).

2.4. Results of Dual Culture Tests

Results obtained from dual culture tests differed significantly depending on the culture medium used (malt extract medium (MEA) or malt extract medium amended with spruce phloem extract (MEA + SPE)). Significant differences between the inter-inhibition levels were detected for the blue-stain fungi (Table 4).

Table 4. Inhibition (%) of radial growth in dual culture test *.

Inhibiting Fungus	Medium	Inhibition of Radial Growth Rate (%)		
		C. polonica	*O. bicolor*	*O. penicillatum*
Ceratocystis polonica	MEA		12.08 ± 1.88	78.91 ± 11.47
	MEA + SPE		49.31 ± 10.31 [a]	46.77 ± 20.28 [a]
Oprhiostoma bicolor	MEA	98.89 ± 1.11		43.28 ± 10.99
	MEA + SPE	24.68 ± 9.55 [a]		41.63 ± 4.75 [a]
Ophiostoma penicillatum	MEA	12.43 ± 4.88	65.14 ± 22.07	
	MEA + SPE	49.27 ± 10.87 [a]	66.89 ± 15.68 [a]	
Beauveria bassiana	MEA	50.77 ± 12.32	22.16 ± 3.84	94.11 ± 5.33
	MEA + SPE	45.54 ± 6.27 [a]	24.02 ± 8.33 [a]	91.58 ± 8.03
Lecanicillium fungicola	MEA	82.42 ± 9.45 [a]	38.34 ± 11.66	100 [a]
	MEA + SPE	86.82 ± 13.15 [a]	56.72 ± 15.21	100 [a]
Metarhizium anissopliae	MEA	58.62 ± 15.27 [a]	17.89 ± 5.16	62.19 ± 13.04 [a]
	MEA + SPE	57.44 ± 20.33 [a]	21.14 ± 8.87	60.73 ± 21.04 [a]
Musicillium theobromae	MEA	59.46 ± 10.19 [a, b]	78.45 ± 14.37 [a, c]	46.28 ± 11.17 [b, c]
	MEA + SPE	32.29 ± 14.03 [a, b]	53.67 ± 22.02 [a, c]	36.66 ± 6.04 [b, c]
Plectosphaerella cucumerina	MEA	46.55 ± 5.09	14.56 ± 4.08	90.01 ± 4.17
	MEA + SPE	44.10 ± 16.99 [a]	18.23 ± 2.78 [a]	89.65 ± 10.20

* MEA: Malt extract medium, MEA + SPE: Malt extract medium amended with spruce phloem extract. Results were presented as means of three tests ± SD (standard deviation). Unmarked values are significantly different ($p < 0.05$). For each inhibiting fungus, inhibition values (in different medium and type of fungi (*C. polonica, O. bicolor* and *O. penicillatum*)) with no significant difference were marked by the same letters ([a, b, c]) ($p > 0.05$).

The most active antagonist on the MEA agar medium was *O. bicolor*, whose colonies developed very rapidly and suppressed the growth other ophiostomatoid fungi, especially *C. polonica*. On MEA medium, *O. bicolor* inhibited radial growth of *C. polonica* and *O. penicillatum* by about 99% and 43%, respectively, while *C. polonica* radial growth of both *O. bicolor* and *O. penicillatum* was inhibited by an average of 12.08 and 78.91%, respectively (Table 4). On MEA medium, other fungi studied, including fungicolous *L. fungicola*, entomopathogenic *B. bassiana* and *M. anissopliae*, were resistant to the blue-stain fungi tested and showed high concurrence peculiarities when grown on MEA medium in dual cultures. In this investigation, *L. fungicola* was the most active against the blue-stain fungi. This fungus completely (100%) inhibited growth of the *O. penicillata* and suppressed colony development of *C. polonica* and *O. bicolor* by approximately 82.42% and 38.34%, respectively (Table 4). *O. penicillatum* was the strain most susceptible to *L. fungicola* as well as to fungal entomopathogens, while *O. bicolor* was the most resistant to these fungi on MEA in the dual culture tests. Very strong inhibition of the radial growth rate of the blue-stain fungi was caused by *B. bassiana* and *M. anisopliae*. *B. bassiana* inhibited growth of *C. polonica, O. bicolor*, and *O. penicillatum* by an average of 50.77, 22.16, and 94.11%, respectively (Table 4). Sterile zones (3–5 mm wide) were found on MEA in dual *M. anisopliae* and *C. polonica* cultures (Figure 4). The growth inhibition percentage induced by *M. anissopliae* ranged from 17.89 to 62.19% for *O. bicolor* and *O. penicillatum*, respectively (Table 4). Results also confirmed high *P. cucumerina* antagonistic peculiarities against the blue-stain fungi, especially against

O. penicillatum (~90%). *M. theobromae* was significantly less active; however, its activity markedly increased after two to three weeks of incubation, the when mycelium and sporulation structures of the impacted fungi were intensively degraded (Figure 4). Additional illustrations of the growth of tested fungal colonies are shown in Figures S1–S5 in Supplementary Materials.

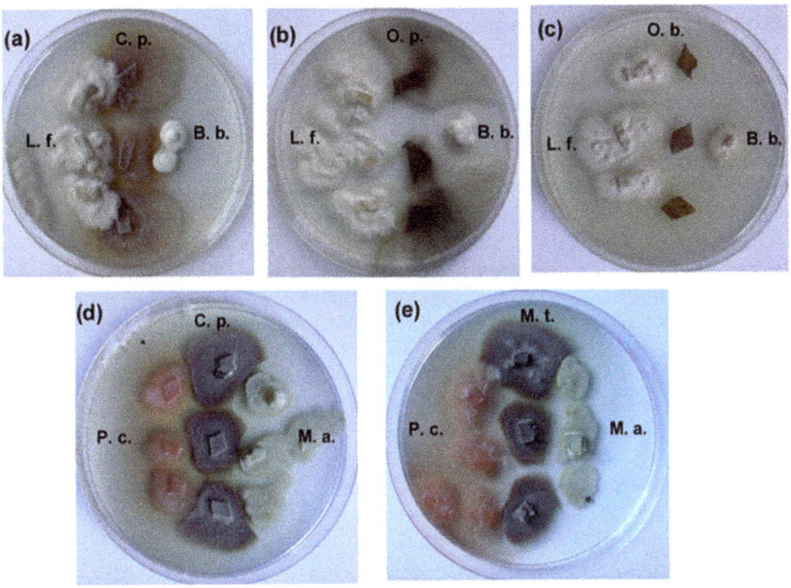

Figure 4. Antagonistic effects of fungi after 10 days' growth on 2% MEA from (**a**–**e**): C. p.—*Ceratocystis polonica*, O. b.—*Ophiostoma bicolor*, O. p.—*Ophiostoma penicillatum* (syn. *Grosmannia penicillata*), B. b.—*Beauveria bassiana*, L. f.—*Lecanicillium fungicola*, P. c.—*Plectosphaerella cucumerina*, M. t.—*Musicillium theobromae*, and M. a.—*Metarhizium anissopliae*. The most representative images were selected from each of at least three replicates ($n \geq 3$).

In dual culture tests, a different situation was detected when fungal cultures were grown on malt extract medium amended with spruce phloem extract (MEA + SPE). The antagonistic abilities of the *C. polonica* strain changed controversially: *O. bicolor* inhibition increased 4-fold (from 12.08% to 49.31% inhibition), while *C. polonica* partially lost activity against *O. penicillatum* (inhibition activity decreased from 78.91% to 46.77%) (Table 4). Proportionally, the antagonistic activity of *O. bicolor* against *C. polonica* decreased from an average of 98.89 to 24.68% on MEA and MEA + SPE media, respectively. The ability of *O. bicolor* to suppress the radial growth of *O. penicillatum* was almost similar on both culture media. On the MEA + SPE medium, inhibition of *C. polonica* growth rate induced by *O. penicillatum* markedly increased (from 12.43% to 49.27%) (Table 4).

Only *P. cucumerina* kept its antagonistic peculiarities against blue-stain fungi in the dual cultures on MEA + SPE medium. The fungus was stimulated by spruce phloem extracts in MEA medium in control plates. Conversely, *M. theobromae* was inhibited by spruce phloem extracts in the control, and thus its antagonistic peculiarities against blue-stain fungi on this medium decreased by 10–25% as compared with those on MEA medium.

The fungal entomopathogens *B. bassiana* and *M. anissopliae* grew more slowly on the malt extract medium with spruce phloem extract amendments; however, their activity almost did not change in dual culture tests against blue-stain fungi. However, the radial growth rate of the *L. fungicola* strain was stimulated by SH extracts, and its antagonistic abilities against blue-stain fungi increased, with the exception of *O. penicillatum* (100%—inhibition did not change).

3. Discussion

Some recent publications concerning bacterial and fungal communities associated with the *Ips typographus* insect have considerably enhanced our understanding of these microbial ecosystems [62–65]. The bark beetle, its associated fungi, and fungal pathogen invasion are all actually related to the host's defensive chemistry [66–68]. After infection of the host, fungi use a variety of strategies to gain access to the host's nutrients [69]. Biotrophic fungi acquire nutrients directly from living cells by penetrating them and causing little visible damage [70]. Necrotrophic fungi, in contrast, produce enzymes and toxins to kill plant cells, and then the fungi feed on the nutrients from the dead tissue [71]. Additionally, potential antifungal defense compounds of the plant may contact with necrotrophs [47]. In the case of Norway spruce infestation with *C. polonica*, the plants act by increasing their total terpene content and accumulating monoterpenes with antifungal properties [45,47,61,72,73]. The correlation between terpene content and fungal resistance is strengthened by the data showing that trees that survive *C. polonica* inoculation have much higher terpene concentrations than trees killed by the fungus [73]. This can be explained by several reasons. If microorganisms can improve the fitness of pests by facilitating their nutrient uptake, they must be resistant to terpenes; if the microorganisms reduce the toxicity of host defence compounds (that is, they might be able to transform compounds to be less toxic), they must be resistant to chemical defence.

Our study is the first report concerning the antimicrobial activity of SH (composed mainly of *trans-isomer*) regarding blue-stain fungus and other microorganisms associated with bark beetle *I. typographus* and its development habitat (galleries created in the phloem). Antimicrobial activity of SH against some strains of microorganisms was detected; however, high SH concentrations (up to 500–1000 μg/disc or mL^{-1}) were necessary in the broth agar disc diffusion and broth macro-dilution methods. SH was less effective than antibiotics, with a narrow spectrum (affecting only few microorganisms used in the present study as indicators for antimicrobial activity) and with small inhibition zones in the agar diffusion method. SH was found to have low toxicity in the agar diffusion method, whereas it showed high toxicity in the broth macro-dilution method. The reason for this may be that in the broth macro-dilution method, the fungal spores are in direct contact with dissolved SH molecules, which are able to exhibit a greater effect than in the agar diffusion method. As SH is insoluble in water, some re-crystallisation may occur in the medium prepared in water. It is well known that the agar diffusion method has its accuracy impaired as the hydrophobic nature of most EOs or their components prevents the uniform diffusion of these substances through agar medium, which may account for differences in the obtained results.

From the data obtained by the broth macro-dilution method in this study, it can be seen that SH has a significant influence on growth of microbial strains, which is in accordance with the published data regarding EOs containing appreciable amounts of SH [12,20,28,29,34,37–40].

B. subtilis was the most susceptible to all tested SH concentrations, while *P. aeruginosa* was the least susceptible—no SH concentration inhibited its growth. Our results indicated greater susceptibility on the part of the Gram-positive bacteria (*B. subtilis* and *S. aureus*), which has been also reported by other authors regarding EOs containing SH [12,20,36,38].

The weak antibacterial activity against Gram-negative bacteria (*E. coli* and *P. aeruginosa*) can be explained by the presence of an outer membrane. Hydrophilic polysaccharide chains act as a barrier to hydrophobic essential oils and do not allow them to enter and have antibacterial activity. In addition, the resistance of *P. aeruginosa* may be due to its ability to utilise terpenes for its growth [74], or it may be related to the possible resistance genes in plasmids, which can inactivate SH, having antimicrobial potential. High resistance of *P. aeruginosa* against essential oils is well documented [75,76].

An EO from *Origanum majorana*, containing appreciable amounts of both isomers of SH (25.18 and 5.44% of *trans-* and *cis-*, respectively) was assessed against *S. aureus*, and *E. coli* strains; MIC values of 0.125–0.250% and 30–61 μM were obtained, respectively [12]. In the efflux pump inhibitory assay, this EO exhibited substantial activity, especially for the *E. coli* strain. In the case of *S. aureus* strains, the EO and SH exhibited moderate potency on the drug-resistant phenotype. SH was found to be an effective inhibitor of biofilm formation (inhibition 36–86%) in *E. coli* and *S. aureus*, while the EO was ineffective on these strains. In contrast to this, biofilms formed by *E. coli* and *S. aureus* were significantly inhibited by the EO [12]. However, research on the antimicrobial properties of EOs commonly used as condiments in Brazil against *Clostridium perfringens* revealed an MIC = 5.0 mg/mL for marjoram EO with appreciable SH content [38].

Additionally, an antimicrobial activity of EOs with the most characteristic components *trans*-sabinene hydrate and terpinen-4-ol, obtained from several *Origanum* species cultivated in Poland, was evaluated against human respiratory pathogens, such as *S. aureus, Haemophilus influenzae, H. parainfluenzae,* and *Pseudomonas aeruginosa* [20]. *O. majorana* EO was the most active in the MIC assay and had the highest inhibitory rate in the anti-biofilm assay against all strains in the above study.

In another study [36], a well diffusion assay revealed that EOs from *O. majorana* and *O. vulgare* (containing 10.26 and 27.48% of *cis*-sabinene hydrate, respectively) were active against both the tested Gram-positive, viz., *B. subtilis, Micrococcus luteus,* and *S. aureus;* and Gram-negative, viz., *E. coli, Klebsiella pneumoniae,* and *P. aeruginosa,* bacteria. MIC values (v/v) indicated the highest efficacy of *O. majorana* EO against *B. subtilis* (0.5%), *M. luteus* (1%), and *S. aureus* (1%), while *O. vulgare* was most efficient against *E. coli* (2%) and *K. pneumoniae* (2%).

EOs from Tunisian *A. absinthium* L. were tested for their antibacterial and antifungal activity against 10 indicator microorganisms including seven pathogenic bacterial references (*E. coli, S. typhimurium, S. aureus, P. aeruginosa, A. hydrophila, L. monocytogenes,* and *B. cereus*), and against three fungus species (*A. flavus, A. niger* and *C. albicans*); and displayed antimicrobial activity against all tested strains with variable degrees. For Gram-negative bacterial strains, comparable levels of antibacterial activities were observed (MIC range from 12.5 to 25% v/v) for the oil containing of 11.83% (*Z*)-sabinene hydrate; the highest activity was recorded against the bacteria *P. aeruginosa* [39].

Fungi, especially filamentous fungi, were more resistant to SH than bacteria were. *C. albicans* was the most sensitive yeast, and *A. niger* as well as *Trichoderma* sp. were the most resistant fungi. Blue-stain fungus *O. bicolor* was the most susceptible fungus in both the disc diffusion and broth macro-dilution methods as compare to other blue-stain fungi. The pioneer *Picea* tree tissue invader *C. polonica* was more resistant to SH than *O. bicolor* and *O. penicillatum*. It was determined that spores from the blue-stain fungi were the most susceptible to SH. No inhibition was found in the growing mycelium. Conversely, some stimulatory effects such as increased radial growth and melanin synthesis were observed, especially in the case of *O. penicillatum* cultures (Figure 1).

SH induced changes in the morphology of blue-stain fungi: dominance of one stage with elimination of the other. It must be noted that blue-stain fungi and saprotrophic fungi were in a strong antagonistic relationship in this investigation. Moreover, saprotrophic fungi were also resistant to SH.

Fungal entomopathogens (*Beauveria bassiana*, (Bals.-Criv) Vuill. and *Metarhizium anissopliae* (Metschn.) Sorokin) were among the fungi distributed in *I. typographus* galleries; they were found on the larva cadavers. Thus, it was interesting to determine their relationship with blue-stain fungi in an in situ experiment. As was mentioned above, phytopathogens are well known to alter plant chemistry. However, even though several studies have considered the effects of plant chemistry on insect pathogens, knowledge on how phytopathogenic fungi may influence herbivores' vulnerability to entomopathogens is almost completely lacking. Contradictory results in studies with fungal entomopathogens have been found [77–79]. It has been suggested that this might reflect differences in their dependence on host insects [80,81]. Entomopathogens should be considered important natural enemies of bark beetles, and their importance has been discussed regarding other herbivores [82].

In our study, two fungi, *M. theobromae* and *P. cucumerina,* isolated from the *I. typographus* galleries and their phloem and one strain from the genus *Lecanicillium* W. Gams & Zare [*L. fungicola* (Preaus) Zare & W. Gams], isolated from *I. typographus* cadavers, were resistant to SH and very active antagonists to blue-stain fungi when grown on standard MEA medium (Figure 4). Their antagonistic properties weakened when phloem extract medium was used for the investigation of the dual cultures, suggesting that they are not pioneer sapwood invaders and develop using partially degraded phloem and/or secondary metabolites from other fungi. Despite this, *M. theobromae* and *P. cucumerina* inhibited development of the blue-stain fungi and overgrew their mycelium and sporulation structures (Figure 4). Only a few studies have addressed the question of how a decrease in host plant suitability might affect the efficiency of entomopathogens. *O. majorana* EOs containing SH exhibited strong antifungal properties against rice seed-borne fungi, such as *Bipolaris orzyae, Curvularia lunata, Fusarium verticilliodies,* and *F. graminearum* [18]. Additionally, *Mentha spicata* EO (content of SH: 7.04%) showed strong antifungal activity to plant-pathogenic fungi, such as *Fusarium oxysporum* f. sp. *radicis-lycopersici* (Sacc.) W.C. Synder & H.N. Hans, *Rhizoctonia solani* J.G. Kuhn. *Alternaria solani,* and *Verticillium dahliae* Kleb; and against selected bacterial strains of *Xanthomonas* spp. [29].

In our investigation, the results of the paired cultures indicated the possibility that they are associated with bark beetle–plant–fungal pathogen systems. If they inhibit the growth of blue-stain fungi, which are hypothesized as its feeding source, they thus influence the development of insects indirectly through feeding. Some explanation could be found in an investigation conducted by Rostás, M. et al., in which the duration of larval development from hatching to pupation increases by about 9% when *Phaedon cochleariae* (Chrysomelidae) larvae feed upon fungus-infected Chinese cabbage leaves. Higher larva mortality under prolonged development was induced by the entomopathogenic fungus *Metarhizium anisopliae* (Metsch.) Sorok. [83]. *I. typographus* larvae feeding on healthy tree tissues could also survive entomopathogen attacks; while feeding on diseased tree tissues, this ability can be lost. Other factors must be also considered, such as, e.g., the induction of defensive plant compounds by the phytopathogen. The effects of plant allelochemicals influencing insect susceptibility to entomopathogens are known [83]. Artificial diets containing plant secondary metabolites may enhance insect mortality caused by entomopathogens. Thus, knowledge about *I. typographus* fungal pathogens is valuable too, and investigations could be continued in the future.

4. Materials and Methods

4.1. Sabinene Hydrate (Dissolution and Preparation for Bioassays)

A commercial synthetic SH (analytical standard, ≥97.0% (GC), composed of isomers, containing a predominant quantity of *trans*-sabinene hydrate, Sigma-Aldrich, Merck KGaA, Darmstadt, Germany) was used for the investigations. SH, being insoluble in water, was dissolved in ethanol (96%). Stock solutions of sabinene hydrate [10% (100 mg/mL) or 20% (200 mg/mL)] were prepared, from which half-and-half dilutions in a range of sabinene hydrate concentrations (6.25, 12.50, 25.00, 50.00, 100.00, and 200.0 mg/mL) were used for in vitro treatments against test organisms.

4.2. Test Organisms

The selected test organisms used to evaluate the antifungal and antibacterial activity of the sabinene hydrate were as follows:

(a) blue-stain fungi: *Ceratocystis polonica* (Siem.) C. Moreau 1994-169/113, *C. polonica* BIGTC-2133, *Ophiostoma bicolor* Davidson & Wells BIGTC-2133, and *O. penicillatum* (Grosmann.) Siemaszko (syn. *Grosmannia penicillata* (Grosmann) Goid) 2006-209/44/2;

(b) other mycelial fungi, which were isolated from *Ips typographus* Linnaeous (Coleoptera, Curculionidae, Scolytinae) galleries in *Picea abies* L. stemps and from its discolorated sapwood, such as *Musicillium theobromae* (Turconi) Zare & W. Gams (syn. *Stachylidium theobromae* Turconi, *Verticillium theobromae* E.W. Mason & S. Hughes BIGTC-

20132 and *Plectosphaerella cucumerina* (Lindt.) W. Gams BIGTC-136, *Aspergillus niger* Tiegh. BIGTC-9823, *Penicillium notatum* Wehmer BIGTC-8914, and *Trichoderma* sp. BIGTC-2131;

(c) yeasts *Candida albicans* BIGTC-MK2, *C. parapsilosis* BIGTC-MK9, *C. krusei* BIGTC-MK3 (Blastomycetes, Cryptococcales, Cryptococcaceae) and *Saccharomyces cerevisiae* BIGTC-MK11 (Saccharomycetes, Saccharomycetales, Saccharomycetaceae) phylogenetically related to the Ascomycota, as well as *Rhodotorula muscilaginosa* BIGTC-056 (Urediomycetes, Sporidiales) phylogenetically related to Basidiomycota;

(d) Gram-positive bacteria *Staphylococcus aureus* BIGTC-BK06 and *Bacillus subtilis* BIGTC-BK09;

(e) Gram-negative bacteria *Escherichia coli* BIGTC-BK08 and *Pseudomonas aeruginosa* BIGTC-BK19.

All cultures were obtained from the Microorganism Culture Collection of Nature Research Centre (Vilnius, Lithuania), except three strains, *C. polonica* 1994-169/113, *O. bicolor*, and *G. penicillata* 2006-209/44/2, which were received from the KTH Royal Institute of Technology, Stockholm, Sweden.

As reference compounds, chloramphenicol and nystatin-dihydrate were used for treatments with bacteria and fungi, respectively.

4.3. Preparation of Test Organisms

The cultures of test organisms were maintained in agar slants at 4 °C (bacteria in nutrient agar (NA), fungi in 2% malt extract agar (MEA), and yeasts in Sabourad agar (SA); all media were purchased from Liofilchem SRL, Roseto degli Abruzzi (TE), Italy). To obtain stock cultures, fungi were pre-cultured on 2% MEA at 25 °C for four weeks (Ophiostomatoid fungi) and 7 days (other fungi), yeasts—on SA for 3 days, and bacteria—on NA for 2 days. Fungal conidia were taken from the slants using sterile saline (0.9% NaCl, *w*/*v*) containing 0.05% Tween 80. Mycelia were removed by filtration through sterile gauze, and the filtrate was adjusted up to 1–2 × 10^5 conidia mL^{-1}. Bacterial and yeast cells were picked from freshly grown slant cultures using 10 mL of sterile saline, and decimal cell solutions were prepared in the sterile saline up to 10^7 and 10^6 colony-forming units (CFU) mL^{-1} (bacteria and yeasts, respectively).

4.4. In Vitro Antifungal and Antibacterial Activity Testing

The CLSI (Clinical and Laboratory Standards Institute) method for antimicrobial susceptibility testing was modified for sabinene hydrate testing. We used two preliminary methods: the agar diffusion method for all strains of microorganisms and the disc volatilization method (vapor phase activity) for microbial strains selected as the most sensitive in the agar diffusion method. Additionally, direct SH activities (minimal inhibition concentrations, MICs) against bacteria and yeasts tested were detected by the micro-broth dilution method; additionally, SH direct activity against the fungi was determined. Activity of SH against spore (or conidium) germination was evaluated for bacterial and yeast strains. A standard antibiotics, nystatine-dihydrate (ROTH, Carl Roth GmbH + Co., Karlsruhe, Germany), was used to control the sensitivity of the tested fungi; chloramphenicol (ROTH, Carl Roth GmbH + Co., Germany) was applied to control the sensitivity of the tested bacteria. Concentrations were explored depending on the method used. Turbidity measurements of the medium were not performed.

4.4.1. Agar Disk Diffusion Method

The evaluation of SH activity against test strains of microorganisms was carried out by the disc diffusion method, which is normally used as a preliminary check and to select between different oils and their constituents. Solidified 2% MEA, SA, and NA (for fungi, yeasts, and bacteria, respectively) media were used for the SH activity treatments. Media were inoculated with 100 µL inoculums of appropriate microorganisms (10^7, 10^6, and 105 CFU mL^{-1} suspension concentrations of bacteria, yeasts, and fungi respectively) and were spread over the plates using a sterile rod display in order to obtain a uniform microbial growth on both control and test plates. After the inoculums' absorption by agar, sterile filter discs (Whatman no 1, 5 mm diameter) were impregnated with 10 µL solutions of sabinene hydrate (at 6.25, 12.50, 25.00, 50.00, 100.00, and 200.00 mg/mL concentration in 96% ethanol). These preparations corresponded to SH concentrations of 0.0625, 0.125, 0.25, 0.50, 1.0, and 2.0 mg per disc, respectively. Filter discs moistened with ethanol alcohol were placed on the seeded Petri dish as a negative control. Filter discs impregnated with nystatine-dihydrate (30 mg/mL corresponding 30 µg/disc) for fungi and chloramphenicol (30 mg/mL, corresponding 30 µg/disc) for bacteria were used as a reference control.

All Petri dishes were sealed with sterile laboratory parafilm to avoid the eventual evaporation of SH. The dishes were left for 30 min at room temperature to allow the diffusion of oil, and then were incubated for 24 h for bacteria at 30 °C, for 48 h for yeasts, and 48–98 h for fungi at 25 °C. After the incubation period, the mean diameter of the inhibition halo where the test microorganisms did not grow (clearly visible inhibition zone) or the growth was partly inhibited was measured in millimeters.

4.4.2. Broth Macro-Dilution Tests

The minimal inhibitory concentration (MIC) values were determined for bacterial and yeast strains using the macro-well dilution method as described [84]. Bacterial strains were cultured for 18 h at 30 °C in Müller-Hinton broth (MHB, Liofilchim, Roseto Degli Abruzzi (TE), Italy); yeasts were cultured for 48 h at 25 °C in 2% malt extract broth (MEB, Liofilchem, Italy). Then, test cultures were suspended in sterile saline (0.9% NaCl) and diluted to produce a final density of 2.5×10^6 cfu mL^{-1} for the bacteria and 1.5×10^5 cfu mL^{-1} for the yeasts.

The 24-well plates were prepared by dispensing into each well 490 µL of appropriate nutrient broth. An aliquot (10 µL) of SH, initially prepared at a 10% concentration (100 mg/mL; *w*/*v* ethanol, was added to each of the first wells, followed by 2-fold serial dilution to obtain concentrations in a range from 1.0 to 0.0625 mg/mL *w*/*v* (corresponding from 0.1% to 0.000625% *w*/*v* concentrations). The prepared inoculums of the test cultures were separately added to the wells (500 µL each). The final volume in each well was 1 mL. The last well, containing 500 µL of MHB (or MEB) without test substance and 500 µL of the inoculum, was used as a negative control. Standard antibiotics, tested at concentrations ranging (chloramphenicol) from 50.0 µg/mL to 1.5625 µg/mL and (nystatine-dihydrate) from 30.0 µg/mL to 0.9375 µg/mL, were used as positive controls. Ethanol was not tested because the even highest concentration used in the plate well was equal 0.096 % (10 µL ethanol (96%) per 1 mL well content = 0.096%). Culture medium + test sample of the sabinene hydrate was used as the sterility control. The plates were covered with a sterile plate sealer and incubated at 30 °C (bacteria) and 25 °C (yeasts) for 18–24 h and 48 h, respectively. Growth of the bacteria and yeasts was indicated by the presence of turbidity and/or white fur at the bottom of the well. The minimum inhibition concentrations (MICs) were determined as the lowest concentration preventing visible growth. Additionally, viability was proven by making subcultures from 50 µL from each well showing no turbidity and negative control on nutrient agar (NA; Liofilchem, Italy) or SA medium. For each strain, the growth conditions were checked and plates were incubated as described above.

Fungal strains in the macro-broth dilution method were treated by some modifications of the method. Fungi spore inoculums, corresponding approximately 1.0–1.5×10^4 conidia mL^{-1}, were prepared as stocks, from which 0.1 mL aliquots were transferred into each plate well containing either 2% MB medium or 2% MB amended with an appropriate sabinene hydrate concentration. Plates were incubated for 4–8 h, and then 100 mL^{-1} of each well content was sub-cultured for 24–48 h on 2% MEA medium (three replicate plates were used per well). After incubation, the number of growing colonies in the control and SH treated variants was counted. Growth inhibition percentage was calculated by comparing the number of CFUs in the SH-treated culture with that of the control. Spores which did not form colonies were considered as having lost their viability. Microscopic observations were made to determine growth (germination and germ tube length) retardation under SH impact.

4.4.3. Disc Volatilization Method (Vapor Phase Activity)

This method was used to evaluate the activity of SH vapor from impregnated paper discs against the blue-stain fungal strains isolated from *P. abies* sapwood and two fungal strains associated with *I. typographus* galleries, the same strains which were used in the disc diffusion method. Agar plugs of actively growing fungi (blue-stain fungi after 2 weeks and other fungi after 7 days' growth on the 2% MEA) were placed in the center of the Petri dish (covered with 2% MEA). Different aliquots (10 μL, 20 μL, and 30 μL) of the SH solution were added to 6 mm sterile blank paper discs placed in the center of the cover of the glass Petri dish (6 cm diameter). The dishes were sealed with laboratory parafilm to avoid eventual evaporation of SH followed by incubation. The volume of the dish in which SH vapor was distributed was 9 cm^3. Blanks were prepared by adding 10 μL of ethanol alcohol to the paper discs. Practically, vapor from either of the SH contents (1 g, 2 g, or 3 g per dish) evaporated into the dish atmosphere above the disc. The effectiveness of SH was calculated as a percentage inhibition of the linear fungus growth (in mm) compare to the control (disc with appropriate content of water). Each assay in these experiments was repeated three times and the results (inhibition %) were expressed as average values ± SD (standard deviation).

4.4.4. Dual Culture Tests

Agar plugs (5 mm diameter) from two actively growing test fungi (blue-stain fungi after 2 weeks and other fungi after 7 days growth on the MEA medium were placed at the different ends of the Petri dish dishes, covered with either of MEA medium or MEA amended with spruce phloem-extract (MEA + SPE)). Dishes were incubated at 25 °C in the dark. The radial growth of mycelium (in mm) was measured daily and compared with that in the MEA and MEA + SPE plates simultaneously inoculated with each fungus only as control.

Percent of test fungus inhibition by the other fungi was evaluated and expressed as calculated percent inhibition (*PI*):

$$PI = \frac{C - T}{C} \times 100$$

where C is the growth of the test fungus (mm) in the absence of the other fungi; *T* is the growth of the test fungus (mm) in the presence of the opposite fungus.

4.5. Statistical Analysis

The obtained data were statistically processed and expressed as means and standard deviation (SD) values, using the XLSTAT program (trial version, Addinsoft 2014, Paris, France). Convergence of results was based on at least three independent measurements. Evaluation of statistically significant differences between tested parameters was performed by one-way ANOVA statistical analysis. Differences between obtained values were compared using Student's *t*-test, at a significance level of $\alpha = 0.05$. IBM SPSS Statistics software (Version 28.0.1.1(15), New York, NY, USA) was applied to calculate the *p*-values. Statistically significant differences were set at p values lower than 0.05.

5. Conclusions

The current study has made a contribution to knowledge regarding the in situ antimicrobial properties of sabinene hydrate (SH), which is a quite common secondary metabolite in plants. For the first time, the effects of SH (composed mainly of *trans*-isomer) were revealed against the following microorganisms: blue-stain fungi (*Ceratocystis polonica*, *Ophiostoma bicolor*, *O. penicillatum*), frequently originating from bark beetle galleries; three fungal strains (*Musicillium theobromae*, *Plectosphaerella cucumerina*, and *Trichoderma* sp.), isolated from sapwood under bark beetle galleries (*Ips typographus*) on spruce (*Picea abies*) stems; and *Verticillium fungicola*, isolated from diseased *I. typographus* larvae. Additionally, monoterpenoid activity was tested and compared against two saprophytic fungi (*Aspergillus niger* and *Penicillium notatum*), two Gram-positive (*Bacillus subtilis* and *Staphylococcus aureus*), and two Gram-negative bacteria (*Escherichia coli* and *Pseudomonas aeruginosa*); and five yeasts (*Candida albicans*, *C. krusei*, *C. parapsilosis*, *Saccharomyces cerevisiae*, and *Rhodotorula muscilaginosa*). The antimicrobial effects were evaluated over a range of SH concentrations in three types of contact tests, namely solid and vapor diffusion and the macro-broth dilution method. SH was less effective than antibiotics, such as chloramphenicol and nystatin-dihydrate, in the agar diffusion method. SH was found to have low toxicity in the agar diffusion method against the micro-organisms tested, whereas it showed a high toxicity in the broth macro-dilution method. In solid agar disc diffusion tests, Gram-positive bacteria were more susceptible to SH than Gram-negative bacteria, followed by yeasts and fungi. The most resistant to SH in both the disc diffusion and broth macro-dilution methods were *P. aeruginosa*, *A. niger*, and *Trichoderma sp.* strains. Blue-stain fungi and fungi isolated from the *Picea* sapwood were the most resistant among the fungal strains tested. The values of the minimum inhibition concentrations generated by SH and determined using the disc volatilization method depended on the tested fungus species. SH showed a more or less important role in the development of microbial inhibition. The Gram-positive bacteria *B. subtilis* and *S. aureus* were the organisms most susceptible to SH, followed by Gram-negative bacterium, *E. coli* and two yeasts, *C. albicans* and *C. kruei*. The strains of *C. parapsilosis* were the yeasts most resistant to SH. Further research may be focused on evaluating the bioactivity of SH against other pathogenic microorganisms and/or investigation of antimicrobial properties of another isomer (*cis*-) of this monoterpenoid.

The investigation of antimicrobial properties of plant secondary metabolites is important for the development of a new generation of fungicides. In general, this study has provided new comprehension regarding the application of SH as a natural product derived from plants. The use of renewable products offers great prospects for more economical, environmentally friendly, and effective development of industry and agriculture.

Supplementary Materials: The following supporting information can be downloaded at https://www.mdpi.com/article/10.3390/molecules29174252/s1, Figure S1: *Ceratocystis polonica*: (a) colonies after 14 days' growth on 2% MEA medium; (b,d) synnemata in culture; (c,e,f) synnemata and conidia in preparates; (g) micro ascus. Scales are indicated in pictures. Figure S2: *Ophiostoma penicillatum* (syn. *Grosmannia penicillata*): (a–c) colonies after 14 days' growth on 2% MEA, PDA and SA media, respectively; (d) synnemata in culture; (e) conidiogenesis in culture; (f) synnemata in culture; (g,h) *Leptographium* state; (a–c) scales are 10 μm; other scales are 100 μm. Figure S3: *Musicillium theobromae*: (a) colonies after 10 days' growth on 2% MEA; (b–d) conidiophores and conidial masses in culture; (e,f) conidiophores and conidial masses (heads) in preparates; (g) aggregates from mycelium in culture; (h,i) conidiophores and conidia. Scales are indicated in pictures. Figure S4: *Plectosphaerella cucumerina*: (a) colonies after 10 days' growth on 2% MEA; (b–d) hyphae, conidiophores, and conidia in culture; (e,f) conidiophores and conidia in preparates. Scales are indicated in pictures. Figure S5: *Ceratocystis polonica* colonies after 6 days' growth on: (a) MEA medium, (b) mineral medium without glucose and with phloem extract medium, and (c) mineral medium with phloem. *Ophiostoma penicillatum* (syn. *Grosmannia penicillata*) colonies after 6 days' growth on: (d) MEA medium, (e) mineral medium without glucose and with phloem extract medium, and (f) mineral medium with phloem.

Author Contributions: Conceptualization, A.J. and I.N.; methodology, D.P.; investigation, D.P.; resources, A.J.; data curation, A.J. and I.N.; writing—original draft preparation, A.J.; writing—review and editing, A.J.; supervision, A.J. All authors have read and agreed to the published version of the manuscript.

Funding: This research received no external funding.

Institutional Review Board Statement: Not applicable.

Informed Consent Statement: Not applicable.

Data Availability Statement: Data are contained within the article and Supplementary Materials.

Conflicts of Interest: The authors declare no conflicts of interest.

References

1. Rehman, R.; Hanif, M.A.; Mushtaq, Z.; Al-Sadi, A.M. Biosynthesis of essential oils in aromatic plants: A review. *Food Rev. Int.* **2016**, *32*, 117–160. [CrossRef]
2. Hallachan, T.W.; Croteau, R. Monoterpene biosynthesis: Demonstration of a geranyl pyrophosphate: Sabinene hydrate cyclase in soluble enzyme preparations from sweet marjoram (*Majorana hortensis*). *Arch. Biochem. Biophys.* **1988**, *264*, 618–631. [CrossRef]
3. Arsenijević, J.; Marković, J.; Šoštarić, I.; Ražić, S. A chemometrics as a powerful tool in the elucidation of the role of metals in the biosynthesis of volatile organic compounds in Hungarian thyme samples. *Plant Physiol. Biochem.* **2013**, *71*, 298–306. [CrossRef]
4. Krause, S.T.; Köllner, T.G.; Asbach, J.; Degenhardt, J. Stereochemical mechanism of two sabinene hydrate synthases forming antipodal monoterpenes in thyme (*Thymus vulgaris*). *Arch. Biochem. Biophys.* **2013**, *529*, 112–121. [CrossRef]
5. González-Mas, M.C.; Rambla, J.L.; López-Gresa, M.P.; Blázquez, M.A.; Granell, A. Volatile compounds in *Citrus* essential oils: A comprehensive review. *Front. Plant Sci.* **2019**, *10*, 12. [CrossRef] [PubMed]
6. Aguilar-Hernández, M.G.; Sánchez-Bravo, P.; Hernández, F.; Carbonell-Barrachina, Á.A.; Pastor-Pérez, J.J.; Legua, P. Determination of the volatile profile of lemon peel oils as affected by rootstock. *Foods* **2020**, *9*, 241. [CrossRef]
7. Flamini, G.; Najar, B.; Leonardi, M.; Ambryszewska, K.E.; Cioni, P.L.; Parri, F.; Melai, B.; Pistelli, L. Essential oil composition of *Salvia rosmarinus* Spenn. wild samples collected from six sites and different seasonal periods in Elba Island (Tuscan Archipelago, Italy). *Nat. Prod. Res.* **2020**, *36*, 1919–1925. [CrossRef]
8. Matulyte, I.; Marksa, M.; Ivanauskas, L.; Kalvėnienė, Z.; Lazauskas, R.; Bernatonienė, J. GC-MS analysis of the composition of the extracts and essential oil from *Myristica fragrans* seeds using magnesium aluminometasilicate as excipient. *Molecules* **2019**, *24*, 1062. [CrossRef]
9. Adiani, V.; Gupta, S.; Chatterjee, S.; Variyar, P.S.; Sharma, A. Activity guided characterization of antioxidant components from essential oil of Nutmeg (*Myristica fragrans*). *J. Food Sci. Technol.* **2013**, *52*, 221–230. [CrossRef]
10. Kapoor, I.P.S.; Singh, B.; Singh, G.; De Heluani, C.S.; De Lampasona, M.P.; Catalan, C.A.N. Chemical composition and antioxidant activity of essential oil and oleoresins of nutmeg (*Myristica fragrans* Houtt.) fruits. *Int. J. Food Prop.* **2013**, *16*, 1059–1070. [CrossRef]
11. Danin, A.; Ravid, U.; Umano, K.; Shibamoto, T. Essential oil composition of *Origanum ramonense* Danin leaves from Israel. *J. Essent. Oil Res.* **1997**, *9*, 411–417. [CrossRef]
12. Ghazal, T.S.A.; Schelz, Z.; Vidács, L.; Szemerédi, N.; Veres, K.; Spengler, G.; Hohmann, J. Antimicrobial, multidrug resistance reversal and biofilm formation inhibitory effect of *Origanum majorana* extracts, essential oil and monoterpenes. *Plants* **2022**, *11*, 1432. [CrossRef] [PubMed]
13. Arafat, K.; Al-Azawi, A.M.; Sulaiman, S.; Attoub, S. Exploring the anticancer potential of *Origanum majorana* essential oil monoterpenes alone and in combination against non-small cell lung cancer. *Nutrients* **2023**, *15*, 5010. [CrossRef] [PubMed]
14. Dudai, N.; Larkov, O.; Chaimovitsh, D.; Lewinsohn, E.; Freiman, L.; Ravid, U. Essential oil compounds of *Origanum dayi* Post. *Flavour. Fragr. J.* **2003**, *18*, 334–337. [CrossRef]
15. Tabanca, N.; Özek, T.; Baser, K.H.C. Comparison of the essential oils of *Origanum majorana* L. and *Origanum* x *majoricum* Cambess. *J. Essent. Oil Res.* **2004**, *16*, 248–252. [CrossRef]
16. Raina, A.P.; Negi, K.S. Essential oil composition of *Origanum majorana* and *Origanum vulgare* ssp. *hirtum* growing in India. *Chem. Nat. Compd.* **2012**, *47*, 1015–1017. [CrossRef]
17. Lukas, B.; Schmiderer, C.; Novak, J. Essential oil diversity of European *Origanum vulgare* L. (Lamiaceae). *Phytochemistry* **2015**, *119*, 32–40. [CrossRef]
18. Mohamed, A.A.; El-Hefny, M.; El-Shanhorey, N.A.; Ali, H.M. Foliar application of bio-stimulants enhancing the production and the toxicity of *Origanum majorana* essential oils against four rice seed-borne fungi. *Molecules* **2020**, *25*, 2363. [CrossRef] [PubMed]
19. Simirgiotis, M.J.; Burton, D.; Parra, F.; López, J.; Muñoz, P.; Escobar, H.; Parra, C. Antioxidant and antibacterial capacities of *Origanum vulgare* L. essential oil from the Arid Andean region of Chile and its chemical characterization by GC-MS. *Metabolites* **2020**, *10*, 414. [CrossRef]
20. Piasecki, B.; Balázs, V.L.; Kieltyka-Dadasiewicz, A.; Szabó, P.; Kocsis, B.; Horváth, G.; Ludwiczuk, A. Microbiological studies on the influence of essential oils from several *Origanum* species on respiratory pathogens. *Molecules* **2023**, *28*, 3044. [CrossRef]
21. Kandoudi, W.; Radácsi, P.; Gosztola, B.; Zámboriné Németh, É. Elicitation of medicinal plants in vivo—Is it a realistic tool? The effect of methyl jasmonate and salicylic acid on Lamiaceae species. *Horticulturae* **2022**, *8*, 5. [CrossRef]
22. Farouk, A.; Mohsen, M.; Ali, H.; Shaaban, H.; Albaridi, N. Antioxidant activity and molecular docking study of volatile constituents from different aromatic Lamiaceous plants cultivated in Madinah Monawara, Saudi Arabia. *Molecules* **2021**, *26*, 4145. [CrossRef]
23. Satyal, P.; Murray, B.L.; McFeeters, R.L.; Setzer, W.N. Essential oil characterization of *Thymus vulgaris* from various geographical locations. *Foods* **2016**, *5*, 70. [CrossRef] [PubMed]
24. Bumbulytė, G.; Būdienė, J.; Būda, V. Essential oils and their components control behaviour of yellow mealworm (*Tenebrio molitor*) larvae. *Insects* **2023**, *14*, 636. [CrossRef]

25. Groendahl, E.; Ehlers, B.K.; Keefover-Ring, E. A new cis-sabinene hydrate chemotype detected in large thyme *Thymus pulegioides* L. growing wild in Denmark. *J. Essent. Oil Res.* **2008**, *20*, 40–41. [CrossRef]
26. Kim, S.-W.; Lee, H.-R.; Jang, M.-J.; Jung, C.-S.; Park, I.-K. Fumigant toxicity of Lamiaceae plant essential oils and blends of their constituents against adult rice weevil *Sitophilus oryzae*. *Molecules* **2016**, *21*, 361. [CrossRef]
27. Trendafilova, A.; Todorova, M.; Ivanova, V.; Zhelev, P.; Aneva, I. Essential oil composition of ten species from sect. Serpyllum of genus Thymus growing in Bulgaria. *Diversity* **2023**, *15*, 759. [CrossRef]
28. Wiese, N.; Fischer, J.; Heidler, J.; Lewkowski, O.; Degenhardt, J.; Erler, S. The terpenes of leaves, pollen, and nectar of thyme (*Thymus vulgaris*) inhibit growth of bee disease-associated microbes. *Sci. Rep.* **2018**, *8*, 14634. [CrossRef]
29. Bayan, Y.; Küsek, M. Chemical composition and antifungal and antibacterial activity of *Mentha spicata* L. volatile oil. *Cien. Inv. Agr.* **2018**, *45*, 64–69. [CrossRef]
30. Kumar, A.; Yadav, L.B.S.; Ahmad, J.; Dubey, N.; Puri, S. Chemical composition of commercial *Juniperus communis* L. leaf oil. *J. Essent. Oil Bear. Plants* **2013**, *10*, 310–313. [CrossRef]
31. Zheljazkov, V.D.; Astatkie, T.; Jeliazkova, E.A.; Tatman, A.O.; Schlegel, V. Distillation time alters essential oil yield, composition and antioxidant activity of female *Juniperus scopulorum* trees. *J. Essent. Oil Res.* **2013**, *25*, 62–69. [CrossRef]
32. Cornwell, C.P.; Leach, D.N.; Wyllie, S.W. The origin of terpinen-4-ol in the steam distillates of *Melaleuca argentea*, *M. dissitiflora* and *M. linariifolia*. *J. Essent. Oil Res.* **1999**, *11*, 49–53. [CrossRef]
33. Valdivieso-Ugarte, M.; Gomez-Llorente, C.; Plaza-Díaz, J.; Gil, Á. Antimicrobial, antioxidant, and immunomodulatory properties of essential oils: A systematic review. *Nutrients* **2019**, *11*, 2786. [CrossRef]
34. Chouhan, S.; Sharma, K.; Guleria, S. Antimicrobial activity of some essential oils—Present status and future perspectives. *Medicines* **2017**, *4*, 58. [CrossRef]
35. Swamy, M.K.; Akhtar, M.S.; Sinniah, U.R. Antimicrobial properties of plant essential oils against human pathogens and their mode of action: An updated review. *Evid. Based Complement. Alternat. Med.* **2016**, *2016*, 3012462. [CrossRef]
36. Rathore, S.; Mukhia, S.; Kumar, R.; Kumar, R. Essential oil composition and antimicrobial potential of aromatic plants grown in the mid-hill conditions of the Western Himalayas. *Sci. Rep.* **2023**, *13*, 4878. [CrossRef]
37. Santoyo, S.; Cavero, S.; Jaime, L.; Ibañez, E.; Señoráns, F.J.; Reglero, G. Supercritical carbon dioxide extraction of compounds with antimicrobial activity from *Origanum vulgare* L.: Determination of optimal extraction parameters. *J. Food Prot.* **2006**, *69*, 369–375. [CrossRef]
38. Radaelli, M.; da Silvaa, B.P.; Weidlich, L.; Hoehne, L.; Flach, A.; Mendonc, L.A.; da Costa, A.; Ethur, E.M. Antimicrobial activities of six essential oils commonly used as condiments in Brazil against *Clostridium perfringens*. *Braz. J. Microbiol.* **2016**, *47*, 424–430. [CrossRef]
39. Riahi, L.; Ghazghazi, H.; Ayari, B.; Aouadhi, C.; Klay, I.; Chograni, H.; Cherif, A.; Zoghlami, N. Effect of environmental conditions on chemical polymorphism and biological activities among *Artemisia absinthium* L. essential oil provenances grown in Tunisia. *Ind. Crops Prod.* **2015**, *66*, 96–102. [CrossRef]
40. Paudel, P.N.; Satyal, P.; Satyal, R.; Setzer, W.N.; Gyawali, R. Chemical composition, enantiomeric distribution, antimicrobial and antioxidant activities of *Origanum majorana* L. essential oil from Nepal. *Molecules* **2022**, *27*, 6136. [CrossRef]
41. Semenzato, G.; Del Duca, S.; Vassallo, A.; Zaccaroni, M.; Mucci, N.; Greco, C.; Padula, A.; Castronovo, L.M.; Chioccioli, S.; Pistelli, L.; et al. Exploring the nexus between the composition of essential oil and the bacterial phytobiome associated with different compartments of the medicinal plants *Origanum vulgare* ssp. *vulgare*, *O. vulgare* ssp. hirtum, and *O. heracleot*. *Ind. Crops Prod.* **2023**, *191*, 115997. [CrossRef]
42. Ghosh, S.K.; Ishangulyyeva, G.; Erbilgin, N.; Bonello, P. Terpenoids are involved in the expression of systemic-induced resistance in Austrian pine. *Plant Cell Environ.* **2024**, *47*, 2206–2227. [CrossRef]
43. Rahmani, R.; Hedenström, E.; Schroeder, M. SPME collection and GC-MS analysis of volatiles emitted during the attack of male *Polygraphus poligraphus* (Coleoptera, Curcolionidae) on Norway spruce. *Z. Für Naturforschung C* **2015**, *70*, 265–273. [CrossRef]
44. Toffolatti, L.; Maddalena, G.; Passera, A.; Casati, P.; Bianco, P.A.; Quaglino, F. 16-Role of terpenes in plant defense to biotic stress. In *Biocontrol Agents and Secondary Metabolites*; Applications and Immunization for Plant Growth and Protection; Woodhead publishing: Sawston, UK, 2021; pp. 401–417. [CrossRef]
45. Zhao, T.; Krokene, P.; Björklund, N.; Långström, B.O.; Solheim, H.; Christiansen, E.; Borg-Karlson, A.-K. The influence of *Ceratocystis polonica* inoculation and methyl jasmonate application on terpene chemistry of Norway spruce, *Picea abies*. *Phytochemistry* **2010**, *71*, 1332–1341. [CrossRef]
46. Wadke, N.; Kandasamy, D.; Vogel, H.; Lah, L.; Wingfield, B.D.; Paetz, C.; Wright, L.P.; Gershenzon, J.; Hammerbacher, A. The bark-beetle-associated fungus, *Endoconidiophora polonica*, utilizes the phenolic defence compounds of its host as a carbon source. *Plant Physiol.* **2016**, *171*, 914–931. [CrossRef] [PubMed]
47. Hammerbacher, A.; Schmidt, A.; Wadke, N.; Wright, L.P.; Schneider, B.; Joerg Bohlmann, J.; Brand, W.A.; Fenning, T.M.; Gershenzon, J.; Paetz, C. A common fungal associate of the spruce bark beetle metabolizes the stilbene defenses of Norway spruce. *Plant Physiol.* **2013**, *162*, 1324–1336. [CrossRef]
48. Zhao, T.; Kandasamy, D.; Krokene, P.; Chen, J.; Gershenzon, J.; Hammerbacher, A. Fungal associates of the tree-killing bark beetle, *Ips typographus*, vary in virulence, ability to degrade conifer phenolics and influence bark beetle tunneling behavior. *Fungal Ecol.* **2019**, *38*, 71–79. [CrossRef]

49. Kandasamy, D.; Zaman, R.; Nakamura, Y.; Zhao, T.; Hartmann, H.; Andersson, M.N.; Hammerbacher, A.; Gershenzon, J. Conifer-killing bark beetles locate fungal symbionts by detecting volatile fungal metabolites of host tree resin monoterpenes. *PLoS Biol.* **2023**, *21*, e3001887. [CrossRef]
50. Lehmanski, L.M.A.; Kandasamy, D.; Andersson, M.N.; Netherer, S.; Alves, E.G.; Huang, J.; Hartmann, H. Addressing a century-old hypothesis–do pioneer beetles of *Ips typographus* use volatile cues to find suitable host trees? *New Phytol.* **2023**, *238*, 1762–1770. [CrossRef]
51. Blažytė-Čereškienė, L.; Apšegaitė, V.; Radžiutė, S.; Mozūraitis, R.; Būda, V.; Pečiulytė, D. Electrophysiological and behavioural responses of *Ips typographus* (L.) to *trans*-4-thujanol—A host tree volatile compound. *Ann. For. Sci.* **2016**, *73*, 247–256. [CrossRef]
52. Schiebe, C.; Unelius, C.R.; Ganji, S.; Binyameen, M.; Birgersson, G.; Schlyter, F. Styrene, (+)-*trans*-(1R,4S,5S)-4-thujanol and oxygenated monoterpenes related to host stress elicit strong electrophysiological responses in the bark beetle *Ips typographus*. *J. Chem. Ecol.* **2019**, *45*, 474–489. [CrossRef] [PubMed]
53. Jirošová, A.; Kalinová, B.; Modlinger, R.; Jakuš, R.; Unelius, C.R.; Blaženec, M.; Schlyter, F. Anti-attractant activity of (+)-*trans*-4-thujanol for Eurasian spruce bark beetle typographus: Novel potency for females. *Pest Manag. Sci.* **2022**, *78*, 1992–1999. [CrossRef] [PubMed]
54. Trubin, A.; Mezei, P.; Afratakhti, K.Z.; Surovy, P.; Jakuš, R. Northernmost European spruce bark beetle *Ips typographus* outbreak: Modelling tree mortality using remote sensing and climate data. *For. Ecol. Manag.* **2022**, *505*, 119829. [CrossRef]
55. Baños-Quintana, A.P.; Gershenzon, J.; Kaltenpoth, M. The Eurasian spruce bark beetle *Ips typographus* shapes the microbial communities of its offspring and the gallery environment. *Front. Microbiol.* **2024**, *15*, 1367127. [CrossRef]
56. Yamaoka, Y.; Wingfield, M.J.; Takahashi, I.; Solheim, H. Ophiostomatoid fungi associated with the spruce bark beetle *Ips typographus* f. *aponicus* in Japan. *Mycol. Res.* **1997**, *1001*, 1215–1227. [CrossRef]
57. Yamaoka, Y.; Takahashi, I.; Iguchi, K. Virulence of ophiostomatoid fungi associated with the spruce bark beetle *Ips typographus* f. *japonicus* in Yezo spruce. *J. For. Res.* **2000**, *5*, 87–94. [CrossRef]
58. Kirisits, T. Fungal associates of European bark beetles with special emphasis on the opiostomatoid fungi. In *Bark and Wood Boring Insects in Living Trees in Europe, a Synthesis*; Lieutier, F., Day, K.R., Battisti, A., Gregoire, J.-C., Evans, H.F., Eds.; Kluwer, Acad: Dordrecht, The Netherlands, 2004; pp. 181–236. [CrossRef]
59. Bidart-Bouzat, M.G.; Imeh-Nathaniel, A. Global change effects on plant chemical dfenses against insect herbivores. *J. Integr. Plant Biol.* **2008**, *50*, 1339–1354. [CrossRef]
60. Kurz, W.A.; Dymond, C.C.; Stinson, G.; Rampley, G.J.; Neilson, E.T.; Carroll, A.L.; Ebata, T.; Safranyik, L. Mountain pine beetle and forest carbon feedback to climate change. *Nature* **2008**, *452*, 987–990. [CrossRef] [PubMed]
61. Krokene, P. Chapter 5—Conifer defense and resistance to bark beetles. In *Bark Beetles*; Vega, F.E., Hofstetter, R.W., Eds.; Academic Press: Cambridge, MA, USA; Elsevier: Amsterdam, The Netherlands, 2015; pp. 177–207. [CrossRef]
62. Fang, J.X.; Zhang, S.F.; Liu, F.; Zhang, X.; Zhang, F.B.; Guo, X.B.; Zhang, Z.; Zhang, Q.H.; Kong, X.B. Differences in gut bacterial communities of *Ips typographus* (Coleoptera: Curculionidae) induced by enantiomer-specific alpha-pinene. *Environ. Entomol.* **2020**, *49*, 1198–1205. [CrossRef]
63. Chakraborty, A.; Purohit, A.; Khara, A.; Modlinger, R.; Roy, A. Life-stage and geographic location determine the microbial assemblage in Eurasian spruce bark beetle, *Ips typographus* L. (Coleoptera: Curculionidae). *Front. Forest. Glob. Chang.* **2023**, *6*, 1176160. [CrossRef]
64. Moussa, A.; Nones, S.; Vannucchi, P.E.; Shahzad, G.I.R.; Dittmer, J.; Corretto, E.; Schebeck, M.; Faccoli, M.; Battisti, A.; Stauffer, C.; et al. The bacterial community of the European spruce bark beetle in space and time. *bioRxiv* **2023**. [CrossRef]
65. Veselská, T.; Švec, K.; Kostovčík, M.; Peral-Aranega, E.; Garcia-Fraile, P.; Křížková, B.; Havlíček, V.; Saati-Santamaría, Z.; Kolařík, M. Proportions of taxa belonging to the gut core microbiome change throughout the life cycle and season of the bark beetle *Ips typographus*. *FEMS Microbiol. Ecol.* **2023**, *99*, fiad072. [CrossRef] [PubMed]
66. Wermelinger, B. Ecology and management of the spruce bark beetle *Ips typographus*–a review of recent research. *For. Ecol. Manag.* **2004**, *2002*, 67–82. [CrossRef]
67. Netherer, S.; Kandasamy, D.; Jirosová, A.; Kalinová, B.; Schebeck, M.; Schlyter, F. Interactions among Norway spruce, the bark beetle *Ips typographus* and its fungal symbionts in times of drought. *J. Pest Sci.* **2021**, *94*, 591–614. [CrossRef]
68. Tanin, S.M.; Kandasamy, D.; Krokene, P. Fungal interactions and host tree preferences in the spruce bark beetle *Ips typographus*. *Front. Microbiol.* **2021**, *12*, 695167. [CrossRef]
69. Johns, L.E.; Goldman, G.H.; Ries, L.N.A.; Brown, N.A. Nutrient sensing and acquisition in fungi: Mechanisms promoting pathogenesis in plant and human hosts. *Fung. Biol. Rev.* **2021**, *36*, 1–14. [CrossRef]
70. Fei, W.; Liu, Y. Biotrophic fungal pathogens: A critical overview. *Appl. Biochem. Biotechnol.* **2023**, *195*, 1–16. [CrossRef]
71. Liao, C.-J.; Hailemariam, S.; Sharon, A.; Mengiste, T. Pathogenic strategies and immune mechanisms to necrotrophs: Differences and similarities to biotrophs and hemibiotrophs. *Curr. Opin. Plant Biol.* **2022**, *69*, 102291. [CrossRef]
72. Zeneli, G.; Krokene, P.; Chistiansen, E.; Krekling, T.; Gershenzon, J. Methyl jasmonate treatment of mature Norway spruce (*Picea abies*) trees increases the accumulation of terpenoid resin components and protects against infection by *Ceratocystis polonica*, a bark beetle-associated fungus. *Tree Physiol.* **2006**, *26*, 977–988. [CrossRef]
73. Novak, M.; Urbanek Krajnc, A.; Lah, L.; Zupanec, N.; Kraševec, N.; Križman, M.; Bohlmann, J.; Komel, R. Low-density *Ceratocystis polonica* inoculation of Norway spruce (*Picea abies*) triggers accumulation of monoterpenes with antifungal properties. *Eur. J. Forest Res.* **2014**, *133*, 573–583. [CrossRef]

74. Förster-Fromme, K.; Höschle, B.; Mack, C.; Bott, M.; Armbruster, W.; Jendrossek, D. Identification of genes and proteins necessary for catabolism of acyclic terpenes and leucine/isovalerate in *Pseudomonas aeruginosa*. *Appl. Environ. Microbiol.* **2006**, *72*, 4819–4828. [CrossRef] [PubMed]
75. Van, L.T.; Hagiu, I.; Popovici, A.; Marinescu, F.; Gheorghe, I.; Curutiu, C.; Ditu, L.M.; Holban, A.-M.; Sesan, T.E.; Lazar, V. Antimicrobial efficiency of some essential oils in antibiotic-resistant *Pseudomonas aeruginosa* isolates. *Plants* **2022**, *11*, 2003. [CrossRef]
76. Iseppi, R.; Mariani, M.; Condò, C.; Sabia, C.; Messi, P. Essential Oils: A natural weapon against antibiotic-resistant bacteria responsible for nosocomial infections. *Antibiotics* **2021**, *10*, 417. [CrossRef]
77. Deka, B.; Baruah, C.; Babu, A. Entomopathogenic microorganisms: Their role in insect pest management. *Egypt. J. Biol. Pest Control* **2021**, *31*, 121. [CrossRef]
78. Altinok, H.H.; Altinok, M.A.; Koca, A.S. Modes of action of entomopathogenic fungi. *Curr. Trends Nat. Sci.* **2019**, *8*, 117–124. Available online: http://natsci.upit.ro (accessed on 18 June 2024).
79. Bugti, G.A.; Bin, W.; Memon, S.A.; Khaliq, G.; Jaffar, M.A. Entomopathogenic fungi: Factors involved in successful microbial control of insect pests. *J. Entomol.* **2020**, *17*, 74–83. Available online: https://scialert.net/abstract/?doi=je.2020.74.83 (accessed on 8 July 2024). [CrossRef]
80. Qu, S.; Wang, S. Interaction of entomopathogenic fungi with the host immune system. *Dev. Comp. Immunol.* **2018**, *83*, 96–103. [CrossRef]
81. Davis, T.S.; Stewart, J.E.; Mann, A.; Bradley, C.; Hofstetter, R.W. Evidence for multiple ecological roles of *Leptographium abietinum*, a symbiotic fungus associated with the north American spruce beetle. *Fungal Ecol.* **2019**, *38*, 62–70. [CrossRef]
82. Elliot, S.L.; Sabelis, M.W.; Janssen, A.; Van Der Geest, L.P.S.; Beerling, E.A.M.; Fransen, J. Can plants use entomopathogens as bodyguards? *Ecol. Lett.* **2000**, *3*, 228–235. [CrossRef]
83. Rostás, M.; Simon, M.; Hilker, M. Ecological cross-effects of induced plant responses towards herbivores and phytopathogenic fungi. *Basic Appl. Ecol.* **2003**, *4*, 43–62. [CrossRef]
84. Zgoda, J.P.; Porter, J.R. A convenient microdilution method for screening natural products against bacteria and fungi. *Pharm. Biol.* **2001**, *39*, 221–225. [CrossRef]

molecules

MDPI

Article

Teadenol B as a Component of Microorganism-Fermented Tea Extract Inhibited Breast Cancers by Promoting Autophagy

Ying Zhao [1,†], Zhang-Gui Ding [2,3,4,5,6,†], Yu-Jie Yan [1], Rui Yang [2,3,4], Miao-Miao Qi [1], Shu-Kang Pan [2,3,4], Ji-Ling Xie [2,3,4], Yu-Hui Sun [1] and Jin Xiang [1,*]

1 Ministry of Education Laboratory of Combinatorial Biosynthesis and Drug Discovery, School of Pharmaceutical Science, Wuhan University, Wuhan 430071, China; zying1305@whu.edu.cn (Y.Z.); yanyujie524@163.com (Y.-J.Y.); qmmwhu@126.com (M.-M.Q.); yhsun@whu.edu.cn (Y.-H.S.)

2 Pu-erh Tea Fermentation Engineering Research Center of Yunnan Province, Kunming 650271, China; dzg@ynu.edu.cn (Z.-G.D.); yangrui_xyz@163.com (R.Y.); psk.happy@163.com (S.-K.P.); xiejl520@126.com (J.-L.X.)

3 Key Laboratory of Pu-erh Tea Processing Technology, Ministry of Agriculture and Rural Affairs, Kunming 650271, China

4 Yunnan Dayi Microbial Technology Co., Ltd., Kunming 650271, China

5 Yunnan Institute of Microbiology, School of Life Sciences, Yunnan University, Kunming 650091, China

6 Key Laboratory for Southwest Microbial Diversity of the Ministry of Education, Yunnan University, Kunming 650091, China

* Correspondence: xiangjin@whu.edu.cn

† These authors contributed equally to this work.

Abstract: Breast cancer is a significant threat to life and health, which needs more safe and effective drugs to be explored. Teadenol B is a characteristic chemical component of microbial fermented tea. This study discovered that teadenol B could exhibit obvious inhibitory effects on all four different clinical subtype characteristics of breast cancer cells. Proteomic studies show that deoxycytidine triphosphate deaminase (DCTD), which could block DNA synthesis and repair DNA damage, had the most significant and consistent reduction in all four types of breast cancer cells with the treatment of teadenol B. Considering MDA-MB-231 cells exhibit poor clinical prognosis and displayed substantial statistical differences in KEGG pathway enrichment analysis results, we investigated its impact on the size and growth of MDA-MB-231 triple-negative breast tumors transplanted into nude mice and demonstrated that teadenol B significantly suppressed tumor growth without affecting body weight significantly. Finally, we found that the conversion of LC3-I to LC3-II in MDA-MB-231 increased significantly with teadenol B treatment. This proved that teadenol B could be a strong autophagy promotor, which explained the down-regulation of DCTD to some extent and may be the potential mechanism underlying teadenol B's anti-breast cancer effects. This finding provides new evidence for drinking fermented tea to prevent breast cancer and highlights the potential of teadenol B as a novel therapeutic option for breast cancer prevention and treatment, necessitating further investigations to clarify its exact target and the details involved.

Keywords: teadenol B; breast cancer; autophagy

1. Introduction

Breast cancer is the most common malignant disease in women [1], affecting more than 1 million women worldwide, with a significant increase in the number of cases worldwide, and patients tend to be younger [2]. Breast cancer cells are clinically classified according to whether they express three proteins: estrogen receptor (ER), progesterone receptor (PR), and human epidermal growth factor receptor 2 (HER2). It is usually divided into luminal A (ER/PR+/HER2−), luminal B (ER+/PR+/HER2+, or ER+/PR+/HER2− grade 3) [3,4], HER2 positive type (ER−/PR−/HER2+), and three negative type (ER−/PR−/HER2−) [5]. Among them, triple-negative breast cancer is characterized by a high mitosis rate, high lymphocytic infiltration rate, high grade, large tumor size, high recurrence rate, and high mortality rate. It is a type of breast cancer with the worst prognosis in clinical treatment at present, and it is urgent to develop new therapeutic methods [6,7]. According to different clinical tumor subtypes, it mainly includes the following three therapies: endocrine therapy, anti-HER2-targeted therapy, and chemotherapy [8–10]. At present, the clinical drugs for the treatment of breast cancer are easy to tolerate and have large side effects on the body, resulting in poor treatment effects [9]. Therefore, it is essential to develop safe and effective new breast cancer prevention and treatment drugs.

Fermented Pu-erh tea is a microbially fermented tea that can play a positive role in maintaining the health of the body [11–13] and has the effects of anti-fatigue [14,15], reducing blood lipid [16–18] and preventing cancers [19–21]. It contains many bioactive substances, mainly polyphenols, catechins, flavonoids, phenolic acids, tea pigments, saponins, polysaccharides, alkaloids, vitamins, amino acids, organic acids, and other chemical components that have been studied and reported [22]. Most of the substances are common substances in tea [23], and very few compounds have been reported to be isolated only from ripe Pu-erh tea. Thus, researching the biological activity of the characteristic chemical components in Pu-erh tea is fundamental for studying the functional mechanism of Pu-erh tea.

Teadenol B (Figure 1) is a characteristic chemical component of ripe Pu-erh tea, which was first disclosed by Japanese scholars in 2011 and isolated from the metabolites of fermented tea by Aspergillus fungi. It has been reported to promote adiponectin secretion and inhibit protein tyrosine phosphatase 1B expression [24].

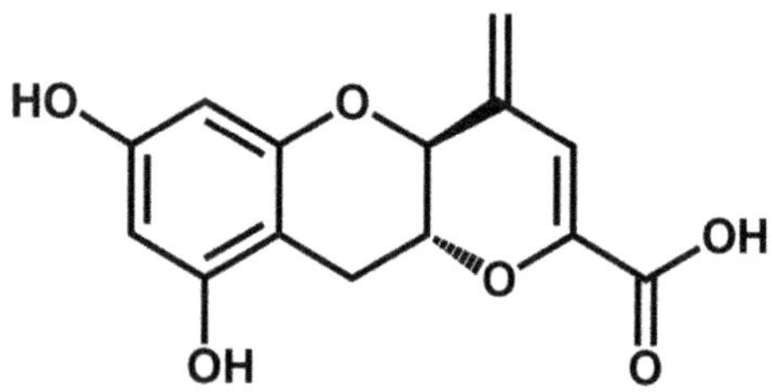

Figure 1. Chemical structure of teadenol B.

Total synthesis of teadenol B was reported in 2016 [25]. It has been reported that teadenol A, which was isolated simultaneously, can bind and activate G protein-coupled receptor 120 to enhance the expression of glucagon-like peptide 1. Although related patents have been applied for teadenol B in many countries and regions [26–28], no other functional activities of teadenol B have been reported at present [29]. We extracted teadenol B from fermented tea and identified its chemical structure as described in our patent [28]. In the bioactivity detection of teadenol B, we first found that it showed an inhibitory effect on breast cancer cells and subsequently launched a series of cell, proteome, and animal studies to explore its role in preventing and treating breast cancer tumors and related mechanisms.

2. Results and Discussion

2.1. *Teadenol B Has Inhibitory Activity on Breast Cancer Cells*

To explore whether teadenol B has therapeutic effects on breast cancer, four breast cancer cell lines were selected as research objects in this study according to receptor phenotypic characteristics, namely MDA-MB-231 (receptor phenotypic characteristics ER−, PR−, HER2−), MDA-MB-453 (receptor phenotypic characteristics ER−, PR−, HER2+), MCF-7 (receptor phenotypic characteristics ER+, PR+/−, HER2−), and BT474 (receptor phenotypic characteristics ER+, PR+/−, HER2+). Breast cancer cells were treated with a range of concentrations of teadenol B for 24 h, and the cell viability was detected by adding an MTT solution. As shown in Figure 2, MDA-MB-231 cell viability was significantly inhibited by teadenol B ($p < 0.01$) after its concentration reached 20 μg/mL. For MDA-MB-

453 cells, the cell survival rate decreased when the concentration of teadenol B reached 10 μg/mL ($p < 0.05$). The cell survival rate decreased significantly ($p < 0.001$) after the concentration of teadenol B reached 50 μg/mL. When teadenol B concentration reached 100 μg/mL, the survival rate of MCF-7 cells decreased significantly ($p < 0.01$). As to BT474 cells, the survival rate decreased significantly after the concentration of teadenol B reached 10 μg/mL ($p < 0.01$).

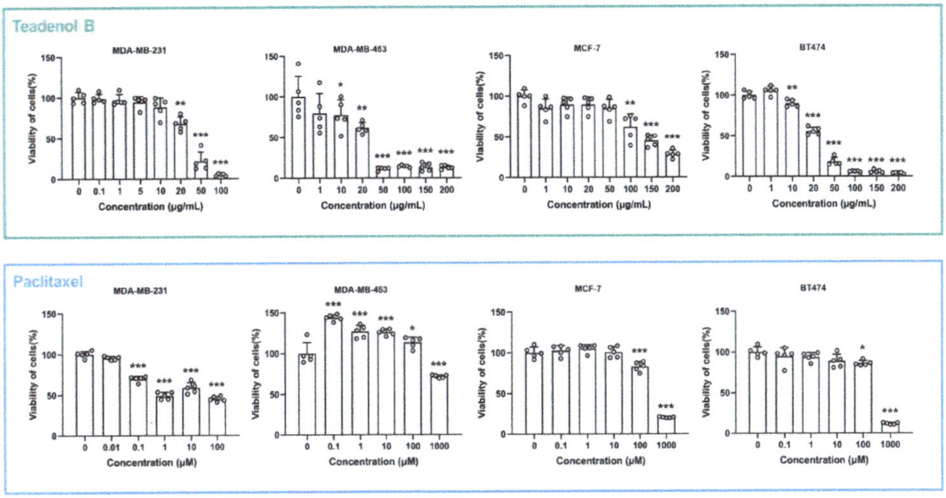

Figure 2. Survival rate of four types of breast cancer cells varied with teadenol B or paclitaxel concentration. The white circles represent the scatter data points for each group. The data are presented as mean ± SD (* $p < 0.05$, ** $p < 0.01$, *** $p < 0.001$, $n = 5$).

Paclitaxel, a chemotherapeutic drug for breast cancers, was used as a positive control drug here. As shown in Figure 2, after the concentration of paclitaxel reached 0.1 μM, the survival rate of MDA-MB-231 cells significantly decreased ($p < 0.001$). Paclitaxel promoted the proliferative activity of MDA-MB-453 cells in the concentration range not exceeding 100 μM. The survival rates of MCF-7 cells and BT474 cells were much higher than 50% even when the concentration of paclitaxel reached 100 μM.

By comparing the half-maximal inhibitory concentration (IC50) of teadenol B and paclitaxel in these four cell types (Table 1), we can see that the IC50 of teadenol B is much lower in MDA-MB-453 and BT474 cells. For MCF-7 cells, the IC50 of teadenol B is roughly at the same level as that of paclitaxel. For MDA-MB-231 cells, the IC50 of teadenol B is higher than paclitaxel, but from the morphology of the dose-response curve, the inhibition of teadenol B increased with concentration more clearly and regularly, which can also be seen in the results of the other three types of breast cancer cells.

Table 1. IC50 of teadenol B and paclitaxel in four types of breast cancer cells.

Cell Line	Receptor Phenotypic Characteristics	Teadenol B		Paclitaxel	
		(μg/mL)	(μM)	(μg/mL)	(μM)
MDA-MB-231	ER−, PR−, HER2−	35	126	64	75
MDA-MB-453	ER−, PR−, HER2+	30	108	>850	>1000
MCF-7	ER+, PR+/−, HER2−	145	525	425	500
BT474	ER+, PR+/−, HER2+	25	90	425	500

2.2. Proteomic Study of the Potential Mechanism of Action of Teadenol B against Breast Cancer

Teadenol B can inhibit the growth of breast cancer cells. To further explore the potential mechanism of its anti-breast cancer action, breast cancer cells, MDA-MB-231, MDA-MB-453, MCF-7, and BT474 were treated with 20 μg/mL teadenol B and their proteins were extracted and treated. The proteins of the teadenol B-treated group were compared with those of the control group using label-free MS. The summary data of all the differentially expressed proteins are shown in Table 2.

Table 2. Statistics of the number of differentially expressed proteins.

Cell Line	Up Regulation ($fc \geq 2$)	Down Regulation ($fc \leq 0.5$)	Differentially Expressed Proteins
MDA-MB-231	473	872	1345
MDA-MB-453	472	1604	2076
MCF-7	272	416	688
BT474	331	932	1263

The Kyoto Encyclopedia of Gene and Genome (KEGG) access database (www.kegg.jp/kegg/pathway.html, accessed on 17 January 2024) stores the function of gene and genome information, along with visual representations of various cellular biochemical processes. Analyzing the metabolic pathways enriched with differentially expressed proteins allows for an understanding of which pathways experience notable systemic changes under differing experimental conditions. In this study, KEGG pathway analysis was performed on proteins with significant expression differences compared with the control group to discover the biological pathways by which teadenol B interferes with four types of breast cancer cells. Figure 3A lists the enrichment analysis results of the KEGG pathway with the top 10 protein expression differences according to Fisher's precise test.

As shown in Figure 3A, the protein with significant differences in metabolic pathways (hsa01100) was the most significant, and the number of different proteins was the most significant after teadenol B interfered with MDA-MB-231 cells. In MDA-MB-453 cells, the protein with significant differences in expression was also mainly enriched in metabolic pathways (hsa01100), with the highest number of differentially expressed proteins. The difference was also significant, second only to Salmonella infection pathways (hsa05132) and Shigellosis pathways (hsa05131). Teadenol B interferes with MCF-7 cells, and the significantly differentially expressed protein is also mainly enriched in metabolic pathways (hsa01100). The significance of the difference is second only to other types of O-glycan biosynthesis pathways (hsa00514) and colorectal cancer pathways (hsa05210), but the difference is the weakest compared with the other three types of breast cancer cells. Teadenol B interferes with BT474 cells, and the most significant difference is between the chronic myeloid leukemia pathway (hsa05220) and the human T-cell leukemia virus (hsa05166), and the number of the different proteins in these two pathways is not very different from its pathway.

After teadenol B treatment, the four types of cells had multiple proteins with the same changes in metabolic pathways (Figure 3B). The expression of lipin 2 (LPIN2), glutamate-cysteine ligase modifier subunit (GCLM), and deoxycytidine triphosphate deaminase (DCTD) decreased. The expression of coenzyme Q3 (COQ3) increased. Among them, DCTD is closely related to anticancer effects, which shows the most significant changes in all four types of breast cancer cells with the treatment of teadenol B.

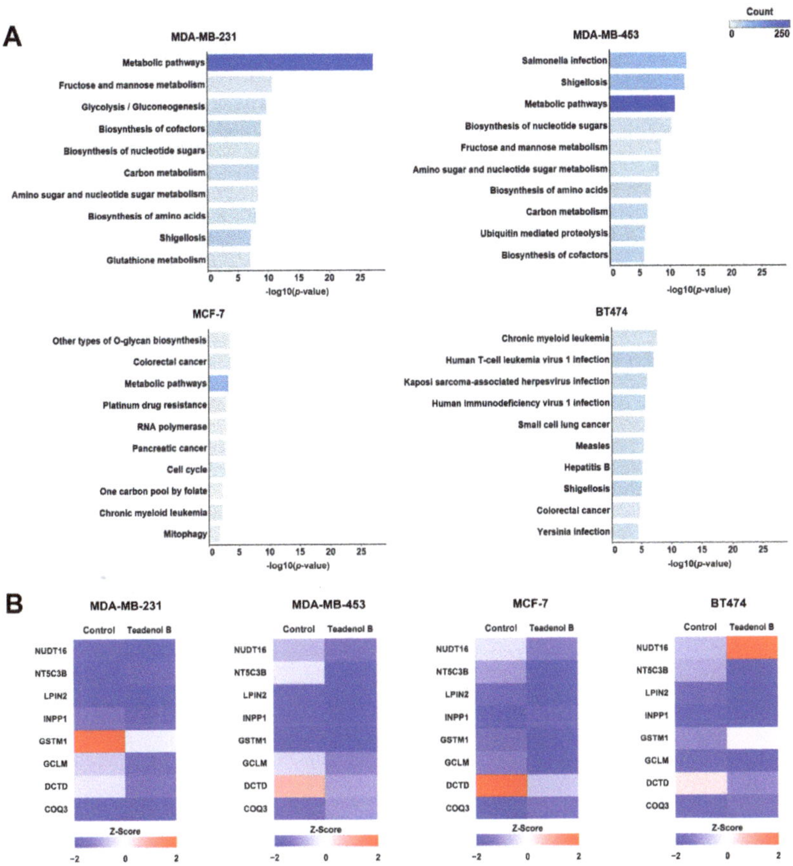

Figure 3. Teadenol B inhibits cancer cell growth by affecting key proteins on metabolic pathways in breast cancer cells. (**A**) KEGG pathway enrichment analysis of teadenol B intervention on differential protein expression in four breast cancer cells. The *p*-value is the scoring value of Fisher's exact test. The smaller the *p*-value is, the larger the value of the horizontal axis -log10 (*p*-value), which means that the difference between the sample group and the control group in the corresponding longitudinal KEGG pathway is more significant. The count represents the number of differentially expressed proteins on the KEGG pathway. (**B**) The heat map showed differences in the expression of common proteins in the metabolic pathways, and teadenol B had a notable effect on the four breast cancer cells.

2.3. Teadenol B Inhibits the Growth of Transplanted Tumors in Nude Mice

Triple-negative breast cancer is characterized by a high mitosis rate, high lymphocytic infiltration rate, high grade, large tumor size, high recurrence rate, and high mortality rate. It is a type of breast cancer with the worst prognosis in clinical treatment at present, and it is urgent to develop new therapeutic methods. KEGG pathway analysis results (Figure 3A) showed that among the four different breast cancer cells above, MDA-MB-231 cells had the most significant difference in protein expression and the largest number of different proteins produced by the intervention of teadenol B. Therefore, triple-negative breast cancer cell MDA-MB-231 was selected as the animal study object to further explore the effect of teadenol B on the growth status, size, and toxicity of transplanted tumors in nude mice.

Cultured MDA-MB-231 breast cancer cells were injected into the axillary region of 2 nude mice with a prepared cell suspension (containing approximately 5×10^6 cells) in a volume of 0.1 mL. Once the tumors reached a certain size, they were dissected into small fragments and transplanted into an additional 20 nude mice. Four weeks after tumor transplantation, the model group received intragastric administration of 0.5% CMC-Na at a dose of 10 mL/kg, while the treatment group was administered teadenol B at a dose of 75 mg/kg every three days for four weeks (Figure 4A). Results demonstrated that breast tumor volume significantly decreased after two weeks of treatment (Figure 4B), indicating effective inhibition of breast tumor growth in nude mice by gastric administration of teadenol B. Moreover, the rate of increase in breast tumor weight was significantly reduced after four weeks of treatment (Figure 4C), confirming excellent anti-breast cancer activity exhibited by teadenol B. Furthermore, no statistically significant difference was observed in body weight changes between the control group receiving an equivalent volume of solvent via oral gavage and the group treated with teadenol B (Figure 4D). These findings preliminarily suggest that this dosage and route do not induce significant toxic reactions.

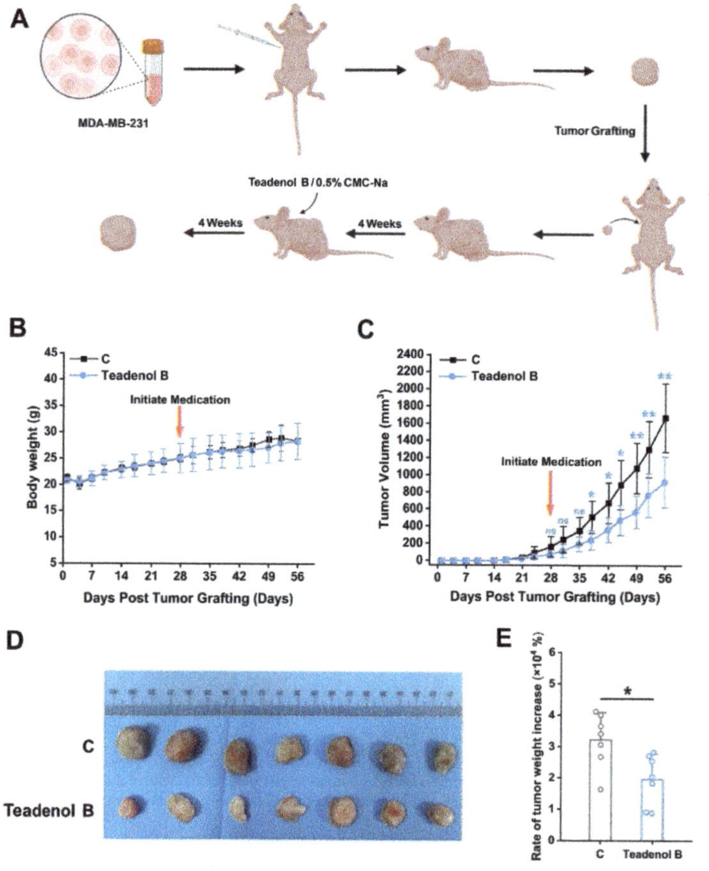

Figure 4. Inhibitory effect of teadenol B on the transplanted tumor in nude mice. (**A**) Flowchart of tumor transplantation and drug treatment in nude mice; (**B**) changes in body weight of nude mice over time. The data are presented as mean ± SD ($p > 0.05$, $n = 7$); (**C**) the changes in breast tumor volume with time in nude mice were statistically significant from 2 to 4 weeks after administration. The data are presented as mean ± SD (ns, $p > 0.05$; * $p < 0.05$, ** $p < 0.01$, $n = 7$); (**D**) at week 8, mice were sacrificed for extract untreated and teadenol B-treated tumor tissues; (**E**) the effect of administration of teadenol B on the rate of breast tumor weight increase was statistically significant after four weeks of administration. The data are presented as mean ± SD (* $p < 0.05$, $n = 7$).

2.4. Teadenol B Inhibits MDA-MB-231 Cells by Inhibiting DCTD as an Autophagy Promotor

According to the proteomic results (Figure 3B), the DCTD protein may be the key protein involved in the inhibition of teadenol B on cancer cell growth. Considering the close relationship between DCTD and apoptosis, we conducted further experiments and found that after treatment with teadenol B, both early and late apoptosis of MDA-MB-231 cells increased, with a more significant increase in early apoptosis. This indicates that teadenol B primarily inhibits cancer cell growth by inducing programmed cell death in MDA-MB-231 cells while maintaining the integrity of the cell membrane (Figure 5A,B). One hour after treatment with teadenol B, there was a slight increase in the expression level of BCL2, but with no statistical difference ($p > 0.05$). We also examined the levels of the uncut forms of caspase-9 and caspase-3 (Figure 5C,D). Compared to the control group treated for 1 h, the expression levels of the uncut form of caspase-9 decreased significantly after 4 h of treatment with teadenol B (40 μg/mL, $p < 0.05$; 80 μg/mL, $p < 0.01$). Compared to the control group treated for the same duration, 80 μg/mL of teadenol B significantly reduced the protein level of the uncut form of caspase-3 ($p < 0.05$). This further demonstrates that teadenol B can induce apoptosis in cells.

As shown in Figure S1, the proteomic results show that teadenol B changes the expression of some proteins in the autophagy pathway. ATG12, ATG3, BCL2, and RELA expression decreased, and mTOR was most significantly down-regulated (Figure S2). Thus, we hypothesized that teadenol B might play a role in promoting autophagy. We examined some autophagy proteins, including the most widely used markers (Figure 5E–G). String analysis results show that these proteins interact with the apoptotic proteins mentioned above (Figure S3). After 4 h of treatment with 40 μg/mL of teadenol B, the protein level of SQSTM1 in MDA-MB-231 cells decreased significantly ($p < 0.05$) with a significant increase in the MAP1LC3-II/I ratio ($p < 0.001$), which represents a high degree of conversion from MAP1LC3-I to MAP1LC3-II. Additionally, teadenol B significantly reduced the protein level of DCTD ($p < 0.001$), and this effect was shown to be enhanced with increasing concentration or treatment time of teadenol B. All these results proved that teadenol B was an autophagy promotor, which is consistent with the results of proteomics in Figure S2. The protein level of DCTD decreases (Figure 5E,G), which might be due to the intracellular protein degradation role of autophagy.

2.5. Discussion

Breast cancer is a serious threat to women's lives and health, among which triple-negative breast cancer is a kind of breast cancer with the worst prognosis in clinical treatment. Ripe Pu-erh tea and microbial fermented tea have positive effects on maintaining body health and preventing cancers [20–22]. Identification of the biological activity of the characteristic chemical components of Pu-erh tea is the basis for the study of the functional mechanism of Pu-erh tea. Teadenol B is a common compound in Pu-erh ripe tea and microbial fermented tea. Except for the known adiponectin secretion-promoting activity and protein tyrosine phosphatase 1B expression inhibitory activity, no other activities have been reported [24]. In this study, in the screening process of anti-breast cancer activity using the MTT test, it was found that teadenol B showed inhibitory effects on four types of breast cancer cells corresponding to different clinical subtypes, including MDA-MB-231 triple-negative breast cancer cells. Among them, the inhibitory effect on MDA-MB-231, MDA-MB-453, and BT474 breast cancer cells was stronger, and the inhibitory effect on MCF-7 breast cancer cells was slightly weaker. Furthermore, proteomic studies were conducted to investigate the potential mechanism of action of teadenol B against breast cancer, and it was found that metabolic pathways (hsa01100) were the most significantly different cell signaling pathways under the intervention of teadenol B, which provided information basis for subsequent studies on its anticancer mechanism. Considering that MDA-MB-231 cells had the worst clinical prognosis and showed the most significant statistical difference in the KEGG pathway enrichment analysis results, to further clarify the inhibitory effect of teadenol B on breast cancer, the interventional effect of teadenol B on the size and growth of MDA-MB-231 triple-negative breast cancer grafts in nude mouse animal models was studied. The experimental results showed that teadenol B significantly inhibited the growth of breast cancer in nude mice but had no significant effect on the body weight of nude mice, indicating that teadenol B could inhibit MDA-MB-231 triple-negative breast cancer grafts. There was no obvious toxic reaction.

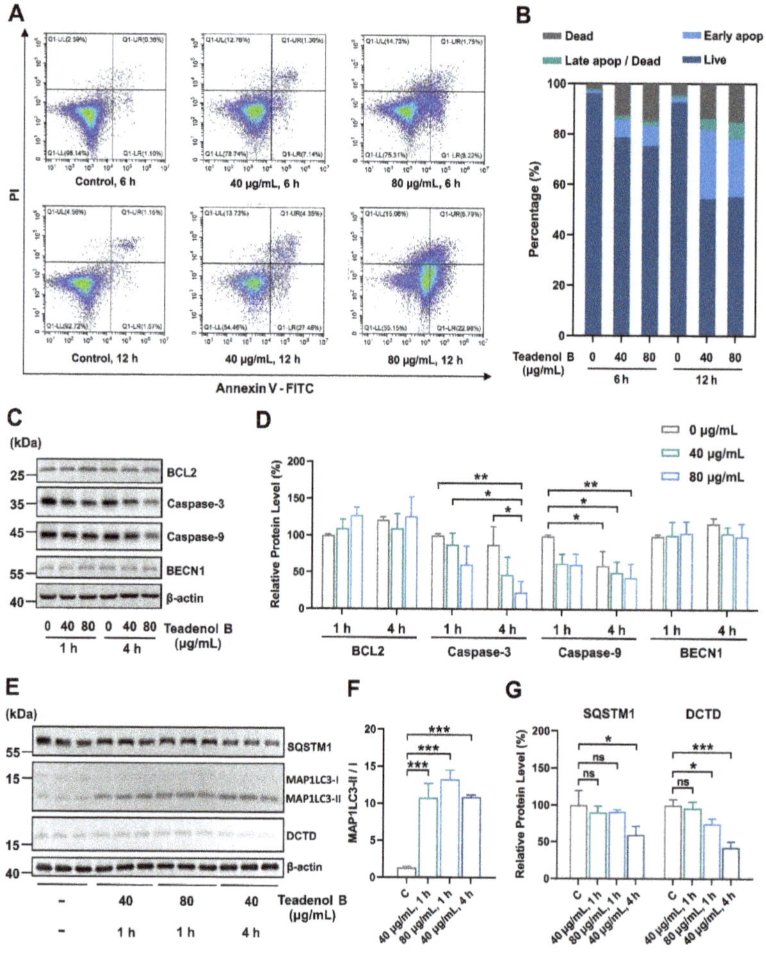

Figure 5. Teadenol B can promote autophagy and reduce the expression level of DCTD to inhibit the growth of MDA-MB-231 cells. (**A**) Teadenol B promotes apoptosis in MDA-MB-231 cells; (**B**) teadenol B mainly promotes early apoptosis in MDA-MB-231 cells; (**C**) changes in the expression levels of apoptosis-related proteins in MDA-MB-231 cells after treatment with teadenol B; (**D**) the semi-quantitative analysis. The data are presented as mean ± SD (* $p < 0.05$, ** $p < 0.01$, $n = 3$); (**E**) changes in the expression levels of autophagy-related proteins and anti-cancer-related proteins in MDA-MB-231 cells after treatment with teadenol B; (**F**,**G**) the semi-quantitative analysis. The data are presented as mean ± SD (ns, $p > 0.05$; * $p < 0.05$, *** $p < 0.001$, $n = 3$).

Through proteomics studies, we found that the metabolic pathway is the most affected by teadenol B. Comparing the results of the detected protein changes in the metabolic pathways, we found that only DCTD's changes were consistent in all four cell types, with significant downregulation. It is speculated that the change in this protein may be one of the reasons for the inhibition of all four types of cancer cells. It has been reported that the degradation of DCTD could block DNA synthesis and the repair of DNA damage [30]. DNA damage can stimulate BH3-only proteins to bind with high affinity to anti-apoptotic BCL2 proteins, activating pro-apoptotic effectors and triggering a cascade of caspase reactions, leading to orderly cell apoptosis [31]. Cell apoptosis is one of the inherent mechanisms in the cell cycle that can promptly eliminate non-functional, harmful, and abnormal cells [32].

Autophagy is one of the important pathways for intracellular protein degradation, and it is closely related to the occurrence and development of cancer. In simple terms, the deficiency of autophagy in cells can lead to the accumulation of misfolded proteins, which can induce carcinogenesis; excessive autophagy can also induce cell apoptosis. Therefore, theoretically, autophagy promotors have potential preventive and therapeutic effects against cancer [33]. Some autophagy promotors, such as rapamycin [34], resveratrol [35], metformin [36], and carnosic acid [37], have been reported to possess anticancer activities. Here, we found that the conversion of MAP1LC3-I to MAP1LC3-II increased extremely significantly with the treatment of teadenol B, which proved teadenol B to be an autophagy promotor that can be used to explain the down-regulation of DCTD to some extent.

3. Materials and Methods

3.1. Cell Culture

All experiments used cells within 20 passages. Both MDA-MB-231 (CELL-C0150, Bioswamp, Wuhan, China) and MDA-MB-453 (CELL-C0152, Bioswamp, Wuhan, China) were cultured in L-15 medium with phenol red (Jinuo, Hangzhou, China) supplemented with 10% fetal bovine serum (FBS, 11011-8611, Sijiqing, Hangzhou, China) in a 37 °C incubator. MCF-7 (CC0302, Cellcook, Guangzhou, China) were cultured in MEM medium with phenol red (MA0217, Meilunbio, Dalian, China) supplemented with 10% FBS and 10 μg/mL insulin (118975, Aladdin, Shanghai, China) at 37 °C in a 5% CO_2 atmosphere. BT474 (CC0310, Cellcook, Guangzhou, China) were cultured in RPMI 1640 medium with phenol red (MA0215, Meilunbio, Dalian, China) supplemented with 10% FBS and 10 μg/mL insulin at 37 °C in a 5% CO_2 atmosphere. The media were replaced with phenol red-free RPMI 1640 medium (11835, TBD, Tianjin, China) before all the experiments were conducted to avoid estrogenic stimulation of the phenol red.

3.2. MTT Assays

The impact of teadenol B on cell viability and proliferation was assessed using MTT assays. Cells (8×10^4 cells/mL) were plated in 96-well plates and incubated overnight at 37 °C with 5% CO_2. The culture medium was replaced with 100 μL phenol red-free and serum-free RPMI-1640 medium, and then the cells were exposed to paclitaxel (P106869, Aladdin, Shanghai, China) or teadenol B, extracted and identified as described in our patent [28], alone for 24 h. The 1H, 13C NMR data of teadenol B are presented in Table S1. The purity of teadenol B is greater than 95%. After washing once with phosphate buffer saline (PBS, MA0015, Meilunbio, Dalian, China), 100 μL of MTT solution (0.5 mg/mL, Kerui, Wuhan, China) was added to each well, and the cells were incubated at 37 °C with 5% CO_2 for 4 h. After aspirating the culture medium, 150 μL dimethylsulfoxide (DMSO, 30072418, SCR, Shanghai, China) was added to each well. The optical density (absorbance) at 570 nm was measured with a microplate reader (Spark, Tecan, Switzerland). Cell viability was determined by calculating the percentage of viable cells in teadenol B-treated samples compared to vehicle control-treated cells, which were considered 100% viable. Each experiment was independently repeated five times.

3.3. Proteomic Sample Preparation

MDA-MB-231 cells were plated into 6-well plates at a density of 5×10^5 cells/mL and incubated at 37 °C with 5% CO_2. After 24 h, the culture medium was replaced with 2 mL phenol red-free and serum-free RPMI-1640 medium, and then the cells were exposed to PEG400 (0.1%) and teadenol B (20 μg/mL) alone for 1 h. After culture, the cells were washed twice with PBS (4 °C) and scraped off the culture dish into a centrifuge tube using a cell scraper. The cell suspension was centrifuged at 1000× g and 4 °C for 1 min, after which the supernatant was removed. Finally, the cells were stored at −80 °C for later testing and analysis.

3.4. Label-Free MS Analysis

Serum-starved cells were exposed to a treatment of 0.1% PEG400 and 20 μg/mL teadenol B for 1 h to explore the effects of teadenol B on breast cancer cells. After washing with cold PBS, the cells were collected and subjected to dialysis, concentration, and quantification using the BCA method. The protein samples were adjusted to an equal concentration, dried, trypsin-digested, and then analyzed using mass spectrometry (Thermo Fisher, Orbitrap Fusion, Waltham, MA, USA). The resulting mass spectrometry raw files were searched against the SwissProt protein database using MaxQuant software (version 1.6.5.0) with a false discovery rate (FDR) $\leq$ 1%. The IBAQ (intensity-based absolute protein quantification) algorithm was employed for quantitative analysis. A comparison of the teadenol B-treated group with the control group was performed to identify proteins with similar differences. Additionally, a pathway analysis based on KEGG was conducted.

3.5. Human Breast Cancer Xenograft Nude Mice Model

Male BALB/c nude mice were purchased from Wuhan Bestcell Model Bio-Tech Co., Ltd. (Wuhan, China). MDA-MB-231 cells were re-suspended in medium and mixed with Matrigel matrix (356231, Corning, New York, NY, USA), resulting in a final cell concentration of 5×10^7 cells/mL, and injected into the armpits of 5 to 6-week-old male nude mice. After the tumors reached approximately 1 cm^3, they were cut into 10 mm^3 pieces and then transplanted into 20 male BALB/c nude mice aged 5 to 6 weeks and weighing 20 to 22 g, respectively. Mice were randomly divided into control and teadenol B groups (10 mice per group). Four weeks after the tumor transplant, oral administration was started. Teadenol B was dissolved in 0.5% sodium carboxymethyl cellulose (CMC-Na, M9317, AbMole, Houston, TX, USA). Teadenol B was given by oral intake at a dose of 75 mg/kg/3d. The administration period was 4 weeks. Tumors were measured at seven-day intervals with a caliper, and tumor volume was calculated using the following formula: volume (mm^3) = $\text{width}^2 \times \text{length} \times 6/\pi$. At the end of the administration cycle, Tumor tissue was taken and weighed to calculate the rate of breast tumor weight increase. All the animal studies obeyed the principles of the 1983 Declaration of Helsinki. They were conducted following the Chinese Regulations for the Administration of Affairs Concerning Experimental Animals and performed in accordance with the Guidelines of the China Animal Welfare Legislation. This study was approved by the Hubei Provincial Science & Technology Department, Wuhan, China (Approval Number: SYXK 2022-0124).

3.6. Western Blot

MDA-MB-231 cells were exposed to 0.1% PEG400 and teadenol B (40, 80 μg/mL) for 1 and 4 h to assess the influence of teadenol B on the expression levels of proteins associated with autophagy. Following treatment, the harvested cells were directly lysed in 200 μL of ice-cold lysis buffer containing protease inhibitors. The resulting lysates were then subjected to centrifugation at 12,000× *g* at 4 °C for 10 min. Subsequently, a loading buffer was added at a 1:1 ratio, and the samples were collected and separated on SDS-polyacrylamide gels. The proteins were then transferred to nitrocellulose filter membranes and washed in Tris-buffered saline (TBS) with 0.1% Tween20 (TBST) 3 times. The membranes were incubated overnight with antibodies for BECN1 (1:10,000, 66665-1-Ig, Proteintech, Chicago, USA), caspase-3 (1:500, A19654, Abclonal, Wuhan, China), caspase-9 (1:500, 10380-1-AP, Proteintech, Chicago, IL, USA), DCTD (1:1000, 68357-1-Ig, Proteintech, Chicago, USA), MAP1LC3 (1:1000 dilution, 14600-1-AP, Proteintech, Chicago, IL, USA), and SQSTM1 (1:2000 dilution, 66184-1-Ig, Proteintech, Chicago, IL, USA), respectively, at 4 °C overnight. The membranes were then washed with TBST and incubated with HRP-conjugated Affinipure Goat Anti-Mouse IgG(H+L) (1:2000 dilution, SA00001-1, Proteintech, Chicago, IL, USA) at 37 °C for 2 h. Finally, the proteins were visualized using an Enhanced HRP-DAB Chromogenic Substrate Kit (4994100, Tiangen, Beijing, China). The antibody β-actin (1:10,000 dilution, 66009-1-Ig, Proteintech, Chicago, IL, USA) was used as the loading control. Each experiment was repeated in triplicate. The quantification of the blots was performed using Photoshop CC 2018.

3.7. *Apoptosis Assay*

Apoptotic activity was assessed using the Annexin V-FITC/PI staining kit (P-CA-201, Procell, Wuhan, China), containing Annexin V-FITC, propidium iodide (PI), and Annexin V Binding Buffer. MDA-MB-231 cells were plated at a density of 5×10^5 cells per well in 6-well plates. Following treatment with the drug, the cells underwent two PBS washes, followed by harvesting and centrifugation at 300× *g* for 5 min. Subsequently, the cells were exposed to 500 μL of 1×Annexin V-FITC Buffer along with 5 μL of Annexin-V and 5 μL of PI for 20 min at room temperature in the absence of light. Annexin staining was quantified using a flow cytometer (CytoFLEX S, Beckman, CA, USA).

3.8. *Statistical Analysis*

The results are reported as the mean ± SD. The statistical analysis of the data was performed using one-way or two-way ANOVA, followed by Tukey's post hoc test as applicable, to assess for any differences. A *p*-value greater than 0.05 indicated no statistically significant difference. Statistical significance was defined as $p < 0.05$, indicating a significant finding. $P < 0.01$ was considered highly significant, while $p < 0.001$ was considered extremely significant.

4. Conclusions

In summary, this study proved the inhibitory effect of teadenol B on the viability of four breast cancer cells, including MDA-MB-231 breast cancer. It preliminarily revealed that its anticancer activity may be related to its inhibitory effect on DCTD as an autophagy promotor, but further research is needed to clarify the details involved in the future. In addition, different types of breast cancer cells have different sensitivity to teadenol B, so the therapeutic value of teadenol B for different breast tumors needs further research. This work provides a new basis for the healthcare efficacy of drinking microbially fermented tea in the prevention and treatment of breast cancer, expands the research scope of the active mechanism and application of teadenol B compound, and also provides a new choice for the development of new drugs for the prevention and treatment of breast cancer.

Supplementary Materials: The following supporting information can be downloaded at: https://www.mdpi.com/article/10.3390/molecules29040872/s1, Figure S1: Differentially expressed proteins related to autophagy pathways in MDA MB 231 cells; Figure S2: Heat map analysis of differentially expressed proteins related to autophagy pathways in MDA MB 231 cells; Figure S3: Interaction analysis of key proteins using STRING database; Table S1: ^{1}H, ^{13}C NMR data for teadenol B (solvent: deuterated dimethyl sulfoxide (DMSO-d_6)).

Author Contributions: Conceptualization, J.X.; investigation, Y.Z., Y.-J.Y., Z.-G.D., R.Y., M.-M.Q., S.-K.P. and J.-L.X.; methodology, Y.Z. and Z.-G.D.; project administration, J.X. and Y.-H.S.; resources, Y.-H.S.; writing—original draft, Y.Z.; writing—review and editing, Y.-J.Y. and J.X.; funding acquisition, Z.-G.D. All authors have read and agreed to the published version of the manuscript.

Funding: This research was funded by the Major Science and Technology Projects of Yunnan Province, grant number 202002AE320001. Xingdian Talent Support Program of Yunnan Province.

Institutional Review Board Statement: All the animal studies obeyed the principles of the 1983 Declaration of Helsinki. They were conducted following the Chinese Regulations for the Administration of Affairs Concerning Experimental Animals and performed in accordance with the Guidelines of the China Animal Welfare Legislation. This study was approved by the Hubei Provincial Science & Technology Department, China (Approval Number: SYXK 2022-0124, 2022-01-24).

Informed Consent Statement: Not applicable.

Data Availability Statement: Data are contained within the article and Supplementary Materials.

Conflicts of Interest: The authors declare no conflict of interest.

References

1. Kolak, A.; Kaminska, M.; Sygit, K.; Budny, A.; Surdyka, D.; Kukielka-Budny, B.; Burdan, F. Primary and secondary prevention of breast cancer. *Ann. Agric. Environ. Med.* **2017**, *24*, 549–553. [CrossRef]
2. McGuire, A.; Brown, J.A.; Malone, C.; McLaughlin, R.; Kerin, M.J. Effects of age on the detection and management of breast cancer. *Cancers* **2015**, *7*, 908–929. [CrossRef] [PubMed]
3. Sviderskiy, V.O.; Blumenberg, L.; Gorodetsky, E.; Karakousi, T.R.; Hirsh, N.; Alvarez, S.W.; Terzi, E.M.; Kaparos, E.; Whiten, G.C.; Ssebyala, S.; et al. Hyperactive CDK2 Activity in Basal-like Breast Cancer Imposes a Genome Integrity Liability that Can Be Exploited by Targeting DNA Polymerase ε. *Mol. Cell* **2020**, *80*, 682–698.e7. [CrossRef] [PubMed]
4. Zhang, Y.; Tian, J.; Qu, C.; Peng, Y.; Lei, J.; Sun, L.; Zong, B.; Liu, S. A look into the link between centrosome amplification and breast cancer. *Biomed. Pharmacother.* **2020**, *132*, 110924. [CrossRef] [PubMed]
5. Zhao, L.; Han, X.; Lu, J.; McEachern, D.; Wang, S. A highly potent PROTAC androgen receptor (AR) degrader ARD-61 effectively inhibits AR-positive breast cancer cell growth in vitro and tumor growth in vivo. *Neoplasia* **2020**, *22*, 522–532. [CrossRef] [PubMed]
6. Qi, M.; Liu, X.; Zhou, Y.; Wang, H.; Zhao, Y.; Ren, J.; Xiang, J. Berberine Inhibits MDA-MB-231 Cells as an Agonist of G Protein-Coupled Estrogen Receptor 1. *Int. J. Mol. Sci.* **2021**, *22*, 11466. [CrossRef] [PubMed]
7. Xiang, J.; Wang, Y.; Su, K.; Liu, M.; Hu, P.C.; Ma, T.; Li, J.X.; Wei, L.; Zheng, Z.; Yang, F. Ritonavir binds to and downregulates estrogen receptors: Molecular mechanism of promoting early atherosclerosis. *Exp. Cell Res.* **2014**, *327*, 318–330. [CrossRef] [PubMed]
8. Harbeck, N.; Gnant, M. Breast cancer. *Lancet* **2017**, *389*, 1134–1150. [CrossRef]
9. Barzaman, K.; Karami, J.; Zarei, Z.; Hosseinzadeh, A.; Kazemi, M.H.; Moradi-Kalbolandi, S.; Safari, E.; Farahmand, L. Breast cancer: Biology, biomarkers, and treatments. *Int. Immunopharmacol.* **2020**, *84*, 106535. [CrossRef]
10. Maughan, K.L.; Lutterbie, M.A.; Ham, P.S. Treatment of breast cancer. *Am. Fam. Physician* **2010**, *81*, 1339–1346.
11. Brody, H. Tea. *Nature* **2019**, *566*, S1. [CrossRef] [PubMed]
12. Yang, C.S.; Wang, Z.Y. Tea and cancer. *J. Natl. Cancer Inst.* **1993**, *85*, 1038–1049. [CrossRef] [PubMed]
13. Trevisanato, S.I.; Kim, Y.I. Tea and health. *Nutr. Rev.* **2000**, *58*, 1–10. [CrossRef] [PubMed]
14. Camfield, D.A.; Stough, C.; Farrimond, J.; Scholey, A.B. Acute effects of tea constituents L-theanine, caffeine, and epigallocatechin gallate on cognitive function and mood: A systematic review and meta-analysis. *Nutr. Rev.* **2014**, *72*, 507–522. [CrossRef] [PubMed]
15. van Dam, R.M.; Hu, F.B.; Willett, W.C. Coffee, Caffeine, and Health. *N. Engl. J. Med.* **2020**, *383*, 369–378. [CrossRef] [PubMed]
16. Sirotkin, A.V.; Kolesárová, A. The anti-obesity and health-promoting effects of tea and coffee. *Physiol. Res.* **2021**, *70*, 161–168. [CrossRef] [PubMed]
17. Jeukendrup, A.E.; Randell, R. Fat burners: Nutrition supplements that increase fat metabolism. *Obes. Rev.* **2011**, *12*, 841–851. [CrossRef]
18. Vázquez Cisneros, L.C.; López-Uriarte, P.; López-Espinoza, A.; Navarro Meza, M.; Espinoza-Gallardo, A.C.; Guzmán Aburto, M.B. Effects of green tea and its epigallocatechin (EGCG) content on body weight and fat mass in humans: A systematic review. *Nutr. Hosp.* **2017**, *34*, 731–737. [CrossRef]
19. Sinha, D.; Biswas, J.; Nabavi, S.M.; Bishayee, A. Tea phytochemicals for breast cancer prevention and intervention: From bench to bedside and beyond. *Semin. Cancer Biol.* **2017**, *46*, 33–54. [CrossRef]
20. Mao, X.; Xiao, X.; Chen, D.; Yu, B.; He, J. Tea and Its Components Prevent Cancer: A Review of the Redox-Related Mechanism. *Int. J. Mol. Sci.* **2019**, *20*, 5249. [CrossRef]
21. Zhao, L.G.; Li, Z.Y.; Feng, G.S.; Ji, X.W.; Tan, Y.T.; Li, H.L.; Gunter, M.J.; Xiang, Y.B. Tea Drinking and Risk of Cancer Incidence: A Meta-Analysis of Prospective Cohort Studies and Evidence Evaluation. *Adv. Nutr.* **2021**, *12*, 402–412. [CrossRef]
22. Zhu, M.Z.; Li, N.; Zhou, F.; Ouyang, J.; Lu, D.M.; Xu, W.; Li, J.; Lin, H.Y.; Zhang, Z.; Xiao, J.B.; et al. Microbial bioconversion of the chemical components in dark tea. *Food Chem.* **2020**, *312*, 126043. [CrossRef]
23. Lv, S.; Wu, Y.; Zhou, J.; Lian, M.; Li, C.; Xu, Y.; Liu, S.; Wang, C.; Meng, Q. The study of fingerprint characteristics of Dayi Pu-Erh tea using a fully automatic HS-SPME/GC-MS and combined chemometrics method. *PLoS ONE* **2014**, *9*, e116428. [CrossRef]
24. Wulandari, R.A.; Amano, M.; Yanagita, T.; Tanaka, T.; Kouno, I.; Kawamura, D.; Ishimaru, K. New phenolic compounds from *Camellia sinensis* L. leaves fermented with *Aspergillus* sp. *J. Nat. Med.* **2011**, *65*, 594–597. [CrossRef]
25. Song, J.-H.; Miyazaki, H.; Yoshida, S. Simple Method for the Preparation of Teadenols A and B by a Combined Process of Submerged Culture with *Aspergillus* sp. and Chromatographic Separation. *Food Sci. Technol. Res.* **2017**, *23*, 91–100. [CrossRef]
26. Yanagita, T.; Ishimaru, K.; Tanaka, T.; Koba, K.; Miyazaki, H.; Aoki, N.; Kawamura, D. Functional Microbially Fermented Tea Extract Containing Polyphenol Derivative and Method for Producing the Same. U.S. Patent US9029110B2, 12 May 2015.
27. Yanagita, T.; Ishimaru, K.; Tanaka, T.; Koba, K.; Miyazaki, H.; Aoki, N.; Kawamura, D. Polyphenol Derivative and Method for Producing the Same. U.S. Patent US8558016B2, 15 October 2013.
28. Liu, J.; Ding, Z.; Gao, L.; Chen, D.; Liu, M.; Tang, S. Methods for Separating Teadenol A and Teadenol B from Fermented Tea. CN Patent No. CN108117558B, 30 October 2020.
29. Nagasawa, T.; Ishimaru, K.; Higashiyama, S.; Hama, Y.; Mitsutake, S. Teadenol A in microbial fermented tea acts as a novel ligand on GPR120 to increase GLP-1 secretion. *Food Funct.* **2020**, *11*, 10534–10541. [CrossRef]

30. Weiner, K.X.B.; Ciesla, J.; Jaffe, A.B.; Ketring, R.; Maley, F.; Maley, G.F. Chromosomal Location and Structural Organization of the Human Deoxycytidylate Deaminase Gene. *J. Biol. Chem.* **1995**, *270*, 18727–18729. [CrossRef]
31. Radha, G.; Raghavan, S.C. BCL2: A promising cancer therapeutic target. *Biochim. Biophys. Acta Rev. Cancer* **2017**, *1868*, 309–314. [CrossRef] [PubMed]
32. Carneiro, B.A.; El-Deiry, W.S. Targeting apoptosis in cancer therapy. *Nat. Rev. Clin. Oncol.* **2020**, *17*, 395–417. [CrossRef] [PubMed]
33. Xiang, J.; Liu, X.; Ren, J.; Chen, K.; Wang, H.L.; Miao, Y.Y.; Qi, M.M. How does estrogen work on autophagy? *Autophagy* **2019**, *15*, 197–211. [CrossRef] [PubMed]
34. Sun, L.; Yan, Y.; Lv, H.; Li, J.L.; Wang, Z.Y.; Wang, K.; Wang, L.; Li, Y.X.; Jiang, H.; Zhang, Y.Y. Rapamycin targets STAT3 and impacts c-Myc to suppress tumor growth. *Cell Chem. Biol.* **2022**, *29*, 373–385. [CrossRef] [PubMed]
35. Abdel-Latif, G.A.; Al-Abd, A.M.; Tadros, M.G.; Al-Abbasi, F.A.; Khalifa, A.E.; Abdel-Naim, A.B. The chemomodulatory effects of resveratrol and didox on herceptin cytotoxicity in breast cancer cell lines. *Sci. Rep.* **2015**, *5*, 12054. [CrossRef] [PubMed]
36. Yang, J.J.; Zhou, Y.L.; Xie, S.D.; Wang, J.; Li, Z.Q.; Chen, L.N.; Mao, M.S.; Chen, C.; Huang, A.H.; Chen, Y.X.; et al. Metformin induces Ferroptosis by inhibiting UFMylation of SLC7A11 in breast cancer. *J. Exp. Clin. Cancer Res.* **2021**, *40*, 206. [CrossRef] [PubMed]
37. Yesil-Celiktas, O.; Sevimli, C.; Bedir, E.; Vardar-Sukan, F. Inhibitory Effects of Rosemary Extracts, Carnosic Acid and Rosma rinic Acid on the Growth of Various Human Cancer Cell Lines. *Plant Food Hum. Nutr.* **2010**, *65*, 158–163. [CrossRef]

molecules

MDPI

Review

An Overview on the Hallucinogenic Peyote and Its Alkaloid Mescaline: The Importance of Context, Ceremony and Culture

Marjolein Doesburg-van Kleffens †, Amy M. Zimmermann-Klemd *,† and Carsten Gründemann

Translational Complementary Medicine, Department of Pharmaceutical Sciences, University of Basel, Campus Rosental–Mattenstrasse 22, CH-4058 Basel, Switzerland; marjolein.doesburg-vankleffens@unibas.ch (M.D.-v.K.); carsten.gruendemann@unibas.ch (C.G.)

* Correspondence: amy.klemd@unibas.ch; Tel.: +41-61-207-61-84

† These authors contributed equally to this work.

Abstract: Peyote (*Lophophora williamsii*) is a cactus that contains various biologically active alkaloids—such as pellotine, anhalonidine, hordenine and mescaline. Here, mescaline induces the psychoactive effects of peyote through the activation of the serotonin 5-HT_{2A} receptor and the subsequent release of calcium (Ca^{2+}) from the endoplasmic reticulum (ER). Moreover, an evaluation of the therapeutic benefits of mescaline is also currently the subject of research. It is important to consider that the outcome of taking a psychedelic drug strongly depends on the mindset of the recipient and the context (set and setting principle), including ceremonies and culture. This overview serves to summarise the current state of the knowledge of the metabolism, mechanism of action and clinical application studies of peyote and mescaline. Furthermore, the benefits of the potential of peyote and mescaline are presented in a new light, setting an example for combining a form of treatment embedded in nature and ritually enriched with our current highly innovative Western medicine.

Keywords: *Lophophora williamsii*; peyote; mescaline; psychoactive; 5-HT_{2A} receptor; set and setting

1. Introduction

Peyote (*Lophophora williamsii*) is a cactus that contains psychoactive alkaloids—mainly mescaline (Figure 1). The ceremonial use of peyote was widespread at the time of Spanish rule in the Aztec Empire and in northern Mexico (around 1520) [1,2]. There are also descriptions of a wide range of medicinal uses, which include the treatment of burns, wounds, fever, rheumatism, snakebites and scorpion stings [3,4]. In the 1960s, the peyote cactus and its psychoactive substance mescaline made big waves. Its use was popular and much discussed in the media. In October 1964, the New York Times published the article "The 'Diabolic Root", which addresses the still very topical question of what is more dangerous: a weakly psychotropic cactus, substances such as tobacco and alcohol, or even narcotic institutions such as advertising and television (—today, the internet and social media would certainly be worth mentioning at this point) [5]. The use of peyote and mescaline was finally banned [6–8]. In 1978, the American Indian Religious Freedom Act authorised members of the Native American Church (NAC) to use peyote for religious purposes. Amendments to the American Indian Religious Freedom Act in 1994 permitted the harvesting, possession and consumption of peyote for "bona fide religious ceremonies" [9]. This was an important step by the Americans towards ending the war on drugs. A central role in this is played by the reform movement "Decriminalize Nature", which has been very successful in decriminalising "herbal medicines" (e.g., psilocybin, ayahuasca and mescaline) [10]. In 1991, the publication of Dr. Alexander Shulgin and Ann Shulgin's "summarised life work" book *PiHKAL* (acronym for phenethylamines I have known and loved): *A Chemical Love Story* [11] caused an uproar, as *PiHKAL* contains an auto bibliographical section as well as detailed instructions for the synthesis of 179 psychedelic phenethylamines (mostly discovered by Dr. Alexander Shulgin)—including mescaline and

MDMA ("ecstasy")—that are still commonly used today. For each substance, there is also information on the recommended effective dose and the subjective effects experienced by the authors.

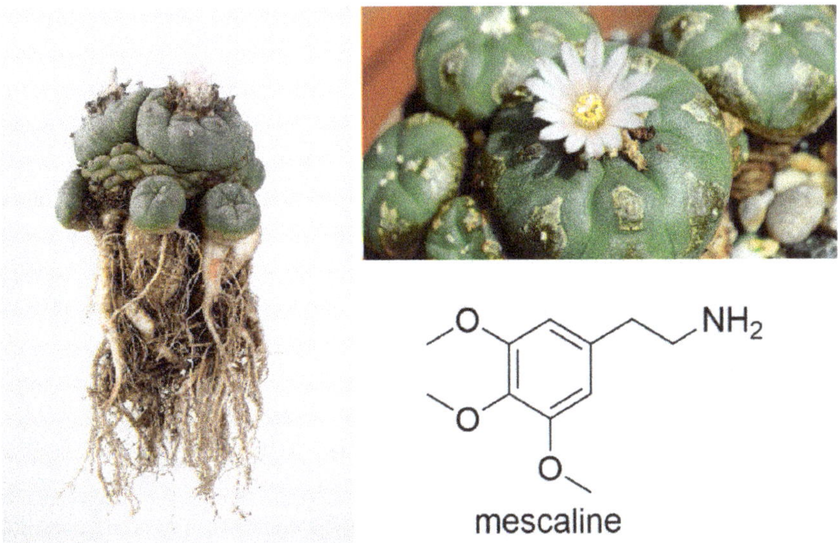

Figure 1. Pictures of the peyote cactus and the structure of its main alkaloid mescaline.

An important question we all have to ask ourselves now, according to an article published in the New York Times, is what a so-called "drug peace" might look like. Is it possible to integrate psychoactive substances into our lives or even use them constructively [12]? Indigenous peoples often manage to integrate psychedelics into their lives as a sacrament, medicine or means of communication. Ritual consumption often seems to protect against drug problems [12]. What is important here is that consumption is not carried out casually and alone, but rarely and then mindfully and together. This approach could serve as a model for integrating psychedelics into everyday life [13].

However, it is particularly important to have a comprehensive knowledge of the mechanism of action, and the potentials and dangers of the substances.

The history of peyote research begins with botanical studies from the 1840s and the listing of peyote in the Mexican pharmacopoeia [14]. Subsequently, in 1887, John Raleigh Briggs published the first study on the effects of mescal buttons [14]. Since then, research into the constituents (e.g., the main alkaloids: mescaline, pellotine, anhalonidine and hordenine), the biological effects and the biosynthesis of the active alkaloids progressed rapidly. The German pharmacologist Louis Lewin (1850–1929) and the chemist and physician Arthur Heffter (1860–1925), as well as the Merck Laboratory in Darmstadt, Germany, provided the decisive insights into alkaloid isolation from peyote in 1897 [14]. Heffter was finally able to show that mescaline, with a half-life of 6 h, was exclusively responsible for the intoxication symptoms associated with peyote consumption [14]. In the 1990s, the mechanism of action of mescaline finally became known. As with other psychedelic agents, the effect of mescaline is based on the binding and activation of the serotonin 5-HT_{2A} receptor [15–18].

Subsequently, the release of calcium (Ca^{2+}) from the endoplasmic reticulum (ER) is mainly induced, but other signalling pathways also seem to play a role (see Section 2) [19–21].

Research is also underway into the potential therapeutic value of mescaline. This step is consequential in light of the increasing acceptance of psychoactive drugs in general and their use for therapeutic purposes (cannabis can be named as a prime example here [22–24]).

Moreover, in the Western world, we are confronted with an increasing number of chronic diseases [25], psychiatric problems [26] and drug addiction [27]. Today, it also becomes more and more evident that there is a link between mental and physical wellbeing. This is also recognised in other medical systems such as traditional Chinese medicine (TCM), Ayurveda and integrative medicine. Data from studies suggest that, on average, people suffering from mental illness have a diminished life expectancy of 10 to 15 years [28–31].

These facts clearly require the establishment of new concepts for dealing with health and illness, self-healing and psychedelic substances, which can strongly influence these processes.

In this overview, we dive into the history and the effects of the peyote cactus and its major hallucinogenic alkaloid, mescaline. Although a single molecule, mescaline is the most active peyote substance; it seems that the whole plant, complemented with non-material factors, is needed for sustainable effects on mental health. We describe the importance of the concept of set and setting; specifically, the context and the ceremony. This could potentially enrich our Western culture, using the traditional application of peyote as an example, with its rich history [32]. In our eyes, this could be the inspiration for a new Western healthcare system.

2. Search Strategy

For this overview, we used a predefined search strategy and included studies published in the PubMed database and the clinicaltrial.gov trial registry (search keyword: Mescaline) up to October 2023. The following keywords were used as search terms with Boolean operators in the PubMed database: Mescaline[tiab] AND psycho-active [tiab], psycho[tiab] AND ritual[tiab], psycho-active[tiab] AND ceremony[tiab], Mescaline[tiab] AND clinic. Only sources and publications in German or English language were considered. Clearly irrelevant studies were eliminated by screening all the titles and abstracts of the publications identified through the database searches conducted. The remaining papers were assessed by reviewing their full-text versions. In addition, the reference lists of all eligible papers were manually reviewed to minimise the risk of overlooking relevant studies. Searches were conducted and data extracted by MDK and AMZK. The extracted data were reviewed by a third author (CG). Discrepancies were resolved through discussions and consensus. The results of the included publications were summarised in a narrative summary.

3. Mescaline—Metabolism, Clinical Reactions and Signalling

Peyote cactus is either eaten or drunk as an infusion (tea). An average intake of 3 to 6 of the cactus buds (approx. 10 to 20 g dry weight) contains a dose of mescaline equivalent to 200–400 mg mescaline sulphate [33] or 178–356 mg mescaline hydrochloride.

The physical responses to mescaline (mescaline hydrochloride: 2.5 mg/kg and 5 mg/kg) in 10 formerly morphine-dependent subjects were increased body temperature, higher systolic blood pressure and pupil diameter, and a lower knee pain threshold. Furthermore, this study described altered visual, temporal and sensory perception after the consumption of mescaline [34]. Another study with 18 volunteers found altered colour perception after the ingestion of 5 mg/kg mescaline [35]. Euphoria was frequently described, but anxiety and panic as well as depression rarely occurred [34]. In some cases, real visual hallucinations or pseudo hallucinations occurred [34]. The peak of the provoked effects was 2–2.5 h after ingestion of the drug [34]. At higher doses (over 400 mg), nausea and vomiting were reported as side effects [36,37]. In studies, lower right hemisphere performance was observed after the ingestion of 500 mg of mescaline-sulfate when the 12 healthy subjects solved a "face/no face" decision task [38–40]. An acute psychotomimetic state occurred 3.5 to 4 h after ingestion of the mescaline [40].

Mescaline (3,4,5-trimethoxy-beta-phenethylamine), responsible for the hallucinogenic effect, is absorbed relatively quickly [41] and distributed to the kidneys and liver, resulting in an increased half-life and a delayed onset of effects [42]. Due to the poor fat solubility of mescaline, transport across the blood–brain barrier is rather poor [33], but brain uptake appears to be relatively rapid according to studies with α-[14C]-mescaline in cats (25 mg/kg) [43]. The brain/plasma ratio one hour after intravenous injection was three and washout after 6 h appeared to be low, so that retention in the brain was long-lasting [43]. This was confirmed by studies with [3H]-mescaline in the brain of marmoset monkeys (*Callithrix jacchus*) [44]. Accumulation in the brain (hippocampus, amygdala, lateral geniculate and anterior cingulate cortex) could still be detected here 18 h after administration (8 mg, i.p.) [44]. It is assumed that the metabolism of mescaline differs organ specifically [45]. In a rabbit model, it was shown that an amine oxidase, which is expressed in the liver and also to a lesser extent in the lungs, plays a central role in the metabolism of mescaline [46]. The amine oxidase oxidatively deaminates mescaline to 3,4,5-trimethoxyphenylacetaldehyde [45]. This aldehyde is non-toxic, but also unstable, so that oxidation to 3,4,5-trimethoxyphenylacetic acid (TMPA) or reduction to the inactive 3,4,5-trimethoxyphenylethanol follows. It can be assumed that the metabolites contribute to the hallucinogenic effect of mescaline, as the peak of the mescaline effect does not correspond to the highest mescaline concentration in the brain. TMPA is demethylated to form the substance 3,4-dihydroxy-5-methoxyphenylacetic acid, which is finally linked to glutamine by the glutamine N-acyltransferase to be excreted as 3,4-dihydroxy-5-methoxyphenacetylglutamine [45]. In vivo studies on mouse livers and brains have shown that conversion of TMPA to 3,4,5-trimethoxybenzoic acid (3,4,5-TMBA) is also possible [47]. In the brain, detoxification of mescaline is assumed to occur mainly through N-acetylation [47]. Studies in mice and rats confirm the formation of N-acetylmescaline, its O-demethylated metabolites N-acetyl-3,5-dimethoxy-4-hydroxy-phenylethylamine and N-acetyl-3,4-dimethoxy-5-hydroxy-phenylethylamine [48]. The process of N-acetylation of mescaline has also been observed in humans [43]. The half-life of mescaline is on average 6 h and 87% is excreted within 24 h and 92% within 48 h [49,50]. In humans, an average of 26.2% of the administered mescaline dose was excreted as TMPA in the urine. However, this value is in all probability dependent on the route of administration (—oral intake with subsequent metabolisation in the liver leads to a higher deamination than with intravenous administration) [51]. In addition to TMPA, minor metabolites such as N-acetyl-3,4-dimethoxy-5-hydroxyphenylethylamine, 3,4,5-trimethoxybenzoic acid, 3,4-dimethoxy-5-hydroxyphenethylamine, and 3,4-dihydroxy-5-methoxyphenacetylglutamine were also detected in human urine [52].

The hallucinogenic effect of mescaline, the active ingredient of peyote, is mainly due to an agonistic effect at the serotonin 5-HT_{2A} receptor [53], to which it has a binding affinity in the low μM range (6.3 μM) [54]. The 5-HT_2 receptors are G protein-coupled receptors (GPCRs) found in the cerebral cortex, *locus coeruleus*, basal ganglia, hippocampus, platelets and vascular smooth muscle [55]. Interestingly, in addition to hallucinogenic 5-HT_{2A} agonists, there are also 5-HT_{2A} agonists (lisuride, ergotamine) that do not produce hallucinogenic effects by activating the 5-HT_{2A} receptor [19]. The model of "biased agonism" provides an explanation for this observation [56,57]. It states that different agonists can stabilise different active conformational states. The subsequent signal transduction is thus dependent on the respective active conformational state. After activation by an agonist, 5-HT_{2A} binds preferentially to $G_{q/11}$ proteins [19,20]. The subsequent activation of PLC triggers the formation of DAG and IP by the hydrolysis of PIP_2, leading to the release of intracellular Ca^{2+} from the endoplasmic reticulum [19,21]. However, the efficiency of this signalling response by hallucinogens is low, which means that other signalling pathways must play a role. Studies have shown that phospholipase A_2 (PLA_2) [58], PLA_2-mediated release of arachidonic acid (AA) [59] and the Gβγ-mediated activation of ERK1/2 as a function of $G_{i/o}$ [58] also play a role in hallucinogenic effects. In addition, studies have shown that the PDZ-binding domain of the 5-HT_{2A} receptor interacts with the protein postsynaptic density 95 (PSD-95), thereby enhancing $G_{q/11}$ binding [60]. Experiments with PDS-95 knockout mice have confirmed that, for instance, the induction of the *c-Fos* genes, and thus the hallucinogenic effect, is dependent on PSD-95 [61]. Downstream, hallucinogenic and non-hallucinogenic 5-HT_{2A} agonists activate different target genes [62].

In HEK293 cells and in the somatosensory cortex of mice, it was shown that treatment with hallucinogenic and non-hallucinogenic drugs leads to comparable gene expression of *c-Fos* and *IkBα*, but that the genes *Egr-1* and *Egr-2* are only induced by hallucinogenic drugs [19,62,63].

High doses of mescaline are known to increase the release and/or reuptake of serotonin, as evidenced by an increased concentration of 5-hydroxyindoleacetic acid (5-HIAA), the major metabolite of serotonin, in the brain [45]. Besides 5-HT_{2A}, mescaline also binds to the serotonin receptor 5-HT_{1A}, the α1-adrenergic receptor, the dopamine receptors D1/2/3 and the trace amine-associated receptor 1 (TAAR1), also all in a low μM range [54]. A low dopamine-releasing activity has also been described for mescaline [64]. The phenylethylamine moiety of mescaline forms the structural basis. However, there is no evidence of dependence on mescaline [45].

4. Mescaline—Chemistry and Synthesis

Mescaline is a ring-substituted amphetamine consisting of phenethylamine substituted at positions 3, 4 and 5 by methoxy groups [65]. It was initially assumed that a slight structural change in the mescaline would destroy the psychoactive effect [66]. In fact, however, a slight structural change leads to much more potent molecules [67]. In their book *PiHKAL*, Dr. Alexander Shulgin and Ann Shulgin describe a 2,5-dimethoxy substitution pattern with a small hydrophobic substituent on C-4 of the benzene ring as optimal in terms of a strong psychedelic effect [11]. Cyclisation of the side chain also proved to be advantageous in terms of potency and interaction with the 5-HT2_A receptor [68].

The biosynthesis of mescaline (and peyote alkaloids in general) in the peyote cactus is not yet fully understood. So far, candidate genes for tyrosine/DOPA decarboxylase, hydroxylases and O-methyltransferases have been discovered in peyote tissue [69].

Various methods have been published for the synthesis of mescaline in the laboratory. Most of the methods are based on the formation of the ethylamine side chain on the corresponding substituted aromatic systems [42]. The two-step reduction of 3,4,5-trimethoxybenzaldehyde yields mescaline [70]. Also, the two-step conversion of substituted hydrocinnamic acids into amides with subsequent Hofmann degradation can be used to synthesise mescaline [71]. Further ways of synthesising mescaline are the basic hydrolysis of benzoylmescaline [72] or synthesis from the bisulphite adduct of the aldehyde [73]. The latter requires substitution of the sulphite moiety, acetylation of the hydroxyl group and catalytic hydrogenation. Last but not least, the reduction of 3,4,5-trimethoxyphenylacetonitrile [74], 3,4,5-trimethoxy-β-nitrostyrene [75] or 3,4,5-trimethoxyacetamide [76] to mescaline has been described. More modern approaches lead to the preparation of the mescaline precursor 3,4,5-trimethoxyacetonitrile [77] or the acetophenone ketal ring opening of 2-methyl-2-(3,4,5-trimethoxyphenyl)-1,3-dioxolane [78].

5. Peyote Alkaloids

Besides mescaline, several other alkaloids have been identified in the peyote cactus (Figure 2 and Table 1). Analogous to mescaline, the concentrations of these alkaloids can vary depending on the part of the plant. In addition, climatic conditions, light availability, soil conditions and harvest time influence the composition of a plant's compounds [79]. Some of the alkaloids do not seem to have any pharmacological activity themselves but enhance the effects of mescaline [45].

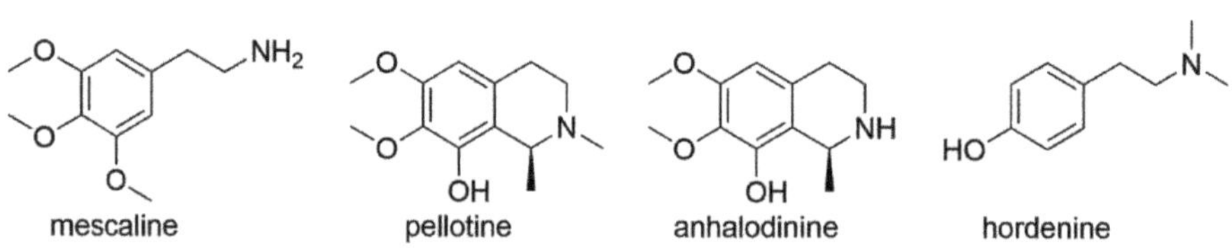

Figure 2. Structures of the main alkaloids of the peyote cactus.

The tyramine N,N-dimethyl derivative hordenine (Figure 2 and Table 1) is structurally similar to neurotransmitters such as dopamine and adrenaline and thus may lead to hypertension and increased respiratory and heart rates, as has already been shown in horses [80] and cats [81]. In addition, hordenine is of forensic interest. When barley grains are malting, hordenine is produced, which is subsequently also present in beer [81]. After beer consumption, hordenine can be detected in blood and urine and can therefore be used as a qualitative and quantitative marker for beer consumption [42,81]. Last but not least, antibiotic properties have been described for hordenine [82].

The second most common alkaloid of the peyote cactus is pellotine (Figure 2 and Table 1). The sleep-inducing effect of pellotine has been well studied. In one study, 49% of the subjects fell asleep 90 min after administration of pellotine (minimum dose 20 mg (s.c.), maximum dose 65 mg (s.c.)) and slept through the night. In 33% of these subjects, a dose of 20 mg (s.c.) was sufficient [83,84]. Another study confirms the sleep-promoting properties of pellotine, but mentions dizziness, nausea, vertigo and vomiting as minor side effects [85]. Further studies concluded that pellotine is also a valuable sleep aid for children [86]. The above-mentioned study results were promising, and pellotine was even marketed for a time by Boehringer und Sohn as a sleep aid [84]. However, the advent of cheaper synthetic barbiturates led to pellotine being taken off the market and not investigated further [87]. A new study that has just been published took up the investigation of pellotine as a sleep-promoting agent. The authors showed that pellotine concentration-dependently decreased locomotion in mice, inhibited REM sleep, and promoted sleep fragmentation [88].

Anhalinine is a mescaline analogue that is also found in the peyote cactus (Figure 2 and Table 1). Anhalinine likewise has stimulant effects by inhibiting cholinergic neuromuscular transmission [89].

Table 1. Alkaloid content of *Lophophora williamsii*, as percent total alkaloid (adapted from [84]).

	Alkaloid Content (Percent Total Alkaloid)
Mescaline	30.0
Pellotine	17.0
Anhalonidine	14.0
Hordenine	8.0

6. Clinical Studies and Therapeutic Potential of Mescaline

The investigation of the therapeutic potential of mescaline began in the 1950s with two studies on schizophrenic patients. After mescaline administration (mescaline sulphate intravenously: 500 and 500/750 mg, respectively), no therapeutic potential for schizophrenia was observed in either of the two studies [37,90]. In 1974, mescaline was then investigated in connection with alcoholism [91]. Participants in the study programme were given the opportunity to take part in NAC peyote meetings, alongside other activities. At these meetings, an average of 500 mg of mescaline was taken in the form of ground peyote powder or tea. Many of the participating American Indians from the Cheyenne and Arapaho Tribes stated that the peyote meetings were essential for overcoming their alcoholism. Increased openness and willingness to communicate were reported as well. A more recent study from 2005 also confirmed the positive effect of peyote on alcoholism [92]. Finally, a recent international study investigated the potential of mescaline in non-clinical settings for mental illnesses such as depression, anxiety, post-traumatic stress disorder (PTSD) and alcohol/drug use disorders [93,94]. Of the 452 participants, mescaline use positively affected 86% of people with depression (n = 184), 80% of people with anxiety (n = 167), 76% of people with PTSD (n = 55), 76% of people with alcohol abuse/disorders (n = 48) and 68% of people with substance abuse/disorders (n = 58). In the study register clinicaltrial.gov, six clinical studies (one, however, withdrawn) investigating mescaline are listed [95]. One completed study (ClinicalTrials.gov ID NCT0484901), with 16 healthy volunteers from Switzerland, investigated the subjective effects of different doses of mescaline using modern psychometric instruments, as well as the involvement of the 5-HT_{2A} receptor in the psychoactive effects of mescaline. Another reported double-blind, placebo-controlled, four-period crossover study with healthy volunteers from Switzerland (ClinicalTrials.gov ID NCT04227756) compared the acute effects of LSD, psilocybin, mescaline and a placebo. One study (ClinicalTrials.gov ID NCT05933213) will assess the effect of mescaline sodium enteric-coated tablets compared to morte-mescaline in the treatment of adult patients with lupus nephritis. The other three studies (ClinicalTrials.gov ID NCT02033707, ClinicalTrials.gov ID NCT05516823, ClinicalTrials.gov ID NCT05180149-withdrawn) will examine the influence of mescaline on the mood and performance of healthy volunteers, as well as the dependence of the use of the drug on the personality and personality perception of the user.

7. Ethnopharmacology

At the time of Spanish rule in the Empire of the Aztecs and Northern Mexico (around 1520), the ceremonial use of peyote was widespread [1,2]. In 1569, the Spanish missionary and ethnologist Bernardino de Sahagún described the use of peyote for religious and medicinal purposes by the indigenous peoples of Mexico in the Codex Florentinus [96]. During the Civil War (1860–1865), peyote was used by American Indians for both ceremonial and medicinal purposes. Medicinal uses were varied and included the treatment of burns, wounds, fever, rheumatism, snakebites and scorpion stings [3,4]. Kiowas used the plant to treat flu, scarlet fever, tuberculosis and venereal diseases. Indian tribes also used the plant to relieve the pain of childbirth, toothache and certain skin conditions [97]. Since the 1870s, the peyote cult has spread among the indigenous cultures of North America and is essential to the rituals of the Native American Church (NAC), founded in 1914 [98,99]. The plant is not conceived as a hallucinogen, but as a "teacher"; there is no distinction between medicine and religion, nor a separation between body and mind [100–102]. Thus, a special religious cult was created around peyote in the Native American Church (NAC) [102–104].

The use of peyote and mescaline was finally banned in the USA (Comprehensive Drug Abuse Prevention and Control Act) in 1970 [6], and in 1971 (Convention on Psychotropic Substances) [7] worldwide [8]. In 1978, the American Indian Religious Freedom Act, was passed to provide legal protection for the Church's use of the plant. Since 1994, the American Indian Religious Freedom Act Amendments have allowed harvesting, possession and consumption of peyote as part of "bona fide religious ceremonies" [9]. The NAC, for whose members, the use of peyote as a sacrament is legal, has grown considerably in recent years, and it is estimated that they now have about 250,000 members in the US and Canada. The church is spreading rapidly, including among tribes where it was not before, such as the Navajo, among whom other religious movements are also on the rise, such as evangelical Christianity. Through the NAC, American indigenous cultural identity is kept alive.

A ritual can be defined as an experience formally structured for the intention of healing or problem-solving [105]. For example, peyote rituals are used to help with alcohol and other addictions. The Navajo deploy the ritual as a powerful healing ceremony, which provides help with trauma and social disruption that is considered more effective than Western psychiatry [105–107].

Peyote ceremonies or rituals are substantially different from a standard psychedelic therapy session because of three important differences. There is little or no talking between participants. The (rhythmic) chanting is intended to alleviate anxiety that may arise from the hallucinatory effects of peyote and is considered an essential success factor in the healing or spiritual (divinatory) process. As a third distinction, rituals usually take place with little light or in the dark. The peyote ceremony differs slightly in this: to receive visions, one stares into the fire (at night) [105].

The peyote ceremony follows meticulous rules. Because sacred rites take place, it cannot be attended by just anyone. A detailed description can be found in Huttlinger and Tanner's 1994 article, the peyote way [108]. In short, the ceremony is led by a "roadman", who is assisted by a drummer, a firekeeper and a cedar-man. The latter is tasked with cleansing the space in a spiritual sense. The participants sit around a fire, in a tipi, and sing peyote songs while staff and rattle are passed around. This goes on all night from evening onwards and can last for about 14 h, during which no one is allowed to go outside, or sleep. The peyote is ingested one hour after the start of the ceremony in the form of powder or as tea. Among a specific group of indigenous Huichol Indians, this is augmented by story-telling, having first made an extensive pilgrimage to the original site of discovery in the so called sacred Wirikuta desert in northern Mexico.

Peyote grows very slowly and only in a limited number of places in southwest Texas and Mexico (Figure 3), where it grows in the desert and prefers limestone soil. Today, more peyote is used than ever before. Harvesting is increased and it is being sold in various countries (although, in certain countries, it is forbidden), thus leading to substantial diminished natural distribution and low-density populations of plants with also smaller size, creating vulnerability and ecological pressure [32].

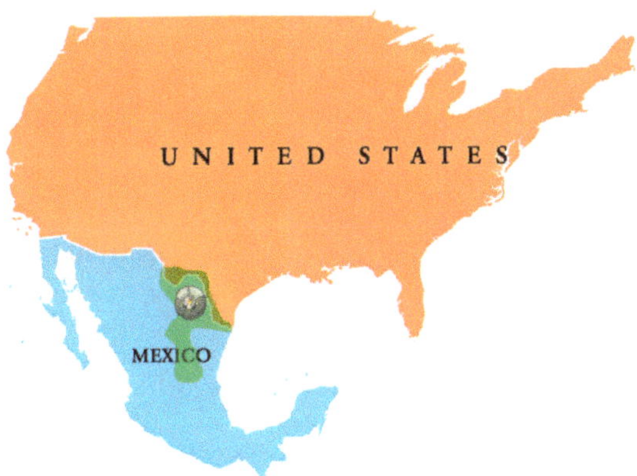

Figure 3. Geographic distribution of peyote (*Lophophora williamsii*) (highlighted in green).

8. Different Ideas about Disease—Chances and Challenges

To make sense of the indigenous peoples' use of Peyote, we need to be aware that there are different concepts regarding health and disease that prevail and reign globally. The way Western medicine considers health and disease is reflected by the WHO definition of health (1948): "Health is a state of complete physical, mental and social well-being and not merely the absence of disease or infirmity" [109] and has undergone unprecedented development over the past two centuries. Whereas previously one's body constitution (which is defined as "the inherent and relatively stable characteristics of individual human beings in morphological structure and function activities" [110]) was seen as the cause of susceptibility to disease, today, genetics, environmental factors and lifestyle are given a major role [111]. Several models exist, all based on the principle of cause (multifactorial or not) and effect (disease). Overall, we can state that today's medicine still looks for explanatory causes [112]. In contrast to this current prevailing mechanistic understanding of medicine, many indigenous peoples and regenerative perspectives assume that health can only be created through a balanced equilibrium [102,108]. That is, our whole way of life and our relationships with our environment and fellow human beings contribute to such balances or imbalances [102]. So, the difference between indigenous and Western medicine is that the former considers all to be embedded in nature, connected with everything. Nowadays, we find this principle also in TCM, Ayurveda and integrative medicine. In Western medicine, this was also the case, until 250 years ago.

When assessing our physical health, we perform measurements and tests. However, concerning mental health problems, it takes courage on the part of both the doctor and the patient to talk about it, as there is still a stigma attached [30,113]. What makes it even more complicated is that the treatment is not just simple giving pill A for disease X and a pill B for disease Y, it usually consists of psychotherapy combined with medication. There is no guarantee that the prescribed treatment will actually work, unfortunately.

Prescribing tablets, however, is often the easier and less complicated approach, also reflected by the high usage of tranquillisers, sleeping pills, anti-depressants and alcohol, increasing every year. Worldwide, three million deaths every year result from the harmful and addictive use of alcohol. This represents 5.3% of all deaths [114]. Not to mention the opioid epidemic which plagues the United States as a serious public health concern [115].

The reason for the use of these kinds of drugs is very aptly described by Aldous Huxley in his 1954 book, *The Doors of Perception*, in which he describes his own experience of taking a small dose of mescaline [116]. Huxley claims that humans will never be able to refrain from chemical intoxicants because most people's lives are perceived as painful and monotonous. This evokes a strong desire to escape suffering—even if only for a moment. This may sound rather melancholic and gloomy, but unfortunately it is probably the daily reality for a large part of humanity, which is evident by the above-mentioned high level of addiction worldwide. Another indication of the mental challenges and the extent of a sense of lostness that people experience is the fact that mental health disorders are the leading cause of morbidity and mortality [13,117].

In Western scientific medicine, the application of mind-altering substances such as the classic hallucinogens is relatively new. Their application is also difficult to reconcile with developments here, which are biomedically and pharmaceutically oriented [13]. One of the aspects that plays a role in this is the so-called set and setting principle: it turns out that the result of the administration of any psychedelic drug is not only determined by the drug, but rather very much depends on the intentions, expectations and general psychological state of being (state) of the receiver (the set). Also crucial is the immediate environment in which the drug is taken (the setting) [118–123]. The indigenous approach assumes that only one's own body carries the potential to regenerate and heal its individual ecosystem. The doctor, healer or therapist can provide a "space" in which healing is possible; the setting, so to speak, that enables healing, when the so-called "set", the factors related to the person that wants to be healed, is also right. In the traditional indigenous approach, however, strengthening one's own healing potential in the harsh living conditions was largely culturally anchored and integral.

It is important to realise that the way of healing using the peyote cactus is also part of a specific worldview, mindset and lifestyle. It is therefore important that we learn to value this ancient traditional view and knowledge and research it further, respectfully and collaboratively [105,124]. This aspect is also addressed by Berlowitz et al. [125], who also advocate this multidisciplinary form of research and argue for bridging knowledge between traditional and Western medicine.

A question that arises is what the difference is between the (lasting) effect of ingesting peyote during a ceremony, and that of ingesting only the active component, the mescaline. In fact, this is the difference between the joint—probably synergistic—effect of the alkaloid mixture contained in the peyote cactus, completed with the so-called set and setting, compared to the effect of "just" the pure active substance. It is unimportant here, whether or not there is a placebo effect, possibly triggered by the presence of the roadman and his helpers, and the whole peyote ceremony [122]. This is what could enrich Western medicine, by creating a culture-specific setting, where healing can take place on multiple levels, making use of rituals more often. The "Western way of rituals" may involve the expertise and guidance of a doctor, in a safe, special, medical environment with good mutual agreements and proper personal preparation, for specific problems.

Here, we took the use of peyote as an example. The risk of addiction to, or dependency on, mescaline usage is nihil, and intoxication produces mild symptoms that are not life-threatening [45]. This does not mean that we advocate the use of peyote, mescaline or other (semi-) natural substances like psilocybin or LSD, or synthetic equivalents with comparable effects, for psychiatric application.

More essential, in our opinion, is that by looking at how various cultures deal with illness, health and medicine, we can gain a broader overview and understanding of how disease can be treated. Ideally, we would like to combine original, proven indigenous knowledge and wisdom with our modern and Western approach and find ways to create the "best of both worlds". An important aspect in all this is the reciprocity principle. Where we in the West could gratefully make use of indigenous wisdom in terms of "set and setting", we could, for instance, share our knowledge in terms of quality and safety (including technique) with them, so that it does not become a one-sided "take", but a shared opportunity for further development, which can benefit all humanity.

9. Future Research Aspects

With this overview, we hoped to present the research from a different perspective in order to offer the possibility of a change in consciousness and thus new chances and paths. How this change in consciousness might look was discussed using the example of peyote and mescaline. The mindset of indigenous people, which includes a connection with the natural world and a strong reliance on one's own body as a "measuring instrument", serves as an orientation here. The setting, which includes rituals and ceremonies, is also essential for the healing effect of the substances used.

A new approach to treatment could be a combination of outer, scientific evidence and internal evidence provided by the body, so that a patient is able, for example, to "feel" if a specific medicine prescribed for a given disease is right or not. There are ways to concretise such internal evidence. Here, it is important to understand that every plant has a potential to influence our body and mind. That is, if you taste peyote or just a "regular European plant" like, for instance, dandelion, a herb like thyme or rosemary, or mistletoe (a special plant used in anthroposophical medicine), you can describe what it does to your body; if you feel warm or cold, light or dark, fresh or exhausted, or other sensory effects. This can be achieved, for example, with the help of validated (sensory, psychological) questionnaires. The knowledge of the effects of plants gained in this way can then be used in the following for health promotion.

10. Conclusions

In short, for the molecular aspects of mescaline, the way it exerts its action in the cells, the signalling pathways that are involved and the effects it elicits in the human body, much has been published since the first description of its use in 1569. Its hallucinogenic effects are mainly due to its binding to the 5-HT_{2A} serotonin receptor.

The highest proportion of mescaline is found in the peyote cactus (*Lophophora williamsii*), which in dried form contains 3–6% of the alkaloid mescaline. The ingestion of this cactus is part of a special (healing) ritual of indigenous peoples in specific parts of Mexico and Northern America. Peyote is classified as a hard drug and its use and possession is illegal (except for the members of the NAC). However, in the last two decades, the interest in the medical use of psychedelics has risen, along with the increasing numbers of complex health challenges we face, as humanity.

In this overview, we looked at the application and the hallucinogenic effects of peyote and its major alkaloid mescaline. Although mescaline and its analogues have advantages (such as more precise dosing and possibly faster hallucinogenic effects), they lack the more sustainable effects of what is reported during peyote rituals. Thus, we think that peyote and its ceremonies serve as an example for a nature-embedded and ritual-enriched way of providing a possible treatment for mental health challenges. Thus, we could search for ways to combine this ancient knowledge with our present highly innovative Western medicine, to be able to develop a more sustainable healthcare system that can be of benefit globally.

Author Contributions: CRediT roles: M.D.-v.K., A.M.Z.-K. and C.G.—conceptualisation; M.D.-v.K. and A.M.Z.-K.—data curation; C.G.—funding acquisition; M.D.-v.K. and A.M.Z.-K.—investigation; M.D.-v.K., A.M.Z.-K. and C.G.—methodology; C.G.—project administration; C.G.—resources; C.G.—supervision; C.G.—validation; M.D.-v.K. and A.M.Z.-K.—visualisation; M.D.-v.K., A.M.Z.-K. and C.G.—roles/writing—M.D.-v.K., A.M.Z.-K. and C.G.—original draft; M.D.-v.K., A.M.Z.-K. and C.G.—writing—review and editing. All authors have read and agreed to the published version of the manuscript.

Funding: MDK: AMZK and CG are financially supported by a PRIAM-based consortium of multiple funders.

Acknowledgments: We would like to thank Jakob K. Reinhardt for his advice on the chemical aspects of this.

Conflicts of Interest: All other authors declare no conflict of interest. The funding sponsors had no role in the design, writing and publishing strategy of the study, or in the collection, analysis, or interpretation of the data.

References

1. Sahagún, B.; Bustamante, C.M. *Historia General de las Cosas de Nueva España*; Imprenta del Ciudadano Alejandro Valdés: Mexico City, Mexico, 1829.
2. Lewin, L. Ueber *Anhalonium lewinii* und andere Cacteen. *Naunyn-Schmiedeberg's Arch. Pharmacol.* **1894**, *34*, 374–391. [CrossRef]
3. Lumholtz, C. *Unknown Mexico: A Record of Five Years' Exploration among the Tribes of the Western Sierra Madre*; Cambridge University Press: Cambridge, UK, 2011; Volume 2.
4. Stork, C.M. Peyote. In *Reference Module in Biomedical Sciences*; Elsevier: Amsterdam, The Netherlands, 2023.
5. The 'Diabolic Root'. *New York Times*, 1 November 1964; 96.
6. US Drug Enforcement Administration Drug Scheduling. Available online: https://web.archive.org/web/20081020210309/http://www.usdoj.gov/dea/pubs/scheduling.html (accessed on 17 October 2023).
7. International Narcotics Control Board List of Psychotropic Substances under International Control. Available online: https://web.archive.org/web/20051205125434/http://www.incb.org/pdf/e/list/green.pdf (accessed on 17 October 2023).
8. Nutt, D. Illegal drugs laws: Clearing a 50-year-old obstacle to research. *PLoS Biol.* **2015**, *13*, e1002047. [CrossRef] [PubMed]
9. 103d United States Congress American Indian Religious Freedom Act Amendments. Available online: https://www.congress.gov/103/statute/STATUTE-108/STATUTE-108-Pg3125.pdf (accessed on 17 October 2023).
10. Decriminalize Nature—Organizer Info & Resources. Available online: https://www.decriminalizenature.org/policy/organizer-info-and-resources (accessed on 17 October 2023).
11. Shulgin, A.T.; Shulgin, A. PIHKAL: Phenethylamines I have known and loved. In *A Chemical Love Story*; Transform Press Berkeley: Berkeley, CA, USA, 1991.
12. Pollan, M. How Should We Do Drugs Now? *New York Times*, 11 July 2021.
13. Ona, G.; Berrada, A.; Bouso, J.C. Communalistic use of psychoactive plants as a bridge between traditional healing practices and Western medicine: A new path for the Global Mental Health movement. *Transcult. Psychiatry* **2021**, *59*, 638–651. [CrossRef] [PubMed]
14. Bruhn, J.G.; Holmstedt, B.R. Early peyote research an interdisciplinary study. *Econ. Bot.* **1973**, *28*, 353–390. [CrossRef]
15. Monte, A.P.; Waldman, S.R.; Marona-Lewicka, D.; Wainscott, D.B.; Nelson, D.L.; Sanders-Bush, E.; Nichols, D.E. Dihydrobenzofuran analogues of hallucinogens. 4. Mescaline derivatives. *J. Med. Chem.* **1997**, *40*, 2997–3008. [CrossRef] [PubMed]
16. Graziano, S.; Orsolini, L.; Rotolo, M.C.; Tittarelli, R.; Schifano, F.; Pichini, S. Herbal Highs: Review on Psychoactive Effects and Neuropharmacology. *Curr. Neuropharmacol.* **2017**, *15*, 750–761. [CrossRef]
17. Aghajanian, G.K.; Marek, G.J. Serotonin and hallucinogens. *Neuropsychopharmacology* **1999**, *21* (Suppl. 2), 16S–23S. [CrossRef]
18. Shulgin, A.T. Mescaline: The chemistry and pharmacology of its analogs. *Lloydia* **1973**, *36*, 46–58.
19. López-Giménez, J.F.; González-Maeso, J. Hallucinogens and Serotonin 5-HT(2A) Receptor-Mediated Signaling Pathways. *Curr. Top. Behav. Neurosci.* **2018**, *36*, 45–73.
20. Hannon, J.; Hoyer, D. Molecular biology of 5-HT receptors. *Behav. Brain Res.* **2008**, *195*, 198–213. [CrossRef]
21. Raymond, J.R.; Mukhin, Y.V.; Gelasco, A.; Turner, J.; Collinsworth, G.; Gettys, T.W.; Grewal, J.S.; Garnovskaya, M.N. Multiplicity of mechanisms of serotonin receptor signal transduction. *Pharmacol. Ther.* **2001**, *92*, 179–212. [CrossRef] [PubMed]
22. Leung, J.; Chan, G.; Stjepanović, D.; Chung, J.Y.C.; Hall, W.; Hammond, D. Prevalence and self-reported reasons of cannabis use for medical purposes in USA and Canada. *Psychopharmacology* **2022**, *239*, 1509–1519. [CrossRef] [PubMed]
23. Kilcher, G.; Zwahlen, M.; Ritter, C.; Fenner, L.; Egger, M. Medical use of cannabis in Switzerland: Analysis of approved exceptional licences. *Swiss Med. Wkly.* **2017**, *147*, w14463. [PubMed]
24. Coughenour, P.; Sadicario, J.S.; Karjane, N.; Parlier-Ahmad, A.B.; Phipps, L.; Svikis, D.S. Prevalence and Social Acceptability of Cannabis, Tobacco, and Alcohol Use in Adult Women. *Womens Health Rep.* **2021**, *2*, 452–458. [CrossRef] [PubMed]

25. Ansah, J.P.; Chiu, C.T. Projecting the chronic disease burden among the adult population in the United States using a multi-state population model. *Front. Public Health* **2022**, *10*, 1082183. [CrossRef]
26. World Health Organization Mental Disorders. Available online: https://www.who.int/news-room/fact-sheets/detail/mental-disorders (accessed on 17 October 2023).
27. Statista Global Drug Use—Statistics & Facts. Available online: https://www.statista.com/topics/7786/global-drug-use/#topicOverview (accessed on 17 October 2023).
28. Collins, E.; Tranter, S.; Irvine, F. The physical health of the seriously mentally ill: An overview of the literature. *J. Psychiatr. Ment. Health Nurs.* **2012**, *19*, 638–646. [CrossRef]
29. Farnam, C.R.; Zipple, A.M.; Tyrrell, W.; Chittinanda, P. Health status risk factors of people with severe and persistent mental illness. *J. Psychosoc. Nurs. Ment. Health Serv.* **1999**, *37*, 16–21. [CrossRef]
30. Belouin, S.J.; Henningfield, J.E. Psychedelics: Where we are now, why we got here, what we must do. *Neuropharmacology* **2018**, *142*, 7–19. [CrossRef]
31. Chapman, D.P.; Perry, G.S.; Strine, T.W. The vital link between chronic disease and depressive disorders. *Prev. Chronic Dis.* **2005**, *2*, A14.
32. Bauml, J.A.; Schaefer, S.B.; Labate, B.C.; Cavnar, C. *Peyote: History, Tradition, Politics, and Conservation*; Bloomsbury Publishing: London, UK, 2016.
33. Laing, R.R. *Hallucinogens: A Forensic Drug Handbook*; Academic Press: Cambridge, MA, USA, 2003.
34. Wolbach, A.; Isbell, H.; Miner, E. Cross tolerance between mescaline and LSD-25 with a comparison of the mescaline and LSD reactions. *Psychopharmacologia* **1962**, *3*, 1–14. [CrossRef]
35. Hartman, A.M.; Hollister, L.E. Effect of mescaline, lysergic acid diethylamide and psilocybin on color perception. *Psychopharmacologia* **1963**, *4*, 441–451. [CrossRef] [PubMed]
36. Cohen, S. Lysergic acid diethylamide: Side effects and complications. *J. Nerv. Ment. Dis.* **1960**, *130*, 30–40. [CrossRef] [PubMed]
37. Denber, H.C.; Merlis, S. Studies on mescaline I. Action in schizophrenic patients: Clinical observations and brain wave patterns, showing effects before and after electric convulsive treatments. *Psychiatr. Q.* **1955**, *29*, 421–429. [CrossRef] [PubMed]
38. Oepen, G.; Fuenfgeld, M.; Harrington, A.; Hermle, L.; Botsch, H. Right hemisphere involvement in mescaline-induced psychosis. *Psychiatry Res.* **1989**, *29*, 335–336. [CrossRef] [PubMed]
39. Hermle, L.; Fünfgeld, M.; Oepen, G.; Botsch, H.; Borchardt, D.; Gouzoulis, E.; Fehrenbach, R.A.; Spitzer, M. Mescaline-induced psychopathological, neuropsychological, and neurometabolic effects in normal subjects: Experimental psychosis as a tool for psychiatric research. *Biol. Psychiatry* **1992**, *32*, 976–991. [CrossRef] [PubMed]
40. Hermle, L.; Gouzoulis-Mayfrank, E.; Spitzer, M. Blood flow and cerebral laterality in the mescaline model of psychosis. *Pharmacopsychiatry* **1998**, *31*, 85–91. [CrossRef]
41. Dasgupta, A. Chapter Five—Challenges in Laboratory Detection of Unusual Substance Abuse: Issues with Magic Mushroom, Peyote Cactus, Khat, and Solvent Abuse. *Adv. Clin. Chem.* **2017**, *78*, 163–186.
42. Kapadia, G.J.; Fayez, M.B.E. Peyote constituents: Chemistry, biogenesis, and biological effects. *J. Pharm. Sci.* **1970**, *59*, 1699–1727. [CrossRef]
43. Cumming, P.; Scheidegger, M.; Dornbierer, D.; Palner, M.; Quednow, B.B.; Martin-Soelch, C. Molecular and Functional Imaging Studies of Psychedelic Drug Action in Animals and Humans. *Molecules* **2021**, *26*, 2451. [CrossRef]
44. Korr, H. Autoradiographic studies on the distribution of 3H-mescaline in the brain of the marmoset, *Callithrix jacchus*. *Psychopharmacologia* **1976**, *46*, 115–117. [CrossRef]
45. Dinis-Oliveira, R.J.; Pereira, C.L.; da Silva, D.D. Pharmacokinetic and Pharmacodynamic Aspects of Peyote and Mescaline: Clinical and Forensic Repercussions. *Curr. Mol. Pharmacol.* **2019**, *12*, 184–194. [CrossRef] [PubMed]
46. Hilliker, K.S.; Roth, R.A. Prediction of mescaline clearance by rabbit lung and liver from enzyme kinetic data. *Biochem. Pharmacol.* **1980**, *29*, 253–255. [CrossRef] [PubMed]
47. Seiler, N.; Demisch, L. Oxidative metabolism of mescaline in the central nervous system. 3. Side chain degradation of mescaline and formation of 3,4,5-trimethoxy-benzoic acid in vivo. *Biochem. Pharmacol.* **1974**, *23*, 259–271. [CrossRef] [PubMed]
48. Musacchio, J.M.; Goldstein, M. The metabolism of mescaline-14-C in rats. *Biochem. Pharmacol.* **1967**, *16*, 963–970. [CrossRef] [PubMed]
49. Charalampous, K.D.; Walker, K.E.; Kinross-Wright, J. Metabolic fate of mescaline in man. *Psychopharmacologia* **1966**, *9*, 48–63. [CrossRef]
50. Dasgupta, A. Chapter 33—Abuse of Magic Mushroom, Peyote Cactus, LSD, Khat, and Volatiles. In *Critical Issues in Alcohol and Drugs of Abuse Testing*, 2nd ed.; Dasgupta, A., Ed.; Academic Press: Cambridge, MA, USA, 2019; pp. 477–494.
51. Charalampous, K.D.; Orengo, A.; Walker, K.E.; Kinross-Wright, J. Metabolic fate of ν-(3,4,5-trimethoxyphenyl)-ethylamine (mescaline) in humans: Isolation and identification of 3,4,5-trimethoxyphenylacetic acid. *J. Pharmacol. Exp. Ther.* **1964**, *145*, 242–246. [PubMed]
52. Páleníсek, T.; Balíková, M.; Bubeníková-Valesová, V.; Horácek, J. Mescaline effects on rat behavior and its time profile in serum and brain tissue after a single subcutaneous dose. *Psychopharmacology* **2008**, *196*, 51–62. [CrossRef] [PubMed]
53. Halberstadt, A.L.; Powell, S.B.; Geyer, M.A. Role of the 5-HT_2A receptor in the locomotor hyperactivity produced by phenylalkylamine hallucinogens in mice. *Neuropharmacology* **2013**, *70*, 218–227. [CrossRef]

54. Rickli, A.; Moning, O.D.; Hoener, M.C.; Liechti, M.E. Receptor interaction profiles of novel psychoactive tryptamines compared with classic hallucinogens. *Eur. Neuropsychopharmacol.* **2016**, *26*, 1327–1337. [CrossRef]
55. Patel, V.; Urban, L.; Vaz, R.J. *Antitargets and Drug Safety*; John Wiley & Sons: Hoboken, NJ, USA, 2015.
56. Vamvakopoulou, I.A.; Narine, K.A.D.; Campbell, I.; Dyck, J.R.B.; Nutt, D.J. Mescaline: The forgotten psychedelic. *Neuropharmacology* **2023**, *222*, 109294. [CrossRef]
57. Urban, J.D.; Clarke, W.P.; von Zastrow, M.; Nichols, D.E.; Kobilka, B.; Weinstein, H.; Javitch, J.A.; Roth, B.L.; Christopoulos, A.; Sexton, P.M.; et al. Functional selectivity and classical concepts of quantitative pharmacology. *J. Pharmacol. Exp. Ther.* **2007**, *320*, 1–13. [CrossRef] [PubMed]
58. Kurrasch-Orbaugh, D.M.; Parrish, J.C.; Watts, V.J.; Nichols, D.E. A complex signaling cascade links the serotonin2A receptor to phospholipase A2 activation: The involvement of MAP kinases. *J. Neurochem.* **2003**, *86*, 980–991. [CrossRef]
59. Berg, K.A.; Maayani, S.; Goldfarb, J.; Scaramellini, C.; Leff, P.; Clarke, W.P. Effector pathway-dependent relative efficacy at serotonin type 2A and 2C receptors: Evidence for agonist-directed trafficking of receptor stimulus. *Mol. Pharmacol.* **1998**, *54*, 94–104. [CrossRef] [PubMed]
60. Xia, Z.; Gray, J.A.; Compton-Toth, B.A.; Roth, B.L. A direct interaction of PSD-95 with 5-HT2A serotonin receptors regulates receptor trafficking and signal transduction. *J. Biol. Chem.* **2003**, *278*, 21901–21908. [CrossRef]
61. Abbas, A.I.; Yadav, P.N.; Yao, W.D.; Arbuckle, M.I.; Grant, S.G.; Caron, M.G.; Roth, B.L. PSD-95 is essential for hallucinogen and atypical antipsychotic drug actions at serotonin receptors. *J. Neurosci.* **2009**, *29*, 7124–7136. [CrossRef]
62. González-Maeso, J.; Weisstaub, N.V.; Zhou, M.; Chan, P.; Ivic, L.; Ang, R.; Lira, A.; Bradley-Moore, M.; Ge, Y.; Zhou, Q.; et al. Hallucinogens recruit specific cortical 5-HT(2A) receptor-mediated signaling pathways to affect behavior. *Neuron* **2007**, *53*, 439–452. [CrossRef] [PubMed]
63. González-Maeso, J.; Yuen, T.; Ebersole, B.J.; Wurmbach, E.; Lira, A.; Zhou, M.; Weisstaub, N.; Hen, R.; Gingrich, J.A.; Sealfon, S.C. Transcriptome fingerprints distinguish hallucinogenic and nonhallucinogenic 5-hydroxytryptamine 2A receptor agonist effects in mouse somatosensory cortex. *J. Neurosci.* **2003**, *23*, 8836–8843. [CrossRef] [PubMed]
64. Trulson, M.E.; Crisp, T.; Henderson, L.J. Mescaline elicits behavioral effects in cats by an action at both serotonin and dopamine receptors. *Eur. J. Pharmacol.* **1983**, *96*, 151–154. [CrossRef]
65. National Center for Biotechnology Information PubChem Compound Summary for CID 4076, Mescaline. Available online: https://pubchem.ncbi.nlm.nih.gov/compound/Mescaline (accessed on 13 November 2023).
66. Reti, L. *Fortschritte der Chemie organischer Naturstoffe*; Zechmeister, L., Ed.; Springer: Wien, Austria, 1950; Volume VI.
67. Cassels, B.K.; Sáez-Briones, P. Dark Classics in Chemical Neuroscience: Mescaline. *ACS Chem. Neurosci.* **2018**, *9*, 2448–2458. [CrossRef]
68. McLean, T.H.; Parrish, J.C.; Braden, M.R.; Marona-Lewicka, D.; Gallardo-Godoy, A.; Nichols, D.E. 1-Aminomethylbenzocycloalkanes: Conformationally restricted hallucinogenic phenethylamine analogues as functionally selective 5-HT2A receptor agonists. *J. Med. Chem.* **2006**, *49*, 5794–5803. [CrossRef]
69. Ibarra-Laclette, E.; Zamudio-Hernández, F.; Pérez-Torres, C.A.; Albert, V.A.; Ramírez-Chávez, E.; Molina-Torres, J.; Fernández-Cortes, A.; Calderón-Vázquez, C.; Olivares-Romero, J.L.; Herrera-Estrella, A. De novo sequencing and analysis of Lophophora williamsii transcriptome, and searching for putative genes involved in mescaline biosynthesis. *BMC Genom.* **2015**, *16*, 657. [CrossRef] [PubMed]
70. Späth, E. Über die Anhalonium-Alkaloide: I. Anhalin und Mezcalin. *Monatshefte Für Chem. Und Verwandte Teile Anderer Wiss.* **1919**, *40*, 129–154. [CrossRef]
71. Slotta, K.; Heller, H. Über β-Phenyl-äthylamine, I. Mitteil.: Mezcalin und mezcalin-ähnliche Substanzen. *Berichte Der Dtsch. Chem. Ges. (A B Ser.)* **1930**, *63*, 3029–3044. [CrossRef]
72. Kindler, K.; Peschke, W. Über neue und über verbesserte Wege zum Aufbau von pharmakologisch wichtigen Aminen III. Über die Synthese von Adrenalin und von adrenalinähnlichen Verbindungen. *Arch. Der Pharm.* **1931**, *269*, 581–606. [CrossRef]
73. Kindler, K.; Peschke, W. Über neue und über verbesserte Wege zum Aufbau von pharmakologisch wichtigen Aminen VI. Über Synthesen des Meskalins. *Arch. Der Pharm.* **1932**, *270*, 410–413. [CrossRef]
74. Hahn, G.; Wassmuth, H. Über β-[Oxyphenyl]-äthylamine und ihre Umwandlungen, I. Mitteil.: Synthese des Mezcalins. *Berichte Der Dtsch. Chem. Ges. (A B Ser.)* **1934**, *67*, 696–708. [CrossRef]
75. Erne, M.; Ramirez, F. Über die Reduktion von β-Nitrostyrolen mit Lithiumaluminiumhydrid. *Helv. Chim. Acta* **1950**, *33*, 912–916. [CrossRef]
76. Banholzer, K.; Campbell, T.W.; Schmid, H. Notiz über eine neue Synthese von Mezcalin, N-Methyl-und N-Dimethylmezcalin. *Helv. Chim. Acta* **1952**, *35*, 1577–1581. [CrossRef]
77. Rose-Munch, F.; Chavignon, R.; Tranchier, J.-P.; Gagliardini, V.; Rose, E. Mescaline synthesis via tricarbonyl (η6-1, 2, 3-trimethoxybenzene) chromium complex. *Inorganica Chim. Acta* **2000**, *300*, 693–697. [CrossRef]
78. Soderquist, J.A.; Kock, I.; Estrella, M.E. Reductive cleavage of acetals and ketals with 9-borabicyclo[3.3. 1]nonane. *Org. Process Res. Dev.* **2006**, *10*, 1076–1079. [CrossRef]
79. Bäumle, S. *Heilpflanzenpraxis Heute: Porträts—Rezepturen—Anwendung*; Urban & Fischer by Elsevier: Munich, Germany, 2006.
80. Frank, M.; Weckman, T.J.; Wood, T.; Woods, W.E.; Tai, C.L.; Chang, S.L.; Ewing, A.; Blake, J.W.; Tobin, T. Hordenine: Pharmacology, pharmacokinetics and behavioural effects in the horse. *Equine Vet. J.* **1990**, *22*, 437–441. [CrossRef] [PubMed]

81. Steiner, I.; Brauers, G.; Temme, O.; Daldrup, T. A sensitive method for the determination of hordenine in human serum by ESI^{+} UPLC-MS/MS for forensic toxicological applications. *Anal. Bioanal. Chem.* **2016**, *408*, 2285–2292. [CrossRef]
82. Zhou, J.-W.; Luo, H.-Z.; Jiang, H.; Jian, T.-K.; Chen, Z.-Q.; Jia, A.-Q. Hordenine: A Novel Quorum Sensing Inhibitor and Antibiofilm Agent against Pseudomonas aeruginosa. *J. Agric. Food Chem.* **2018**, *66*, 1620–1628. [CrossRef] [PubMed]
83. Pilcz, A. Ueber Pellotin. *Klin. Wochenschr.* **1896**, *9*, 1121–1122.
84. Chan, C.B.; Poulie, C.B.M.; Wismann, S.S.; Soelberg, J.; Kristensen, J.L. The Alkaloids from *Lophophora diffusa* and Other "False Peyotes". *J. Nat. Prod.* **2021**, *84*, 2398–2407. [CrossRef] [PubMed]
85. Hutchings, R. Report on the use of pellotine as a sedative and hypnotic. *State Hosp. Bull.* **1897**, *2*, 45–48.
86. Krüger, E. Die Wirkung des Pellotin im Kindesalter. *Klin. Wochenschr.* **1934**, *13*, 376–378. [CrossRef]
87. Perrine, D.M. Visions of the Night-Western Medicine Meets Peyote 1887–1899. *Heffter Rev. Psychedelic Res* **2001**, *2*, 6–52.
88. Poulie, C.B.M.; Chan, C.B.; Parka, A.; Lettorp, M.; Vos, J.; Raaschou, A.; Pottie, E.; Bundgaard, M.S.; Sørensen, L.M.E.; Cecchi, C.R.; et al. In Vitro and In Vivo Evaluation of Pellotine: A Hypnotic Lophophora Alkaloid. *ACS Pharmacol. Transl. Sci.* **2023**, *6*, 1492–1507. [CrossRef]
89. Ghansah, E.; Kopsombut, P.; Maleque, M.A.; Brossi, A. Effects of mescaline and some of its analogs on cholinergic neuromuscular transmission. *Neuropharmacology* **1993**, *32*, 169–174. [CrossRef]
90. Merlis, S. The effects of mescaline sulfate in chronic schizophrenia. *J. Nerv. Ment. Dis.* **1957**, *125*, 432–433. [CrossRef] [PubMed]
91. Albaugh, B.J.; Anderson, P.O. Peyote in the treatment of alcoholism among American Indians. *Am. J. Psychiatry* **1974**, *131*, 1247–1250. [CrossRef] [PubMed]
92. Halpern, J.H.; Sherwood, A.R.; Hudson, J.I.; Yurgelun-Todd, D.; Pope, H.G., Jr. Psychological and cognitive effects of long-term peyote use among Native Americans. *Biol. Psychiatry* **2005**, *58*, 624–631. [CrossRef] [PubMed]
93. Agin-Liebes, G.; Haas, T.F.; Lancelotta, R.; Uthaug, M.V.; Ramaekers, J.G.; Davis, A.K. Naturalistic use of mescaline is associated with self-reported psychiatric improvements and enduring positive life changes. *ACS Pharmacol. Transl. Sci.* **2021**, *4*, 543–552. [CrossRef] [PubMed]
94. Uthaug, M.V.; Davis, A.K.; Haas, T.F.; Davis, D.; Dolan, S.B.; Lancelotta, R.; Timmermann, C.; Ramaekers, J.G. The epidemiology of mescaline use: Pattern of use, motivations for consumption, and perceived consequences, benefits, and acute and enduring subjective effects. *J. Psychopharmacol.* **2022**, *36*, 309–320. [CrossRef] [PubMed]
95. United States National Library of Medicine ClinicalTrials.gov—Search Results: Mescaline. Available online: https://clinicaltrials.gov/study/NCT05180149?intr=Mescaline&rank=6 (accessed on 13 October 2023).
96. Feest, C.F. *Beseelte Welten: Die Religionen der Indianer Nordamerikas*; Herder: Middelburg, The Netherlands, 1998.
97. Shemluck, M. Medicinal and other uses of the Compositae by Indians in the United States and Canada. *J. Ethnopharmacol.* **1982**, *5*, 303–358. [CrossRef] [PubMed]
98. Jones, P.N. The Native American Church, peyote, and health: Expanding consciousness for healing purposes. *Contemp. Justice Rev.* **2007**, *10*, 411–425. [CrossRef]
99. Ronald Reagan Presidential Library Digital Library Collections Folder Title: Native American Church of North America. Available online: https://www.reaganlibrary.gov/public/digitallibrary/smof/publicliaison/blackwell/box-038/40_047_7007844_038_007_2017.pdf (accessed on 10 October 2023).
100. Carvalho, I.; Steil, C.; Gonzaga, F. Learning from a more-than-human perspective. Plants as teachers. *J. Environ. Educ.* **2020**, *51*, 144–155. [CrossRef]
101. Mastinu, A.; Anyanwu, M.; Carone, M.; Abate, G.; Bonini, S.A.; Peron, G.; Tirelli, E.; Pucci, M.; Ribaudo, G.; Oselladore, E.; et al. The Bright Side of Psychedelics: Latest Advances and Challenges in Neuropharmacology. *Int. J. Mol. Sci.* **2023**, *24*, 1329. [CrossRef]
102. Jones, P.N. The American Indian Church and its sacramental use of peyote: A review for professionals in the mental-health arena. *Ment. Health Relig. Cult.* **2005**, *8*, 277–290. [CrossRef]
103. Schultes, R.E. The botanical and chemical distribution of hallucinogens. *Annu. Rev. Plant Physiol.* **1970**, *21*, 571–598. [CrossRef]
104. Schultes, R.E. An overview of hallucinogens in the Western Hemisphere. In *Flesh of the Gods*; Furst, P.T., Ed.; Praeger Publishers: New York, NY, USA, 1972.
105. Metzner, R. Hallucinogenic drugs and plants in psychotherapy and shamanism. *J. Psychoact. Drugs* **1998**, *30*, 333–341. [CrossRef]
106. Garrity, J.F. Jesus, peyote, and the holy people: Alcohol abuse and the ethos of power in Navajo healing. *Med. Anthr. Q.* **2000**, *14*, 521–542. [CrossRef] [PubMed]
107. McClusky, M.S.W. Native American Church Peyotism and the Treatment of Alcoholism. *Newsl. Multidiscip. Assoc. Psychedelic Stud. MAPS* **1997**, *7*, 3–4.
108. Huttlinger, K.W.; Tanner, D. The Peyote way: Implications for Culture Care theory. *J. Transcult. Nurs.* **1994**, *5*, 5–11. [CrossRef]
109. World Health Organization the Constitution. Available online: https://www.who.int/about/accountability/governance/constitution (accessed on 25 October 2023).
110. Yuan, B. Holistic medicine: A new medical system based on body constitution and functional status. *J. Tradit. Chin. Med. Sci.* **2017**, *4*, 3–9. [CrossRef]
111. Risch, N.; Merikangas, K. The future of genetic studies of complex human diseases. *Science* **1996**, *273*, 1516–1517. [CrossRef]
112. Broadbent, A. Causation and models of disease in epidemiology. *Stud. Hist. Philos. Biol. Biomed. Sci.* **2009**, *40*, 302–311. [CrossRef]

113. Longdon, E.; Read, J. 'People with Problems, Not Patients with Illnesses': Using Psychosocial Frameworks to Reduce the Stigma of Psychosis. *Isr. J. Psychiatry Relat. Sci.* **2017**, *54*, 24–28.
114. World Health Organization Alcohol. Available online: https://www.who.int/news-room/fact-sheets/detail/alcohol (accessed on 17 October 2023).
115. Skolnick, P. The Opioid Epidemic: Crisis and Solutions. *Annu. Rev. Pharmacol. Toxicol.* **2018**, *58*, 143–159. [CrossRef]
116. Huxley, A. *The Doors of Perception*; Strelbytskyy Multimedia Publishing: Kyiv, Ukraine, 2021.
117. Collins, P.Y.; Patel, V.; Joestl, S.S.; March, D.; Insel, T.R.; Daar, A.S.; Scientific Advisory, B.; The Executive Committee of the Grand Challenges on Global Mental Health; Anderson, W.; Dhansay, M.A.; et al. Grand challenges in global mental health. *Nature* **2011**, *475*, 27–30. [CrossRef] [PubMed]
118. Metzner, R. (Ed.) *Ayahuasca: Hallucinogens, Consciousness, and the Spirit of Nature*; Running Press: Philadelphia, PA, USA, 1999.
119. Eisner, B. Set, setting, and matrix. *J. Psychoact. Drugs* **1997**, *29*, 213–216. [CrossRef] [PubMed]
120. Olson, J.A.; Suissa-Rocheleau, L.; Lifshitz, M.; Raz, A.; Veissiere, S.P.L. Tripping on nothing: Placebo psychedelics and contextual factors. *Psychopharmacology* **2020**, *237*, 1371–1382. [CrossRef] [PubMed]
121. Hartogsohn, I. Constructing drug effects: A history of set and setting. *Drug Sci. Policy Law* **2017**, *3*, 2050324516683325. [CrossRef]
122. Hartogsohn, I. Set and setting, psychedelics and the placebo response: An extra-pharmacological perspective on psychopharmacology. *J. Psychopharmacol.* **2016**, *30*, 1259–1267. [CrossRef]
123. Soloman, D. *LSD—The Consciousness-Expanding Drug*; Berkley Medallion Book: Berkley, CA, USA, 1966.
124. O'Shaughnessy, D.M.; Berlowitz, I. Amazonian Medicine and the Psychedelic Revival: Considering the "Dieta". *Front. Pharmacol.* **2021**, *12*, 639124. [CrossRef]
125. Berlowitz, I.; O'Shaughnessy, D.M.; Heinrich, M.; Wolf, U.; Maake, C.; Martin-Soelch, C. Teacher plants—Indigenous Peruvian-Amazonian dietary practices as a method for using psychoactives. *J. Ethnopharmacol.* **2022**, *286*, 114910. [CrossRef]

molecules

MDPI

Article

A New Glucosyl Flavone with Inhibitory Activity of Cancer Cell Viability and Other Bioactive Constituents from the Traditional Kurdish Plant *Plantago loeflingii* L.

Hawraz Ibrahim M. Amin [1,2,*], Kamaran Younis M. Amin [3], Chabaco Armijos [4], Faiq H. S. Hussain [5], Zanko Hassan Jawhar [6], Diego Caprioglio [7], Mariella Mella [8] and Giovanni Vidari [5,8,*]

1 Department of Chemistry, College of Science, Salahaddin University-Erbil, Erbil 44001, Iraq
2 Department of Medical Biochemical Analysis, Cihan University-Erbil, Erbil 44001, Iraq
3 Department of Chemistry, College of Education, Salahaddin University-Erbil, Erbil 44001, Iraq; kamaran.younis@su.edu.krd
4 Departamento de Química, Universidad Técnica Particular de Loja, Loja 110107, Ecuador; cparmijos@utpl.edu.ec
5 Department of Medical Analysis, Faculty of Applied Science, Tishk International University, Erbil 44001, Iraq; faiq.hussain@tiu.edu.iq
6 Department of Science, College of Health Science, Lebanese French University, Erbil 44001, Iraq; zanko.jawhar@lfu.edu.krd
7 Department of Pharmaceutical Sciences, University of Eastern Piedmont, Largo Donegani 2, 28100 Novara, Italy; diego.caprioglio@uniupo.it
8 Department of Chemistry, University of Pavia, Via Taramelli 12, 27100 Pavia, Italy; mariella.mella@unipv.it
* Correspondence: hawraz.mohammedamin@su.edu.krd (H.I.M.A.); vidari@unipv.it or giovanni.vidari@tiu.edu.iq (G.V.)

Abstract: A new glucosyl flavone, 5,7,2′,5′-tetrahydroxyflavone 7-*O*-β-D-glucopyranoside, named loeflingiin, together with apigenin 6-*C*-glucoside (isovitexin), coumarins citropten and isompinellin, triterpenoids betulin and betulinic acid, and a mixture of phytosterols β-sitosterol, stigmasterol and campesterol were isolated for the first time from the leaves of wild *Plantago loeflingii* L. (*Plantaginaceae*) collected in the Iraqi Kurdistan region. The plant is used by local people to treat wounds and as a vulnerary remedy. The structures of isolated compounds were determined by spectroscopic analysis. The activities of isovitexin and loeflingiinon the viability of breast (MCF7), ovarian (BG-1), endometrial (Ishikawa), and mesothelioma (IST-MES1) human cancer cells and two normal cell lines were determined with an MTT assay. Notably, the new 7-*O*-glucosyl flavone showed effects higher than cisplatin against the Ishikawa and IST-MESI cell lines. The significant biological activities exhibited by all the compounds isolated from *P. loeflingii* provided scientific evidence to support the use of the plant in the Kurdish traditional medicine.

Keywords: 7-*O*-glucosyl flavone; *Plantago loeflingii* L.; *Plantaginaceae*; antiproliferative activity; Kurdish medicinal plant

1. Introduction

The discovery of the Shanidar IV Neanderthal grave in northern Iraq, and the use of flowers in the burials reveals that herbal medicine was already practiced in the mountains and plains of Kurdistan region of Iraq at least 60,000 years ago [1]. Since that time, traditional medicine and plant remedies have been continuously used by nomadic tribes in Kurdish villages and rural areas, especially in the Erbil province [2,3]; moreover, in the main bazars of major towns, such as Erbil and Sulaymaniya, herbalist shops have been trading and selling natural medicinal products to date (Figure 1) [4].

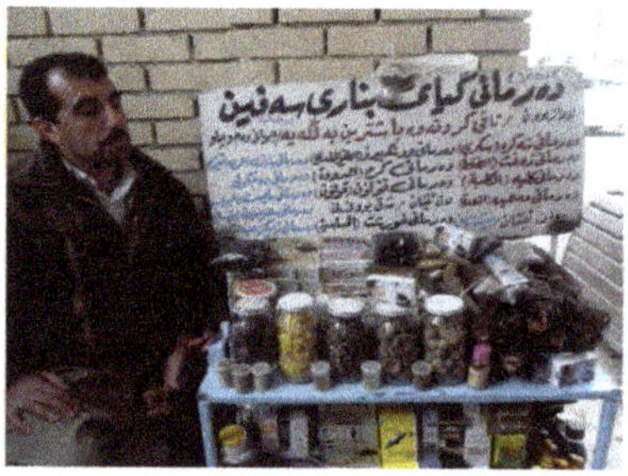

Figure 1. Kurdish seller of traditional remedies (photo taken by H.I.M.A.).

As a matter of fact, it has been found that most of the approximately 1500 plants used in Iraq are valued for their medicinal and aromatic properties. Most medicinal plants are collected from wild habitats, but some are also cultivated [5,6]. However, despite the great use in Kurdistan of herbal remedies, only a few phytochemical investigations have been carried out so far on the isolation and structure determination of the main secondary metabolites expressed in plants grown in Kurdistan. Even rarer are studies aimed at the determination of the bioactivities of isolated compounds. Indeed, the development in the last century by pharmaceutical companies of drug discovery strategies based on synthetic organic chemistry led to a progressive abandonment of the research of new drugs from natural sources. However, with the failure of most of these approaches, the last decades have seen the resurrection of alternative, plant-based drugs [7], as well as the discovery of new potential applications of natural resources [8]. As a result, several plant-originated biomolecules have become economically important commercial products [9]. Moreover, many modern drug-discovery programs include a continuous search for alternative natural products, as well as the re-discovery of underutilized plants and the investigation of plants endemic to little-studied geographical regions, such as those growing in biodiversity-rich developing countries. For these reasons, a few years ago, we started a project directed at the scientific validation of Kurdistan traditional plants and the search of new bioactive metabolites produced by them [2,3,10]. This work is a continuation of this program.

We drew our attention toward the genus *Plantago* L. (family *Plantaginaceae*). This genus encompasses about 270 species of herbs, or rarely subshrubs, that have a terrestrial to an aquatic cosmopolitan distribution, occurring predominantly in temperate and high-altitude tropical regions of the world [11]. The genus is characterized by a wide variety of phytochemical components. Iridoid glycosides, flavonoids, phenolic acids, phenylethanoids, terpenoids, vitamins, alkaloids, and saponins are mainly present in the aerial parts, while unsaturated fatty acids and polysaccharides predominate in the seeds. *Plantago* plants have been used since ancient times as diuretic, anti-inflammatory, and asthmatic drugs in Asia and Europe. The ethnobotanical uses, chemical constituents, and applications of *Plantago* taxa have been described in a few reviews [12,13], with *P. lanceolata*, *P. major*, *P. ovata*, and *P. media* having received the greatest attention from scientists [14–19].

Sixteen *Plantago* species are reported to grow in Iraq [20,21], and nine are native to Kurdistan, where they are distributed in different habitats at altitudes between 820 and 1100 m. The list includes *Plantago loeflingii* L., *P. major* L., *P. lanceolata* L., *P. ovata* Forssk., *P. lagopus* L., *P. cretica* L., *P. bellardii* All., *P. afra* L., and *P. atrata* Hoppe. Antioxidant, anti-inflammatory, cytotoxic, and wound-healing activities are the most prominent biological properties attributed to parts or tissues of some of these plants [19]; although, in vivo studies are lacking, and most of the compounds responsible for the activities are still unknown.

P. loeflingii is an annual plant and grows primarily in the temperate biome, distributed from the Iberian Peninsula to Algeria–Morocco, Lebanon–Syria, Turkey, Iraq, Iran, and Pakistan. In the Iraqi Kurdistan region, the plant (Figure 2A) grows in sandy soils and forests, especially in the Zrarati area (Erbil) at altitudes between 887 and 1076 m (Figure 2B). It is commonly used by local communities to heal wounds and as a vulnerary remedy [5];

however, the phytochemical constituents and the evaluation of biological properties of *P. loeflingii* have not been investigated so far. In this paper, we report, for the first time, the isolation of the main non-volatile constituents from a methanol extract of the aerial parts, including a new *O*-glucosyl flavone, and the evaluation of the effects of two isolated flavonoids on the viability of four human cancer cell lines and two normal ones.

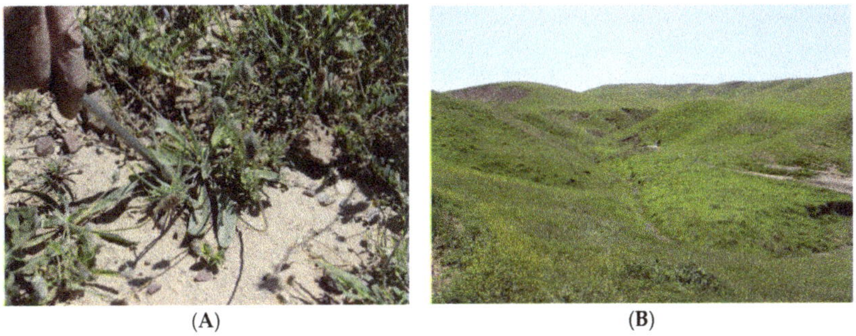

Figure 2. (**A**) *Plantago loeflingii* L.; (**B**) Zrarati area where the plant was collected (photos taken by H.I.M.A.).

2. Results and Discussion

2.1. Phytochemical Investigation

Multiple column chromatographic separations on RP-18 reversed-phase of the residue from a *n*-butanol subextract of a methanol extract of *P. loeflingii* dried leaves afforded nine compounds (Figure 3) belonging to four different families of secondary metabolites: two flavonoid glucosides, 5,7,2′,5′-tetrahydroxyflavone 7-*O*-β-D-glucopyranoside (**1**) and apigenin 6-*C*-β-D-glucopyranoside (isovitexin, **2**); two coumarins, citropten (**3**) and isopimpinellin (**4**); an inseparable mixture of three phytosterols, campesterol (**5**), β-sitosterol (**6**), and stigmasterol (**7**); two lupane triterpenoids, betulin (**8**) and betulinic acid (**9**). The structures of the isolated compounds (Figure 3) were established by spectral data, especially by extensive 1D- and 2D-NMR experiments and, for known compounds, by comparison with the data reported in the literature. The purity (≥95%) of compounds **1–4**, **8**, and **9** was assessed by TLC on silica gel and RP-18 plates (Figure S8 in the Supplementary Information), as well as by NMR spectra (Figures S1–S7).

Compound **1** exhibited UV absorption maxima at 265, 285, and 362 nm and ^{1}H NMR and ^{13}C NMR data which were characteristic of a flavone nucleus [22,23]. Moreover, the IR band at 1655 cm^{-1} confirmed the presence of an α,β-unsaturated carbonyl ketone at C-4 in the ring C of a flavonoid molecule. The ESI-MS spectrum (negative ion mode) of **1** revealed a [M-H]$^-$ ion peak at m/z 447.33, suggesting a MW = 448 and the formula $C_{21}H_{20}O_{11}$, based on elemental analysis, and proton and carbon counts in the NMR spectra. The ^{1}H and ^{13}C NMR spectra (Figures S1 and S3, respectively, in the Supplementary Information), in addition to the signals associated with a flavonoid aglycone, showed signals for a β-glucosyl moiety. This finding was confirmed by the ion peak [$C_{15}H_9O_6$ = M-$C_6H_{11}O_5$]$^-$ at m/z 285 in the ESI-MS spectrum of compound **1**, corresponding to the loss of the sugar unit, and by acid hydrolysis of **1** which afforded D-glucose. The ^{1}H NMR spectrum of **1** exhibited a singlet at δ_H 6.48 (1H) assigned to H-3 of a flavone and an AB system attributed to two coupled protons (see ^{1}H-^{1}H COSY spectrum in Figure S2 in the Supplementary Information) with J = 2.1 Hz which were characteristic of the protons H-6 and H-8 of a 5,7-dihydroxysubstituted flavone [22]. The deshielded nature of these two protons in the ^{1}H NMR spectrum (δ_H 6.46 and 6.77) (Figure 4), in addition to the upfield signal of C-7 (δ_C 164.4) in the ^{13}C NMR spectrum of **1** (Figure 5), indicated [23] the attachment of the glucosyl unit to the HO-7 group of the aglycone (cfr. the NMR signals of H-6, H-8 and C-7 for luteolin (**10**) and luteolin 7-*O*-β-D-glucopyranoside (**11**) in Figures 4 and 5, respectively). On the other hand, the β-bond of O-1″ was suggested by the coupling constant of the anomeric H-1″ signal at δ_H 5.06 ($J_{1''-2''}$ = 8.0 Hz). Moreover, the HMBC correlation (not shown) of H-1″ with C-7 confirmed the attachment of the glucosyl moiety to the HO-7 of the aglycone. Apart from the signals associated with rings A and C, all the other ^{1}H and ^{13}C NMR signals of compound **1** were assigned to the ring B of a flavonoid which, in addition to the C-2-C-1′ bond, was substituted by two phenolic OH groups. In fact, the ^{1}H-NMR and ^{1}H-^{1}H COSY spectra (Figures S1 and S2 in the Supplementary Information) showed the signals of an approximate ABX system formed by three aromatic protons resonating at δ_H 6.66 (d, J = 8.4 Hz, H-3′), 7.35 (dd, J = 8.4 and 2.4 Hz, H-4′), and 7.28 (d, J = 2.4 Hz, H-6′) (Figure 4), respectively. This spin system was in principle assignable either to the three protons of a 3,4-diphenolic ring B, such as that of luteolin (**10**) [24] and luteolin 7-*O*-glucoside (**11**) [25] (Figure 4), or a 2,4-diphenolic ring B, such as that of norartocarpetin (**12**) (Figure 4) [26], or a 2,5-diphenolic ring B, such as that of 5,7,2′,5′-tetrahydroxyflavone (**13**) [27] (Figure 4). However, comparing the chemical shifts of the ring B protons of compound **1** with those of flavonoids **10–13** (Figure 4), we firmly excluded the 2,4-substitution, as in **12**, while the proton patterns of luteolins **10** [24] and **11** [25] were also significantly different from those of compound **1** (Figure 4). Marked differences were also observed between the carbon signals of compounds **1** and **11** [28] in the corresponding ^{13}C NMR spectra in MeOH-d_4 (Figure 5), except for the ring A carbons. This finding clearly indicated that the patterns of substituents in the ring B of glucosides **1** and **11** were different, which resulted in different electronic environments and thus chemical shifts of the carbons in ring C. Based on these data, the structure 5,7,2′,5′-tetrahydroxyflavone 7-*O*-β-D-glucopyranoside was thus assigned to compound **1**, named loeflingiin, which, to our knowledge, is a new natural product. Instead, the corresponding aglycone **13** was isolated from *Bridelia* (Phyllanthaceae) [27], *Scutellaria* (Labiatae) [29,30], and *Euphorbia* (Euphorbiaceae) species [31].

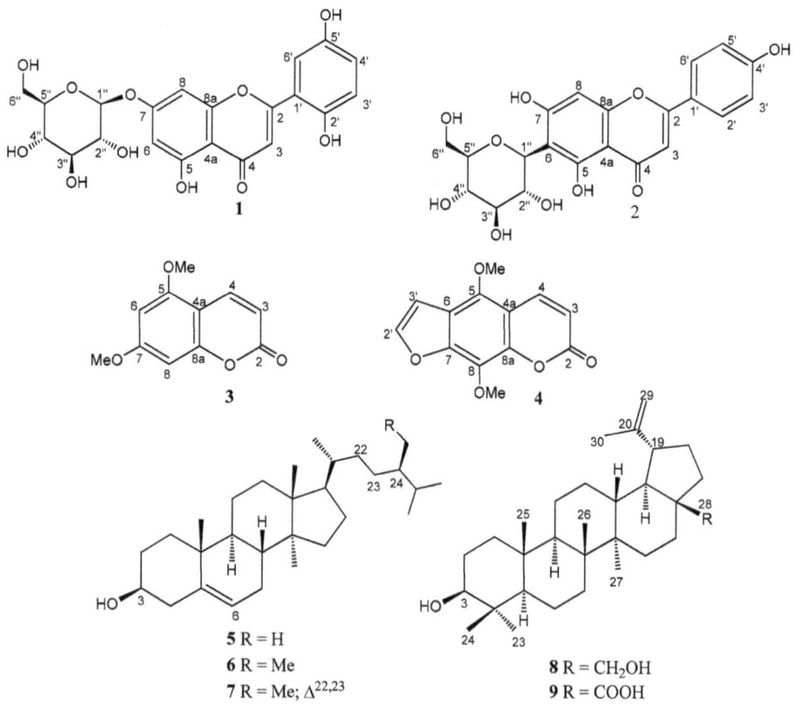

Figure 3. Structures of the compounds isolated from *P. loeflingii* leaves.

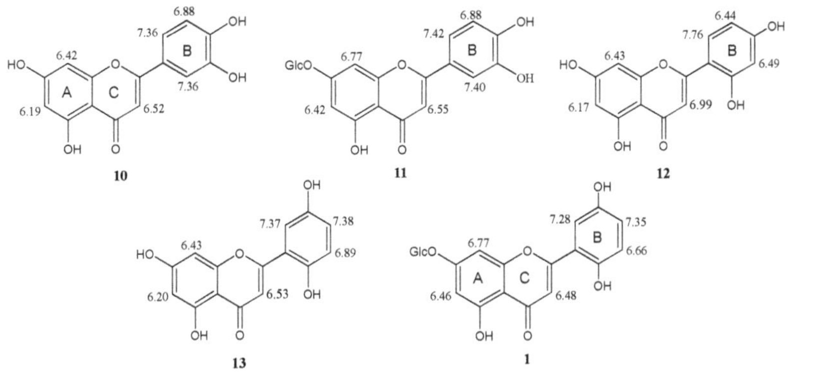

Figure 4. ^{1}H chemical shifts (d_H, ppm) of loeflingiin (**1**), luteolin (**10**) [24], 7-*O*-β-glucosylluteolin (**11**) [25], and 5,7,2′,5′-tetrahydroxyflavone (**13**) [27] in MeOH-d$_4$; norartocarpetin (**12**) in DMSO-d$_6$ [26].

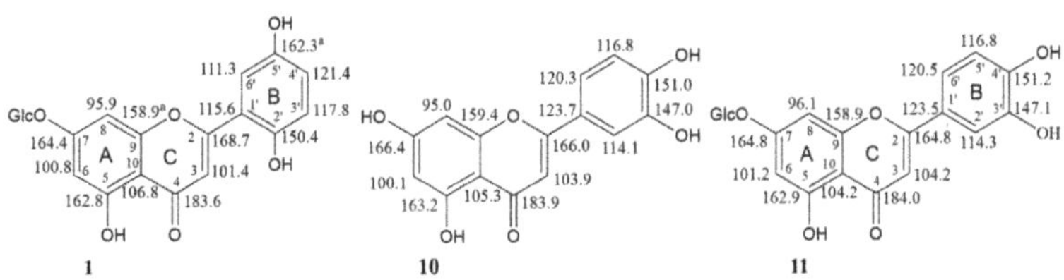

Figure 5. ^{13}C chemical shifts (d_C, ppm) of loeflingiin (**1**), luteolin (**10**) [24], and 7-*O*-β-D-glucosylluteolin (**11**) [28] in MeOH-d$_4$. [a] Assignments can be interchanged.

Contrary to flavonoid **1**, compounds **2–9** (Figure 3) are known. Isovitexin (apigenin-6-C-glucoside) (**2**) has been isolated together with the isomer vitexin (apigenin-8-C-glucoside) from various medicinal plants such as pigeon pea, *Passiflora*, *Crataegus*, and *Ficus* species, bamboo, mimosa, wheat leaves, and many others [32–34]. 5,7-Dimethoxycoumarin (citropten) (**3**) occurs in the essential oils of citrus such as lime, lemon, and bergamot; moreover, it has been isolated from *Euphorbia*, *Zanthoxylum*, *Edgeworthia* (Thymelaeaceae), *Urbanodendron* (Luraceae), *Zingiber* (Zingiberaceae), and *Schisandra* (Schisandraceae) species and many other plants. Isopimpinellin (**4**) is also a quite common plant metabolite, mainly occurring in species belonging to Lamiaceae, Poaceae, Apiaceae, Araliaceae, Zingiberaceae, Rutaceae, Caprifoliaceae, Asteraceae, and Thymelaeaceae families [34]. Sterols **5–7** are widely distributed in nature, in many vegetables, fruits, nuts, and seeds, having a major function to maintain the structure and physiology of cell membranes. Betulin (**8**) and betulinic acid (**9**) are pentacyclic triterpenoids isolated from the bark and sap of birch trees. They also occur as secondary metabolites in hundreds of different plants ubiquitously distributed across the plant kingdom, including *Plantago lanceolata* [34].

In conclusion, to the best of our knowledge, this is the first isolation of isovitexin (**2**), citropten (**3**), and isopimpinellin (**4**) from a species belonging to the genus *Plantago*.

2.2. Biological Activities of Isolated Compounds

All the isolated compounds **2–9** have shown various biological activities, which are summarized below. Isovitexin (**2**), although less studied than vitexin (the 8-C-glucosyl isomer), exerts similar pharmacological effects, partly due to their similar chemical structure [32]. Isovitexin exhibited anti-inflammatory and antioxidant activities on lipopolysaccharide-induced acute lung injury by inhibiting MAPK and NF-κB and activating HO-1/Nrf2 pathways. It inhibits α-glucosidase, an enzyme that is responsible for the breakdown of carbohydrate to sugar and has anti-tumor and neuroprotective effects. Moreover, by inhibition of xanthine oxidase, it may protect cells from oxidative stress [35]. 5,7-Dimethoxycoumarin (citropten)

(**3**) showed antioxidant activity, anti-inflammatory activity in colitis, and antiproliferative effects against the A2058 human melanoma cell line [36]. The furocoumarin isopimpinellin (**4**) exhibited moderate cytotoxicity against Colo-205 tumor cells and inhibited the growth of the human bladder carcinoma cell line E-J in vitro. Moreover, it strongly inhibited insulin-stimulated lipogenesis, induced hepatic GSTs, and was a potent inhibitor of cytochrome P450 1A1/1B1. Oral administration of isopimpinellin blocked DNA adducts formation and skin tumor initiation by 7,12-dimehylbenz[a]anthracene in SENCAR mice and in mouse mammary glands. Phytosterols **5**–**7** have been recommended as food additives, having the potential to reduce blood LDL cholesterol and thus the risk of cardiovascular diseases [37] and benign prostatic hyperplasia [38]. Stigmasterol (**7**) has also been shown to exert anti-angiogenic and anti-cancer effects via the downregulation of TNF-α and VEGFR-2 [39]. The lupane triterpenoids betulin (**8**) and betulinic acid (**9**) exhibited a multitude of biological and pharmacological properties ranging from antimicrobial, antitumor, anti-inflammatory, antimalarial, antiparasitic, and anti-HIV activities and colitis protective effects [40–42]. Moreover, both substances seem to be promising experimental anti-cancer drugs, and betulin (**8**) was found to be a potent antimutagenic agent of skin carcinogenesis. In addition, betulinic acid (**9**) has been reported to reduce oxidative stress and demonstrated an in vivo protective effect on dexamethasone-induced thymocyte apoptosis.

Some flavonoids such as quercetin, fisetin, luteolin (**10**), and luteolin 7-*O*-glucoside (**11**) are potent inhibitors of cell proliferation and angiogenesis [43–45].

In view of our general interest in biologically active flavonoids [46], we performed a standard MTT assay [47–49] to measure the effects of flavonoids loeflingiin (**1**) and isovitexin (**2**) on the metabolic activity of human breast (MCF7), ovarian (BG-1), endometrial (Ishikawa), and mesothelioma (IST-MES1) human cancer cells. For comparison, two normal human healthy cells, i.e., peripheral blood mononuclear (PBM) [50] and human umbilical vein endothelial cells (HUVECs) [51], were also included in the test. The MTT assay detects perturbations in mitochondria and their functions, and thus, it is commonly used to measure the metabolic activity of cells, which serves as an indicator of cell proliferation, vitality, and cytotoxicity [52,53].

The choice of the selected cancer cell lines was mainly dictated by the severity and wide spread of certain types of human cancers, such as breast and ovarian cancers which are the most frequent malignancies in females. Clinically relevant cellular models are essential for understanding cancer physiology at advanced stages. MCF-7 is one of the most widely used metastatic breast cancer cell lines in MTT assays [54], as it represents a more prevalent form of human breast adenocarcinoma. It retains several features of differentiated mammary epithelium and is more likely to express both consistently and discordantly expressed genes. The BG-1 human ovarian adenocarcinoma cell line is one of the most widely used cell lines in ovarian cancer research [55] as it is a representative model of the most common ovarian cancers, providing insights into hormone receptor expression and estrogen responsiveness. Ishikawa cells serve as valuable models for investigating the behavior of endometrial adenocarcinoma (uterine cancer) [56], whose exact causes remain unknown, and for evaluating potential therapies. Research involving IST-Mes1 contributes to our understanding of mesothelioma biology and drug sensitivity [57]. It is part of the Cancer Dependency Map project and the COSMIC cell lines project, aimed at exploring novel therapeutic approaches to combat this rare but aggressive cancer type that originates from the mesothelium.

The activities of loeflingiin (**1**) and isovitexin (**2**) in the MTT assay were compared with *cis*-diamminedichloroplatinum (II) (cisplatin). This complex is a well-known antitumor drug, commonly used to treat ovarian, triple-negative breast cancer (TNBC), mesothelioma, and endometrial cancer, either alone or in combination with other chemotherapeutic agents, such as doxorubicin or taxol.

The IC_{50} values of **1**, **2**, and cisplatin, i.e., the concentrations of tested compounds which reduced cell viability by 50%, were calculated as the means of three MTT assays for each cell line. Optimized conditions of cell viability assays were used [52,53]. The results are reported in Table 1.

Table 1. Results of an MTT assay of cisplatin and compounds **1** and **2** from *Plantago loeflingii*.

	IC_{50} (μM) ± SD					
Compound/Cell Line	**MCF7**	**IST-MES1**	**BG-1 Cells**	**Ishikawa Cells**	**HUVE Cells**	**PBM Cells**
loeflingiin (**1**)	17 ± 2	13 ± 3	4 ± 0.3	6 ± 0.5	>40	>40
isovitexin (**2**)	>50	>50	>50	>50	>50	>50
cisplatin	17 ± 4	10 ± 3	12 ± 3	12 ± 2	-	-

Notably, the 6-*C*-glucoside isovitexin (**2**) was inactive on all the cell lines, while the 7-*O*-glucoside **1** exhibited good activity against all cancer lines, which was significantly higher than cisplatin against the Ishikawa and BG-1 cells (Table 1).

These results require further studies aimed to elucidate the mechanism underpinning loeflingiin's effects on cancer cells. In fact, it is well known that flavonoids, especially luteolin (**10**), which is structurally related to **1**, inhibit cancer cells' growth by targeting different cellular processes such as apoptosis, cell-cycle progression, angiogenesis, and migration [58–61]. It is thus possible that **1** and cisplatin inhibit cell viability through different mechanisms which would explain the different activities observed in the MTT assays. It would also be important to determine the mechanism for loeflingiin's selective effects on cancerous but not normal cells. Our findings seem to confirm that distinct mechanisms for modulating cellular signaling pathways exist in normal cells and in malignant cancer cells [60,61].

3. Materials and Methods

3.1. General Procedures

Preparative medium-pressure liquid chromatographic (MPLC) separations were carried out on a Biotage Isolera instrument (Biotage Italy SRL, Milan, Italy), using a home-made reversed phase cartridge (Merck, Milan, Italy, LiChroprep RP-18, 25–40 mm); TLC: 0.25 mm RP-18 (F254s, Merck, Rahway, NJ, USA), Al-supported plates; visualization under UV light at 254 and 366 nm, directly and after exposure to a 0.5% soln. of vanillin in H_2SO_4/EtOH, 4:1, followed by heating at 100 °C until maximum color development. Reagent-grade solvents, purchased from Carlo Erba (Milan, Italy) or from Aldrich, were used for extraction and chromatographic separations. Optical rotation: PerkinElmer 241 polarimeter (Perkin Elmer, Milan, Italy). Mps were determined on a Fisher-Johns melting point apparatus (Thermo Fisher Scientific, Segrate, Italy) and are uncorrected. All the 1D and 2D NMR experiments were conducted on a Bruker AV300 spectrometer (Bruker Italia SRL, Milan, Italy), at 300 (^{1}H) and 75.47 MHz (^{13}C), respectively. Deuterated solvents (purity 99.8%) were purchased from Sigma-Aldrich (St. Louis, MO, USA). ^{1}H NMR chemical shifts (δ_H, ppm) are relative to the signal at δ_H 7.26 of residual $CHCl_3$ or to the central line of a quintuplet at δ_H 3.31 of residual CD_2HOD in the corresponding fully deuterated solvents [62]; ^{13}C NMR chemical shifts (δ_C, ppm) are relative to the $^{13}CD_3OD$ signal at δ_C 49.0 (central line of a septuplet) [62]; coupling constant (*J*) in Hz; multiplicities of the ^{13}C atoms determined by DEPT experiments. IR spectra: PerkinElmer Paragon 100 PC FT-IR spectrometer; on KBr disks; ν_{max} in cm^{-1}. UV spectra: Lambda 25 UV/Vis spectrophotometer N.3903 (Perkin Elmer instruments, Waltham, MA, USA). ESI-MS experiments were carried out on a Thermo-TSQ mass spectrometer (Thermo Fischer Scientific, Rozzano, Italy) by flow injection analysis (FIA), with electron-spray ionization source (ESI) at 5 kV on TIP capillary. Spectroscopy grade solvents (Merck/Sigma-Aldrich, Milan, Italy) were used.

3.2. Plant Material

Leaves of *P. loeflingii* L. were collected in April 2021 during the flowering season, from the Zrarati district, in the Kurdistan region of Iraq; GPS coordinates: longitude:

36°23′38.54″ N; latitude: 44°16′59.53″ E. A voucher specimen (code no. 7248) was deposited at the Herbarium of Salahaddin University-Erbil (ESUH). The plant was identified by Dr. A. H. Al-khayyat, Professor of botany at the Salahaddin University-Erbil/Iraq. Fresh leaves were cleaned and air-dried under shade at room temperature (20–25 °C) to a constant weight. After drying, the leaves were finely powdered using a laboratory grinding mill to provide a homogeneous powder which was stored in bottles at room temperature until analysis.

3.3. *Extraction and Isolation*

3.3.1. Extraction of *Plantago loeflingii* Leaves

Powdered dried leaves (100 g) were soaked in *n*-hexane (3 × 250 mL) in an Erlenmeyer flask with occasional shaking in an ultrasonic bath for 15 min; subsequently, the leaves were left in the same solvent at room temperature for 1 h. The mixture was filtered through a Whatman filter paper, and the solvent was removed in a rotavapor under reduced pressure to give an oily residue (A, 0.61 g). Subsequently, the defatted leaves were placed in a flask and extracted with methanol (250 mL) in an ultrasonic bath for 15 min and then at room temperature for 1 h under continuous stirring. The process was repeated another two times, and the combined methanol extracts were filtered. Evaporation under reduced pressure in a rotavapor at ≤35 °C afforded crude residue B (10.53 g, 10.5% *w*/*w* dried leaves).

3.3.2. Chromatographic Separation of *Plantago loeflingii* Secondary Metabolites

The residue B (10.5 g) was partitioned between distilled water (250 mL) and CH_2Cl_2 (250 mL) to afford an organic fraction (B1) and an aqueous fraction (B2). The aqueous layer B2 was further partitioned with *n*-butanol (250 mL) to afford, after evaporation, a *n*-butanol soluble residue (B3, 5.7 g). The residual aqueous phase was not examined.

A sample of B3 (1 g) was separated by medium-pressure liquid chromatography (MPLC) on a home-made reversed phase C18 cartridge (100 g). Elution with a gradient of MeOH-H_2O, from 60:40 to 100:0, over 30 min at room temperature, with a flow rate of 20 mL/min, afforded 120 fractions which were analyzed by TLC on RP 18 Al-supported plates (eluent: MeOH-H_2O, 55:45) (Figure S8 in the Supplementary Information). According to the compositions, these fractions were grouped into eight main fractions B3/1–B3/8. Multiple MPLC separations of these fractions over several reversed-phase C18 columns, eluted with various mixtures of MeOH-H_2O, afforded the new glucosyl flavone loeflingiin **1** (7.1 mg), and eight known compounds: apigenin 6-C-glucoside (isovitexin) (**2**) (11 mg), citropten (**3**) (1.8 mg), isopimpinellin (**4**) (0.9 mg), an inseparable mixture (9.5 mg) of campesterol (**5**), β-sitosterol (**6**), and stigmasterol (**7**), betulin (**8**) (30 mg), and betulinic acid (**9**) (50 mg). The structures of the isolated compounds are shown in Figure 3.

3.3.3. Compounds Characterization

Loeflingiin (5,7,2′,5′-tetrahydroxyflavone 7-*O*-β-D-glucopyranoside or 2-(2,5-dihydroxyphenyl)-5,7-dihydroxy-4H-chromen-4-one 7-*O*-β-D-glucopyranoside) (**1**): pale yellow powder; mp around 250 °C (dec.); TLC (RP-18 plate, MeOH/H_2O, 55:45): Rf = 0.42; UV (MeOH) λ_{max} (log e): 265 (4.25), 285 (4.10), 362 (4.08) nm; IR (KBr) ν_{max}: 3400 (broad band, OH), 1655 (conjugated CO), 1625 and 1580 (arom. ring) cm^{-1}; ESI-MS (negative ion mode): *m*/*z* 447.33 $[M-H]^-$ ($C_{21}H_{19}O_{11}^-$). Elemental analysis: calcd. for $C_{21}H_{20}O_{11}$: C, 56.25%; H, 4.50%; found: C, 56.42%; H, 4.63%. ^1H NMR (300 MHz, CD_3OD) aglycone moiety: δ_H (ppm) 7.35 (1H, dd, *J* = 8.4 and 2.4 Hz, H-4′), 7.28 (1H, d, *J* = 2.4 Hz, H-6′), 6.77 (1H, d, *J* = 2.1 Hz, H-8), 6.66 (1H, d, *J* = 8.4 Hz, H-3′), 6.48 (1H, s, H-3), 6.46 (1H, d, *J* = 2.1 Hz, H-6); glucose moiety: δ_H 5.06 (1H, d, *J* = 8.0 Hz, H-1″), 3.93 (1H, dd, *J* = 12.2 and 1.7 Hz, H-6_a″), 3.73 (1H, dd, *J* = 12.0 and 5.4 Hz, H-6_b″), 3.6–3.25 (4H, m's, H-2″, H-3″, H-4″, H-5″). ^{13}C NMR (75 MHz, CD_3OD) aglycone moiety: δ_C (ppm) 183.6 (0, C-4), 168.7 (0, C-2), 164.4 (0, C-7), 162.8 (0, C-5), 162.3 (0, C-5′)[a], 158.9 (0, C-8a)[a], 150.4 (0, C-2′), 121.4 (1, C-4′), 117.8 (1, C-3′), 115.6 (0, C-1′), 111.3 (1, C-6′), 106.8 (0, C-4a), 101.4 (1, C-3), 100.8 (1, C-6), 95.9 (1, C-8); glucose moiey: δ_C 101.6 (1, C-1″), 78.3 (1, C-3″), 77.8 (1, C-5″), 74.8 (1, C-2″), 71.3 (1, C-4″), 62.4 (2, C-6″). [a]Assignments can be interchanged. The numbers in parentheses are the protons attached to the corresponding carbon, which were determined by DEPT experiments.

Isovitexin (apigenin 6-C-β-glucopyranoside or 5,7,4′-trihydroxyflavone-6-C-β-D-glucopyranoside) (**2**): pale-yellow powder; TLC (RP-18 plate, MeOH/H_2O, 60:40): Rf = 0.51; UV (MeOH) λ_{max}: 275, 333 nm; ESI-MS (positive ion mode): *m*/*z* 455.22 $[M + Na]^+$ ($C_{21}H_{20}NaO_{10}^+$); ESI-MS (negative ion mode): *m*/*z* 431.20 $[M-H]^-$ ($C_{21}H_{19}O_{10}^-$). ^{1}H NMR (300 MHz, CD_3OD) aglycone moiety: δ_H (ppm) 7.83 (2H, d, *J* = 8.7 Hz, H-2′ and H-6′), 6.93 (2H, d, *J* = 8.7 Hz, H-3′ and H-5′), 6.59 (1H, s, H-3), 6.50 (1H, s, H-8); glucose moiety: δ_H 4.91 (1H, d, *J* = 10.0 Hz, H-1″), 4.19 (1H, distorted t, H-2″), 3.90 (1H, dd, *J* = 12.2 and 1.7 Hz, H-6_a″), 3.75 (1H, dd, *J* = 12.0 and 5.0 Hz, H-6_b″), 3.52–3.35 (3H, m's, H-3″, H-4″, H-5″). ^{13}C NMR (75 MHz, CD_3OD) aglycone moiety: δ_C (ppm) 184.0 (0, C-4), 166.1 (0, C-2), 164.9 (0, C-7), 162.8 (0, C-4′), 162.0 (0, C-5), 158.7 (0, C-8a), 129.4 (1 and 1, overlapped C-2′ and C-6′), 123.1 (0, C-1′), 117.0 (1 and 1, overlapped C-3′ and C-5′), 109.2 (0, C-6), 105.2 (0, C-4a), 103.8 (1, C-3), 95.2 (1, C-8); glucose moiety: δ_C 82.6 (1, C-5″), 80.1 (1, C-3″), 75.2 (1, C-1″), 72.6 (1, C-2″), 71.8 (1, C-4″), 62.9 (2, C-6″). The numbers in parentheses are the protons attached to the corresponding carbon, which were determined by DEPT experiments. The NMR spectra were consistent with the literature [63]. No rotational isomerism was observed, in accordance with references [64,65].

Citropten (limettin; 5,7-dimethoxycoumarin) (**3**). ^{1}H NMR (300 MHz, $CDCl_3$): δ_H (ppm) 7.97 (1H, d, *J* = 9.7 Hz, H-4), 6.42 (1H, d, *J* = 2.2 Hz, H-8), 6.28 (1H, d, *J* = 2.2 Hz, H-6), 6.16 (1H, d, *J* = 9.7 Hz, H-3), 3.89 (3H, s, *Me*O-5), 3.86 (3H, s, *Me*O-7); ^{13}C NMR (75 MHz, $CDCl_3$) δ_C (ppm) 163.8 (0, C-7), 161.4 (0, C-2), 157.0 (0, C-5), 156.9 (0, C-8a), 138.6 (1, C-4), 111.0 (1, C-3), 104.1 (0, C-4a), 94.9 (1, C-6), 92.9 (1, C-8), 55.9 (3 and 3, CH_3O-5 and CH_3O-7). The NMR spectra were consistent with those reported in the literature [66,67].

Isopimpinellin (5,8-dimethoxypsoralen) (**4**). ^{1}H NMR (300 MHz, $CDCl_3$): δ_H (ppm) 8.12 (1H, d, *J* = 9.7 Hz, H-4), 7.63 (1H, d, *J* = 2.3 Hz, H-2′), 7.0 (1H, d, *J* = 2.3 Hz, H-3′), 6.29 (1H, d, *J* = 9.7 Hz, H-3), 4.17 (2 × 3H, 2 × s, *Me*O-5 and *Me*O-8); ^{13}C NMR (75 MHz, $CDCl_3$): δ_C (ppm) 160.4 (0, C-2), 150.0 (0, C-7), 145.1 (1, C-2′), 144.3 (0, C-5), 143.8 (0, C-8a), 139.3 (1, C-4), 128.1 (0, C-8), 114.9 (0, C-6), 113.0 (1, C-3), 108.0 (0, C-4a), 105.0 (1, C-3′), 61.7 and 60.9 (3 and 3, CH_3O-5 and CH_3O-8). The NMR spectra were consistent with those reported in the literature [68,69].

Phytosterols **5**–**7**. A mixture of chromatographically inseparable phytosterols **5**–**7** was revealed by the ^{1}H NMR spectrum which showed a cluster of singlets, doublets, and triplets between 0.72 and 1.02 ppm, assignable to different Me, Me-CH, and Et groups of sterols, a multiplet at δ_H 3.63 assigned to oxymethine H-3, two double doublets at δ_H 5.04 (1H, *J* = 12.0 and 6.0 Hz) and δ_H 5.20 (1H, *J* = 12.0 and 7.0 Hz), attributed to the olefinic protons H-22 and H-23 of stigmasterol (**7**), and a broad doublet (1H, *J* = 3.0 Hz) at δ_H 5.37, characteristic of the olefinic proton H-6 in sterols **5**–**7**.

Betulin (lup-20(29)-ene-3β,28-diol) (**8**). ^{1}H NMR (300 MHz, $CDCl_3$): δ_H (ppm) 0.76 (3H, s, H_3-24), 0.83 (3H, s, H_3-25), 0.97 and 0.99 (2 × 3H, 2 × s, H_3-23 and H_3-27), 1.02 (3H, s, H_3-26), 1.70 (3H, s, H_3-30), 0.68-2.10 (25H, m's, H_2-1, H_2-2, H-5, H_2-6, H_2-7, H-9, H_2-11, H_2-12, H-13, H_2-15, H_2-16, H-18, H_2-20, H_2-21, *OH*), 2.38 (1H, td, *J* = 10.5 and 5.5 Hz, H-19), 3.21 (1H, dd, *J* = 11.5 and 4.0 Hz, H-3), 3.35 and 3.80 (2 × 1H, 2 × brd, J_{AB} = 10.5 Hz, H-28a and H-28b), 4.60 and 4.70 (2 × 1H, 2 × brs, H-29a and 29b). The ^{1}H NMR spectrum corresponded to that in the literature [42].

Betulinic acid (3β-hydroxylup-20(29)-en-28-oic acid) (**9**). ^{1}H NMR (300 MHz, $CDCl_3$): δ_H (ppm) 0.76 (3H, s, H_3-24), 0.83 (3H, s, H_3-25), 0.95 (3H, s, H_3-26), 0.97 and 0.99 (2 × 3H, 2 × s, H_3-23 and H_3-27), 1.70 (3H, s, H_3-30), 0.68-2.25 (25H, m's, H_2-1, H_2-2, H-5, H_2-6, H_2-7, H-9, H_2-11, H_2-12, H-13, H_2-15, H_2-16, H-18, H_2-20, H_2-21, *OH*), 3.05 (1H, td, *J* = 10.5 and 5.0 Hz, H-19), 3.21 (1H, dd, *J* = 11.5 and 4.0 Hz, H-3), 4.63 and 4.76 (2 × 1H, 2 × brs, H-29a and 29b). The ^{1}H NMR spectrum corresponded to that in the literature [70].

Acid hydrolysis of loeflingiin (**1**). Compound **1** (2 mg) was treated with 10% HC1 (2 mL) in a sealed tube at 100 °C for 4 h. The mixture was extracted with EtOAc, and the aqueous layer was neutralized with Et_3N and freeze-dried. Glucose was identified in the residue from evaporation of the aqueous layer by TLC on a precoated silica gel plate (Silicagel G-60 F_{254}, 0.2 mm, Merck-Sigma Aldrich) using EtOAc/MeOH/H_2O/AcOH (65:15:15:25 *v*/*v*/*v*/*v*) as eluent and authentic glucose as a reference compound. The plate was sprayed with a 0.5% soln. of vanillin in H_2SO_4/EtOH, 4:1 and heated by a hot gun to give a dark brown spot for glucose. The sign of the rotary power of the residue was positive, consistent with D-glucose.

3.3.4. MTT Assay

The inhibition of cell viability by a sample and cisplatin as a reference compound was evaluated through the reduction of the yellow-colored water-soluble salt MTT [3-(4,5-dimethylthiazol-2-yl)-2,5-diphenyltetrazolium bromide] by mitochondrial NAD(P)H-dependent dehydrogenase enzymes in metabolically active cells to a purple-blue formazan salt, which has an absorbance maximum near 570 nm [47]. Metabolically damaged cells lose the ability to convert MTT into formazan. The color change thus serves as a convenient marker of only the viable cells. The darker the solution is, the greater the number of metabolically active cells is, and the measure of the absorbance can be directly related to the number of viable cells.

Cell Cultures and Reagents

Two human normal cells and four human cancer cell lines were used in the MTT test. MCF7 breast cancer cells were maintained in Dulbecco's Modified Eagle's Medium (DMEM)/F-12 and DMEM, respectively, supplemented with heat-inactivated 10% fetal bovine serum (FBS), 100 mg/mL penicillin/streptomycin and 2 mM L-glutamine (Life Technologies and Euroclone S.P.A., Milan, Italy) at 37 °C with 5% CO_2, 95% air and complete humidity. BG-1 ovarian cancer cells were cultured in Roswell Park Memorial Institute (RPMI) 1640 medium (Thermo Fisher Scientific, Segrate, Italy) and DMEM medium, respectively, without Phenol Red, supplemented with 10% FBS, 100 mg/mL penicillin/streptomycin and 2 mM L-glutamine (Life technologies). Ishikawa endometrial cancer cells were maintained in Minimum Essential Medium (MEM, Sigma-Aldrich, Milan, Italy) supplemented with 10% FBS, 100 mg/mL penicillin/streptomycin, and 2 mM L-glutamine and 1% non-essential amino acids solution (Life technologies). Mesothelioma cancer cells IST-MES1 were maintained in Ham's F-10 Nutrient Mixture (Thermo Fisher Scientific) supplemented with 20% FBS, 100 mg/mL penicillin/streptomycin. Thawed human normal peripheral blood mononuclear cells (PMBCs) were cultured in RPMI medium in 5% CO_2 at 37 °C [50]. Human umbilical vein endothelial cells (HUVECs) were purchased from Merck/Sigma-Aldrich (Milan) and cultured in Endothelial Cell Growth Medium (211–500) (Merck/Sigma-Aldrich) according to the seller protocol. Cancer and PBMC cells were obtained from the American Type Culture Collection (ATCC, Manassas, VA, USA), except IST-MES1 cells which were kindly provided by the ICLC (Interlab Cell Line Collection) at Istituto Nazionale per la Ricerca sul Cancro, Genoa, Italy. The cells were used less than six months after resuscitation. MTT stock solution (5 mg/mL in PBS; Sigma–Aldrich) was stored for less than one month in the dark at 4 °C until use.

Cell Viability Assay

An equal number of cells (around 1×10^4) were seeded in quadruplicate in 96-well flat-bottom plates in their regular growth medium (100 μL/well) supplemented with 10% FBS and were grown in the dark at 37 °C under a humidified atmosphere of 5%% CO_2-95% air until 75% confluence. Cells were washed once they had attached; subsequently, they were separately treated for 48 h at 22 °C with 100 μL of loeflingiin (**1**), isovitexin (**2**), and cisplatin solutions at eight concentrations (0.1, 1, 5, 10, 25, 50, 100, 125 μM). Stock solutions (20 mM) for cisplatin, used as a positive control, and the two flavonoids were prepared, just before use, using DMSO (Sigma-Aldrich; stored at −78 °C), further diluted with 1X PBS (ThermoFisher Scientific) to the appropriate concentration. The final concentration of DMSO was adjusted at about 0.6% (*v*/*v*). Medium was removed;

subsequently, cells were washed with PBS and then treated with 50μL of stock MTT solution plus 100 μL of culture medium for each well, except the cell-free blank wells. Cells were incubated for an additional 4 h at 37 °C with 5% CO_2, 95% air, and complete humidity until intracellular purple formazan crystals were visible under a microscope. The MTT solution was carefully replaced with DMSO (100 μL) and glycine buffer (12 μL, pH 10.5) to solubilize the formazan formed. After cells had been lysed at room temperature and purple crystals had completely dissolved, the absorbance (Abs) of the resulting solution was read at 565 nm by an automated microplate reader (Agilent BioTek, Santa Clara, CA, USA). Three independent experiments were performed for each sample concentration, and mean absorbance (Abs) was calculated. The percentage of viable cells was given by the equation $[(Abs_{sample} - Abs_{blank})/Abs_{control} - Abs_{blank})] \times 100$, where the positive control was 100% lysed untreated cells, and blank were cell-free wells containing medium only. Cells are lysed by freeze–thaw and pipetting before addition of the MTT. The values of percent viable cells were plotted versus sample concentrations, and IC_{50} value (μM) was calculated by probit analysis ($p < 0.05$, v2 test) as the concentration of tested sample yielding 50% cell viability or, as a complement, 50% viability inhibition. MTT assays on a control group of cells treated with 1X PBS medium (100 μL) alone and with 1X PBS (100 μL) plus 0.6% (*v*/*v*) DMSO ruled out any effect of medium or DMSO on cell viability.

4. Conclusions

This paper describes the first phytochemical investigation of the secondary metabolites of *P. loeflingii*, which was collected in Iraqi Kurdistan Region, where it is used as an herbal remedy. Eight known compounds were isolated, which belonged to the flavonoid, coumarin, sterol, and triterpenoid families. In addition, a new flavonoid was isolated, whose structure was determined as the 7-*O*-β-D-glucopyranoside of the rare 5,7,2′,5′-tetrahydroxyflavone (**1**) by spectral analysis and acid hydrolysis. The isolated compound significantly reduced the viability of four important human cancer cell lines in a MTT assay. The effects were higher than cisplatin against Ishikawa and BG-1 cells. This activity together with various known biological and pharmacological properties of the other isolated compounds give scientific evidence to the traditional uses of *P. loeflingii* in Kurdistan. The inhibitory mechanism of cell viability by the new flavonoid **1**, as well as the specific effects on human cancer cells compared to normal cells will be the objects of further investigations.

Supplementary Materials: The following supporting information can be downloaded at: https://www.mdpi.com/article/10.3390/molecules29051079/s1, Figure S1: ^{1}H NMR spectrum (300 MHz, CD_3OD) of compound **1**; Figure S2: ^{1}H-^{1}H COSY spectrum of compound **1**; Figure S3: ^{13}C NMR spectrum (75 MHz, CD_3OD) of compound **1**; Figure S4: DEPT spectrum of compound **1**; Figure S5: HSQC spectrum of compound **1**; Figure S6: HSQC spectrum (enlargement) of compound **1**; Figure S7: ESI-MS (negative ion mode) spectrum of compound **1**; Figure S8: TLC chromatograms (RP 18 phase; eluent: MeOH-H_2O, 55:45) of subextract B3 and the fractions resulting from its MPLC separation.

Author Contributions: Conceptualization, H.I.M.A., F.H.S.H. and K.Y.M.A.; methodology, H.I.M.A., D.C., C.A. and Z.H.J.; investigation, H.I.M.A., K.Y.M.A. and M.M.; writing—original draft preparation, H.I.M.A. and C.A.; writing—review and editing, G.V.; supervision, G.V., H.I.M.A. and K.Y.M.A. All authors have read and agreed to the published version of the manuscript.

Funding: This research received no external funding.

Institutional Review Board Statement: Not applicable.

Informed Consent Statement: Not applicable.

Data Availability Statement: All data presented in this study are available in the article and in Supplementary Materials.

Acknowledgments: We are grateful to Abdul Hussain Al Khayyat for the botanical identification and the Universidad Técnica Particular de Loja (UTPL) for supporting open access publication.

Conflicts of Interest: The authors declare no conflicts of interest.

References

1. Solecki, R.S. Shanidar IV, a Neanderthal flower burial in northern Iraq. *Science* **1975**, *190*, 880–881. [CrossRef]
2. Amin, H.I.M.; Ibrahim, M.F.; Hussain, F.H.S.; Sardar, A.S.; Vidari, G. Phytochemistry and ethnopharmacology of some medicinal plants used in the Kurdistan region of Iraq. *Nat. Prod. Commun.* **2016**, *11*, 291–296. [CrossRef]
3. Abdullah, F.O.; Hussain, F.H.S.; Sardar, A.S.; Vita-Finzi, P.; Vidari, G. Phytochemistry and ethnopharmacology of medicinal plants used on Safeen Mountain in the Kurdistan region of Iraq. *Nat. Prod. Commun.* **2016**, *11*, 1923–1927. [CrossRef]
4. Mati, E.; de Boer, H. Ethnobotany and trade of medicinal plants in the Qaysari Market, Kurdish autonomous region, Iraq. *J. Ethnopharmacol.* **2011**, *133*, 490–510. [CrossRef]
5. Handa, S.S.; Rakesh, D.D.; Vasisht, K. *Compendium of Medicinal and Aromatic Plants—Vol. 2-Asia*; United Nations Industrial Development Organization and the International Centre for Science and High Technology (UNIDO-ICS): Trieste, Italy, 2006.
6. Nahida, A. The most medicinal plants used in Iraq: Traditional knowledge. *Adv. Environ. Biol.* **2011**, *5*, 401–406.
7. Atanasov, A.G.; Waltenberger, B.; Pferschy-Wenzig, E.M.; Linder, T.; Wawrosch, C.; Uhrin, P.; Temml, V.; Wang, L.; Schwaiger, S.; Heiss, E.H.; et al. Discovery and resupply of pharmacologically active plant-derived natural products: A review. *Biotechnol. Adv.* **2015**, *33*, 1582–1614. [CrossRef]
8. Süntar, I. Importance of ethnopharmacological studies in drug discovery: Role of medicinal plants. *Phytochem. Rev.* **2020**, *19*, 1199–1209. [CrossRef]
9. Fierascu, R.C.; Fierascu, I.; Ortan, A.; Georgiev, M.I.; Sieniawska, E. Innovative approaches for recovery of phytoconstituents from medicinal/aromatic plants and biotechnological production. *Molecules* **2020**, *25*, 309. [CrossRef] [PubMed]
10. Amin, H.I.M.; Hussain, F.H.S.; Najmaldin, S.K.; Thu, Z.M.; Ibrahim, M.F.; Gilardoni, G.; Vidari, G. Phytochemistry and biological activities of *Iris* species growing in Iraqi Kurdistan and phenolic constituents of the traditional plant *Iris postii*. *Molecules* **2021**, *26*, 264. [CrossRef] [PubMed]
11. Schwarzbach, A.E. Plantaginaceae. In *Flowering Plants Dicotyledons. The Families and Genera of Vascular Plants*; Kadereit, J.W., Ed.; Springer: Berlin/Heidelberg, Germany, 2004; Volume 7, pp. 327–329.
12. Janković, T.; Gordana Zdunić, G.; Beara, I.; Balog, K.; Pljevljakušić, D.; Stešević, D.; Šavikin, K. Comparative study of some polyphenols in *Plantago* species. *Biochem. Syst. Ecol.* **2012**, *42*, 69–74. [CrossRef]
13. Gonçalves, S.; Romano, A. The medicinal potential of plants from the genus *Plantago* (Plantaginaceae). *Ind. Crops Prod.* **2016**, *83*, 213–226. [CrossRef]
14. Fierascu, R.C.F.; Fierascu, I.; Ortan, A.; Paunescu, A. *Plantago media* L.—Explored and potential applications of an underutilized plant. *Plants* **2021**, *10*, 265. [CrossRef] [PubMed]
15. Abate, L.; Bachheti, R.K.; Tadesse, M.G.; Bachheti, A. Ethnobotanical uses, chemical constituents, and application of *Plantago lanceolata* L. *J. Chem.* **2022**, *2022*, 1532031. [CrossRef]
16. Mayer, J.G. Plantain (*Plantago lanceolata*)—Medicinal plant of the year 2014. *Z. Phytother.* **2013**, *34*, 242–243. [CrossRef]
17. Adom, M.B.; Taher, M.; Mutalabisin, M.F.; Amri, M.S.; Abdul Kudos, M.B.; Wan Sulaiman, M.W.A.; Sengupta, P.; Susanti, D. Chemical constituents and medical benefits of *Plantago major*. *Biomed. Pharmacother.* **2017**, *96*, 348–360. [CrossRef] [PubMed]
18. Samuelsen, A.B. The traditional uses, chemical constituents and biological activities of *Plantago major* L. A review. *J. Ethnopharmacol.* **2000**, *72*, 1–21. [CrossRef] [PubMed]
19. Franco, E.A.N.; Sanches-Silva, A.; Ribeiro-Santos, R.; de Melo, N.R. Psyllium (*Plantago ovata* Forsk): From evidence of health benefits to its food application. *Trends Food Sci. Technol.* **2020**, *96*, 166–175. [CrossRef]
20. Townsend, C.C.; Guest, E.R. (Eds.) *Flora of Iraq, Vol. 8: Monocotyledones Excluding Graminae*; Ministry of Agriculture and Agrarian Reform: Baghdad, Iraq, 1985; p. 440.
21. Ghazanfar, S.A.; Edmondson, J.R. (Eds.) *Flora of Iraq, Vol. 5, Part 2: Lythraceae to Campanulaceae*; Ministry of Agriculture and Agrarian Reform: Baghdad, Iraq, 2013; p. 349.
22. Mabry, T.J.; Markham, K.R.; Thomas, K.R. *The Systematic Identification of Flavonoids*; Springer: New York, NY, USA, 1970.
23. Agrawal, P.K.; Rastogi, R.P. ^{13}C NMR spectroscopy of flavonoids. *Heterocycles* **1981**, *16*, 2181–2236.
24. Lin, L.-C.; Pai, Y.-F.; Tsai, T.-H. Isolation of luteolin and luteolin-7-*O*-glucoside from *Dendranthema morifolium* Ramat Tzvel and their pharmacokinetics in rats. *J. Agric. Food Chem.* **2015**, *63*, 7700–7706. [CrossRef]
25. Žemlička, L.; Fodran, P.; Lukeš, V.; Vagánek, A.; Slováková, M.; Staško, A.; Dubaj, T.; Liptaj, T.; Karabín, M.; Birošová, L.; et al. Physicochemical and biological properties of luteolin-7-*O*-β-D-glucoside (cynaroside) isolated from *Anthriscus sylvestris* (L.) Hoffm. *Monatsh. Chem.* **2014**, *145*, 1307–1318. [CrossRef]
26. Jeong, S.H.; Ryu, Y.B.; Curtis-Long, M.J.; Ryu, H.W.; Baek, Y.S.; Kang, J.E.; Lee, W.S.; Park, K.H. Tyrosinase inhibitory polyphenols from roots of *Morus lhou*. *J. Agric. Food Chem.* **2009**, *57*, 1195–1203. [CrossRef]
27. Puja, S.D.; Shahriar, K.R.; Hasan, C.M.; Ahsan, M. Flavonoids from the leaves of *Bridelia stipularis* with in vitro antioxidant and cytotoxicity activity. *Pharmacol. Pharm.* **2020**, *11*, 137–146. [CrossRef]
28. Velázquez Fiza, M.P.; Díaz Lanza, A.M.; Fernández Matellano, L. Polyphenolic compounds from *Plantago lagopus* L. *Z. Naturforsch.* **2000**, *55c*, 877–880. [CrossRef]
29. Zhang, Y.-Y.; Guo, Y.-Z.; Onda, M.; Hashimoto, K.; Ikeya, Y.; Okada, M.; Marumo, M.Y. Four flavonoids from *Scutellaria baicalensis*. *Phytochemistry* **1994**, *35*, 511–514. [CrossRef]
30. Miyaichi, Y.; Hanamitsu, E.; Kizu, H.; Tomimori, T. Studies on the constituents of *Scutellaria* species (XXII). Constituents of the roots of *Scutellaria amabilis* HARA. *Chem. Pharm. Bull.* **2006**, *54*, 435–441. [CrossRef] [PubMed]

31. Magozwi, D.K.; Dinala, M.; Mokwana, N.; Siwe-Noundou, X.; Krause, R.W.M.; Sonopo, M.; McGaw, L.J.; Augustyn, W.A.; Tembu, V.J. Flavonoids from the genus *Euphorbia*: Isolation, structure, pharmacological activities and structure-activity relationships. *Pharmaceuticals* **2021**, *14*, 428. [CrossRef]
32. He, M.; Min, J.-W.; Kong, W.-L.; He, X.-H.; Li, J.-X.; Peng, B.-W. A review on the pharmacological effects of vitexin and isovitexin. *Fitoterapia* **2016**, *115*, 74–85. [CrossRef]
33. Kalinová, J.P.; Vrchotová, N.; Tříska, J. Vitexin and isovitexin levels in sprouts of selected plants. *J. Food Compos. Anal.* **2021**, *100*, 103895. [CrossRef]
34. Natural Product Activity and Species Source (NPASS) Database. Available online: https://bidd.group/NPASS/ (accessed on 20 November 2023).
35. Lin, C.-M.; Chen, C.-T.; Lee, H.-H.; Lin, J.-K. Prevention of cellular ROS damage by isovitexin and related flavonoids. *Planta Med.* **2002**, *68*, 365–367. [CrossRef]
36. Wolny, D.; Chodurek, E.; Dzierzewicz, Z. Antiproliferative effect of valproic acid and 5,7-dimethoxycoumarin against A2058 human melanoma cells. *Acta Pol. Pharm.* **2014**, *71*, 1056–1059. [PubMed]
37. Cabral, C.E.; Klein, M.R. Phytosterols in the treatment of hypercholesterolemia and prevention of cardiovascular diseases. *Arq. Bras. Cardiol.* **2017**, *109*, 475–482. [CrossRef]
38. Kim, T.H.; Lim, H.J.; Kim, M.S.; Lee, M.S. Dietary supplements for benign prostatic hyperplasia: An overview of systematic reviews. *Maturitas* **2012**, *73*, 180–185. [CrossRef]
39. Kangsamaksin, T.; Chaithongyot, S.; Wootthichairangsan, C.; Hanchaina, R.; Tangshewinsirikul, C.; Svasti, J. Lupeol and stigmasterol suppress tumor angiogenesis and inhibit cholangiocarcinoma growth in mice via downregulation of tumor necrosis factor-α. *PLoS ONE* **2017**, *12*, e0189628. [CrossRef]
40. Hordyjewska, A.; Ostapiuk, A.; Horecka, A.; Kurzepa, J. Betulin and betulinic acid: Triterpenoids derivatives with a powerful biological potential. *Phytochem. Rev.* **2019**, *18*, 929–951. [CrossRef]
41. Lou, H.; Li, H.; Zhang, S.; Lu, H.; Chen, Q. A review on preparation of betulinic acid and its biological activities. *Molecules* **2021**, *26*, 5583. [CrossRef] [PubMed]
42. Kaur, P.; Arora, S.; Singh, R. Isolation, characterization and biological activities of betulin from *Acacia nilotica* bark. *Sci. Rep.* **2022**, *12*, 9370. [CrossRef] [PubMed]
43. Fotsis, T.; Pepper, M.S.; Aktas, E. Flavonoids, dietary-derived inhibitors of cell proliferation and in vitro angiogenesis. *Cancer Res.* **1997**, *57*, 2916–2921. [PubMed]
44. Seelinger, G.; Merfort, I.; Wölfle, U.; Schempp, C.M. Anti-carcinogenic effects of the flavonoid luteolin. *Molecules* **2008**, *13*, 2628–2651. [CrossRef] [PubMed]
45. Kawaii, S.; Tomono, Y.; Katase, E.; Ogawa, K.; Yano, M. Antiproliferative activity of flavonoids on several cancer cell lines. *Biosci. Biotechnol. Biochem.* **1999**, *63*, 896–899. [CrossRef] [PubMed]
46. Amin, H.I.M.; Hussain, F.H.S.; Maggiolini, M.; Vidari, G. Bioactive constituents from the traditional Kurdish plant *Iris persica*. *Nat. Prod. Commun.* **2018**, *13*, 1127–1128. [CrossRef]
47. Mosmann, T. Rapid colorimetric assay for cellular growth and survival: Application to proliferation and cytotoxicity assays. *J. Immunol. Methods* **1983**, *65*, 55–63. [CrossRef] [PubMed]
48. Alley, M.C.; Scudiere, D.A.; Monks, A.; Hursey, M.L.; Czerwinski, M.J.; Fine, D.L.; Abbott, B.J.; Mayo, J.G.; Shoemaker, R.H.; Boyd, M.R. Feasibility of drug screening with panels of human tumor cell lines using a microculture tetrazolium assay. *Cancer Res.* **1988**, *48*, 589–601. [PubMed]
49. Kumar, P.; Nagarajan, A.; Uchil, P.D. Analysis of Cell Viability by the MTT Assay. *Cold Spring Harb. Protoc.* **2018**, *2018*. [CrossRef] [PubMed]
50. Riedhammer, C.; Halbritter, D.; Weissert, R. Peripheral blood mononuclear cells: Isolation, freezing, thawing, and culture. In *Multiple Sclerosis. Methods in Molecular Biology*; Weissert, R., Ed.; Humana Press: New York, NY, USA, 2014; Volume 1304. [CrossRef]
51. Vakili Zahir, N.; Nakhjavani, M.; Hajian, P.; Shirazi, F.H.; Mirzaei, H. Evaluation of silibinin effects on the viability of HepG2 (Human hepatocellular liver carcinoma) and HUVEC (Human Umbilical Vein Endothelial) cell lines. *Iran. J. Pharm. Res.* **2018**, *17*, 261–267.
52. Ghasemi, M.; Turnbull, T.; Sebastian, S.; Kempson, I. The MTT assay: Utility, limitations, pitfalls, and interpretation in bulk and single-cell analysis. *Int. J. Mol. Sci.* **2021**, *22*, 12827. [CrossRef]
53. Larsson, P.; Engqvist, H.; Biermann, J.; Rönnerman, E.W.; Forssell-Aronsson, E.; Kovács, A.; Karlsson, P.; Helou, K.; Parris, T.Z. Optimization of cell viability assays to improve replicability and reproducibility of cancer drug sensitivity screens. *Sci. Rep.* **2020**, *10*, 5798. [CrossRef]
54. Ahmadian, S.; Barar, J.; Saei, A.A.; Fakhree, M.A.; Omidi, Y. Cellular toxicity of nanogenomedicine in MCF-7 cell line: MTT assay. *J. Vis. Exp.* **2009**, *26*, 1191. [CrossRef]
55. Kang, N.-H.; Hwang, K.-A.; Lee, H.-R.; Choi, D.-W.; Choi, K.-C. Resveratrol regulates the cell viability promoted by 17β-estradiol or bisphenol A via down-regulation of the cross-talk between estrogen receptor α and insulin growth factor-1 receptor in BG-1 ovarian cancer cells. *Food Chem. Toxicol.* **2013**, *59*, 373–379. [CrossRef]
56. Tsai, C.-C.; Chang, Y.-H.; Chang, C.-C.; Cheng, Y.-M.; Ou, Y.-C.; Chien, C.-C.C.; Hsu, Y.-C. Induction of apoptosis in endometrial cancer (Ishikawa) cells by *Pogostemon cablin* aqueous extract (PCAE). *Int. J. Mol. Sci.* **2015**, *16*, 12424–12435. [CrossRef]

57. Orengo, A.M.; Spoletini, L.; Procopio, A.; Favoni, R.E.; De Cupis, A.; Ardizzoni, A.; Castagneto, B.; Ribotta, M.; Betta, P.G.; Ferrini, S.; et al. Establishment of four new mesothelioma cell lines: Characterization by ultrastructural and immunophenotypic analysis. *Eur. Respir. J.* **1999**, *13*, 527–534. [CrossRef] [PubMed]
58. Ko, W.G.; Kang, T.H.; Lee, S.J.; Kim, Y.C.; Lee, B.H. Effects of luteolin on the inhibition of proliferation and induction ofapoptosis in human myeloid leukaemia cells. *Phytother. Res.* **2002**, *16*, 295–298. [CrossRef]
59. Singh Tuli, H.; Rath, P.; Chauhan, A.; Sak, K.; Aggarwal, D.; Choudhary, R.; Sharma, U.; Vashishth, K.; Sharma, S.; Kumar, M.; et al. Luteolin, a potent anticancer compound: From chemistry to cellular interactions and synergetic perspectives. *Cancers* **2022**, *14*, 5373. [CrossRef]
60. Lin, Y.; Shi, R.; Wang, X.; Shen, H.M. Luteolin, a flavonoid with potential for cancer prevention and therapy. *Curr. Cancer Drug Targets* **2008**, *8*, 634–646. [CrossRef]
61. Horinaka, M.; Yoshida, T.; Shiraishi, T.; Nakata, S.; Wakada, M.; Nakanishi, R.; Nishino, H.; Matsui, H.; Sakai, T. Luteolin induces apoptosis via death receptor 5 upregulation in human malignant tumor cells. *Oncogene* **2005**, *24*, 7180–7189. [CrossRef] [PubMed]
62. Gottlieb, H.E.; Kotlyar, V.; Nudelman, A. NMR Chemical shifts of common laboratory solvents as trace impurities. *J. Org. Chem.* **1997**, *62*, 7512–7515. [CrossRef] [PubMed]
63. Ersöz, T.; Harput, Ü.Ş.; Saragoğlu, İ.; Çaliş, I.; Ogihara, Y. Phenolic compounds from *Scutellaria pontica*. *Turk. J. Chem.* **2002**, *26*, 581–588.
64. Zhou, G.; Yan, R.; Wang, X.; Li, S.; Lin, J.; Liu, J.; Zhao, Z. The overlooked rotational isomerism of C-glycosyl flavonoids. *Phytochem. Rev.* **2019**, *18*, 443–461. [CrossRef]
65. Davoust, D.; Massias, M.; Molho, D. 13C-NMR investigation of flavonoid C-β-D-glucosides. Detection of a conformational equilibrium. *Org. Magn. Reson.* **1980**, *13*, 218–219. [CrossRef]
66. Osborne, A.G. ^{13}C NMR Spectral studies of some methoxycoumarin derivatives. A re-assignment for citropten (limettin) and an examination of peri-proximity effects for the methyl-methoxy and methoxy-methyl couples. *Magn. Reson. Chem.* **1989**, *27*, 348–354. [CrossRef]
67. Lee, H.-S.; Eun-Nam Kim, E.-N.; Jeong, G.-S. Ameliorative effect of citropten isolated from *Citrus aurantifolia* peel extract as a modulator of T cell and intestinal epithelial cell activity in DSS-induced colitis. *Molecules* **2022**, *27*, 4633. [CrossRef]
68. Qiu, H.; Xiao, X.; Li, G. Separation and purification of furanocoumarins from *Toddalia asiatica* (L.) Lam. using microwave-assisted extraction coupled with high-speed counter-current chromatography. *J. Sep. Sci.* **2012**, *35*, 901–906. [CrossRef] [PubMed]
69. O'Neill, T.; Johnson, J.A.; Webster, D.; Gray, C.A. The Canadian medicinal plant *Heracleum maximum* contains antimycobacterial diynes and furanocoumarins. *J. Ethnopharmacol.* **2013**, *147*, 232–237. [CrossRef] [PubMed]
70. Yili, A.; Mutalipu; Aisa, H.A.; Isaev, M.I. Betulinic acid and sterols from *Astragalus altaicus*. *Chem. Nat. Compd.* **2009**, *45*, 592–594. [CrossRef]

molecules

MDPI

Article

Non-Volatile Component and Antioxidant Activity: A Comparative Analysis between *Litsea cubeba* Branches and Leaves

Wei Dai [1], Boyi Li [2], Yanli Xiong [2], Liping Dai [1], Yuan Tian [3], Liangqian Zhang [3], Qi Wang [3,*] and Guoqiang Qian [2,*]

[1] Teaching and Experimental Center, Guangdong Pharmaceutical University, Guangzhou 510006, China; dai_gdpu_2018@gdpu.edu.cn (W.D.)

[2] School of Chinese Medicine, Guangdong Pharmaceutical University, Guangzhou 510006, China; xiongyanli106@163.com (Y.X.)

[3] Key Laboratory of Xinjiang Phytomedicine Resource and Utilization, Ministry of Education, School of Pharmacy, Shihezi University, Shihezi 832003, China

* Correspondence: wq_pha@shzu.edu.cn (Q.W.); tgqqian@gdpu.edu.cn (G.Q.)

Abstract: *Litsea cubeba*, which is found widely distributed across the Asian region, functions as both an economic tree and a medicinal plant with a rich historical background. Previous investigations into its chemical composition and biological activity have predominantly centered on volatile components, leaving the study of non-volatile components relatively unexplored. In this study, we employed UPLC-HRMS technology to analyze the non-volatile components of *L. cubeba* branches and leaves, which successfully resulted in identifying 72 constituents. Comparative analysis between branches and leaves unveiled alkaloids, organic acids, and flavonoids as the major components. However, noteworthy differences in the distribution of these components between branches and leaves were observed, with only eight shared constituents, indicating substantial chemical variations in different parts of *L. cubeba*. Particularly, 24 compounds were identified for the first time from this plant. The assessment of antioxidant activity using four methods (ABTS, DPPH, FRAP, and CUPRAC) demonstrated remarkable antioxidant capabilities in both branches and leaves, with slightly higher efficacy observed in branches. This suggests that *L. cubeba* may act as a potential natural antioxidant with applications in health and therapeutic interventions. In conclusion, the chemical composition and antioxidant activity of *L. cubeba* provides a scientific foundation for its development and utilization in medicine and health products, offering promising avenues for the rational exploitation of *L. cubeba* resources in the future.

Keywords: *Litsea cubeba*; non-volatile component; antioxidant activity; UPLC-HRMS

1. Introduction

Litsea cubeba, a member of the Lauraceae family in the *Litsea* genus, thrives primarily in China, India, Thailand, and various Asian countries [1]. Despite occupying a mere 0.04% of China's wild forest area, the *L. cubeba* tree stands out for its rich plant resources [2]. Recognized for its economic significance, *L. cubeba* has been an integral part of traditional Chinese folk medicine for generations. Its roots, stems, leaves, flowers, and fruits have been employed for medicinal purposes, offering remedies for dispelling wind and cold, reducing swelling, and alleviating pain [1,3].

A considerable amount of research has delved into unraveling the chemical constituents and biological activities of *L. cubeba*, with a predominant focus on its volatile components, especially the essential oil. The fruit and leaves of *L. cubeba*, rich in essential oils, exhibit a diverse composition of monoterpenes and sesquiterpenes [4]. Notably, citral predominates, widely used in toothpaste, soap, perfumes, and various pharmaceutical and chemical products [5–7]. While volatile components have received significant attention, there remains a noteworthy gap in exploring non-volatile components. Over 150 non-volatile components, including alkaloids, lignans, flavonoids, and terpenoids, have been identified in *L. cubeba*. Alkaloids and lignans, constituting over half of these components, emerge as prominent contributors with significant pharmacological activities [8–11]. Aporphine alkaloids, in particular, have demonstrated hypoglycemic, anti-inflammatory, and anti-cancer effects [12]. Despite these promising findings, research on non-volatile components remains comparatively limited, overshadowed by the predominant focus on essential oils. The imperative for an in-depth exploration of *L. cubeba*'s active ingredients and their potential pharmacological effects is evident.

Oxidative stress, implicated in the onset and progression of numerous diseases, poses a significant threat to human health, particularly in the context of neurodegenerative and cardiovascular diseases [13]. Addressing this challenge involves exploring exogenous antioxidants or enhancing endogenous antioxidant defenses. Plants, recognized as valuable repositories of secondary metabolites, emerge as promising sources of natural antioxidants. Studies underscore the potential of *L. cubeba* as a natural antioxidant, with its essential oil showcasing robust antioxidant activity [14,15]. Extracts from *L. cubeba* bark, including methanol, chloroform, *n*-butanol, and water extracts, also exhibit antioxidant activity [16].

Given the abundant resources of *L. cubeba*, and the relatively limited research on its non-volatile components, there is a need for a more comprehensive exploration to facilitate the rational development and utilization of this plant resource. This is particularly crucial for uncovering its broader medicinal value, with a specific focus on discovering its potential as a robust antioxidant. This study endeavors to bridge this knowledge gap, focusing on the branches and leaves of *L. cubeba*. Employing UPLC-HRMS, we aim to comprehensively identify non-volatile components in the methanol extract. The antioxidant activity will be assessed through standardized assays, including ABTS (2,2′-azino-bis(3-ethylbenzothiazoline-6-sulphonic acid)), DPPH (1,1-diphenyl-2-trinitrophenylhydrazine), FRAP (ferric reducing antioxidant power), and CUPRAC (cupric reducing antioxidant capacity). By meticulously comparing and analyzing differences in non-volatile components and antioxidant activity, this study aspires to provide a fresh perspective for the rational development and utilization of *L. cubeba* resources, potentially unlocking novel avenues in medicinal research.

2. Results

2.1. UPLC-HRMS Analysis of Non-Volatile Components from *L. cubeba* Branches and Leaves

The chemical composition of the methanol extracts from *L. cubeba* branches and leaves was analyzed using UPLC-Q-Orbitrap HRMS in both positive and negative ion modes. Figures S1–S4 in the Supplementary Materials present the total ion chromatograms of mass spectrometry analysis for the branches and leaves of *L. cubeba*. Detailed identification information for the compounds is provided in Table 1. A total of 72 compounds were identified in *L. cubeba*, comprising 23 alkaloids, 15 flavonoids, 14 organic acids, five amino acids, four alcohols, three carbohydrates, two ketones, two phenols, two esters, one ether, and one phenylpropanoid. Alkaloids, flavonoids, and organic acids emerged as the major chemical constituents of *L. cubeba*. Specifically, 36 and 44 compounds were identified in the branches and leaves of *L. cubeba*, respectively, with 24 compounds being identified for the first time from this plant. The discovery of these compounds significantly contributes to the chemical information available for *L. cubeba*.

Table 1. Compounds identified in the methanol extract of *L. cubeba* branches and leaves by UPLC-HRMS.

No.	RT/min		Compounds	Molecular Formula	Error/ppm	*m/z*	Ion Mode	Compound Types	References
	Leaves	Branches							
1	0.851	–	2-Aminosuccinamic acid	$C_4H_8N_2O_3$	−1.54	131.04599	$[M-H]^-$	alkaloids	[17]
2	0.88	–	Gluconic acid	$C_6H_{12}O_7$	−1.22	195.05079	$[M-H]^-$	carbohydrates	
3	0.89	–	L-Threonic acid	$C_4H_8O_5$	−1.26	135.02972	$[M-H]^-$	organic acids	[18]
4	0.893	–	D-(−)-Fructose	$C_6H_{12}O_6$	−0.76	179.05597	$[M-H]^-$	carbohydrates	[19]
5	0.904	–	D-(-)-Quinic acid	$C_7H_{12}O_6$	−0.89	191.05595	$[M-H]^-$	organic acids	[20]
6	0.908	–	L-Threonine	$C_4H_9NO_3$	−0.3	120.06559	$[M+H]^+$	amino acids	[21]
7	0.915	–	D-Glucosamine	$C_6H_{13}NO_5$	0	180.0867	$[M+H]^+$	carbohydrates	[22]
8	0.918	–	(2R)-2,3-Dihydroxypropanoic acid ★	$C_3H_6O_4$	−1.37	105.01919	$[M-H]^-$	organic acids	[23]
9	0.940	–	DL-Malic acid	$C_4H_6O_5$	−1.53	133.01403	$[M-H]^-$	organic acids	[24]
10	0.950	–	D-Serine ★	$C_3H_7NO_3$	−0.06	106.04986	$[M+H]^+$	amino acids	[25]
11	0.982	–	Proline	$C_5H_9NO_2$	0.5	116.07066	$[M+H]^+$	amino acids	[26]
12	0.998	–	Adenine	$C_5H_5N_5$	0.91	136.06189	$[M+H]^+$	alkaloids	[27]
13	1.019	–	Acetophenone	C_8H_8O	0.54	121.06486	$[M+H]^+$	ketones	[28]
14	–	1.024	4-Methoxycinnamaldehyde	$C_{10}H_{10}O_2$	−0.18	180.10186	$[M+H]^+$	ethers	
15	–	1.140	Higenamine ★	$C_{16}H_{17}NO_3$	0.31	272.1282	$[M+H]^+$	alkaloids	[29]
16	1.219	–	Citric acid	$C_6H_8O_7$	−0.32	191.01967	$[M-H]^-$	organic acids	[30]
17	1.232	–	Nicotinic acid	$C_6H_5NO_2$	0.14	124.03932	$[M+NH_4]^+$	alkaloids	[31]
18	1.238	–	Pipecolic acid	$C_6H_{11}NO_2$	0.45	130.08631	$[M+H]^+$	alkaloids	[32]
19	1.331	–	Methylmalonic acid	$C_4H_6O_4$	−1.03	117.01921	$[M-H]^-$	organic acids	[33]
20	1.335	–	Fumaric acid	$C_4H_4O_4$	−1.05	115.00356	$[M-H]^-$	organic acids	[34]
21	1.373	–	Isoleucine	$C_6H_{13}NO_2$	0.35	132.10195	$[M+H]^+$	amino acids	[35]
22	1.456	–	L-Norleucine	$C_6H_{13}NO_2$	0.41	132.10196	$[M+H]^+$	amino acids	[36]
23	–	1.615	L-N-Acetylphenylalaninol ★	$C_{11}H_{15}NO_2$	−0.04	194.11755	$[M+H]^+$	alkaloids	
24	–	1.989	(-)-Salsoline	$C_{11}H_{15}NO_2$	−0.17	194.11752	$[M+H]^+$	alkaloids	
25	2.089	–	Gentisic acid 5-O-β-glucoside ★	$C_{13}H_{16}O_9$	−0.85	315.07189	$[M-H]^-$	organic acids	
26	–	2.098	Indole-3-acetic acid	$C_{10}H_9NO_2$	−0.03	176.07061	$[M+H]^+$	alkaloids	[37]
27	–	3.396	trans-3-Indoleacrylic acid ★	$C_{11}H_9NO_2$	−0.39	188.07054	$[M+H]^+$	alkaloids	[38]
28	–	5.066	Norisoboldine	$C_{18}H_{19}NO_4$	0.42	314.13882	$[M+H]^+$	alkaloids	[39]
29	5.091	–	3-(4-Hydroxyphenyl)-3-oxopropyl β-D-glucopyranoside	$C_{15}H_{20}O_8$	−0.82	327.10827	$[M-H]^-$	phenols	[40]
30	5.888	5.261	Boldine	$C_{19}H_{21}NO_4$	−0.07	328.15432	$[M+H]^+$	alkaloids	[41]
31	5.486	–	Dihydrophaseic acid ★	$C_{15}H_{22}O_5$	−0.41	281.13933	$[M-H]^-$	organic acids	[42]
32	6.213	6.072	(S)-Boldine	$C_{19}H_{21}NO_4$	0.26	328.15442	$[M+H]^+$	alkaloids	[41]
33	6.636	6.487	Glaufinine	$C_{19}H_{21}NO_4$	0.07	328.15436	$[M+H]^+$	alkaloids	[43]

Table 1. *Cont.*

No.	RT/min		Compounds	Molecular Formula	Error/ppm	*m*/*z*	Ion Mode	Compound Types	References
	Leaves	Branches							
34	6.604	–	Kaempferol 3-sophoroside ★	$C_{27}H_{30}O_{16}$	−0.28	609.14594	$[M-H]^-$	flavonoids	[44]
35	–	6.765	Isocorydine	$C_{20}H_{23}NO_4$	0.26	342.17007	$[M+H]^+$	alkaloids	[45]
36	7.526	7.817	Rutin	$C_{27}H_{30}O_{16}$	−0.69	609.14558	$[M-H]^-$	flavonoids	[41]
37	–	7.117	Isoquercetin	$C_{21}H_{20}O_{12}$	−0.28	463.08796	$[M-H]^-$	flavonoids	[46]
38	7.316	–	Kaempferitrin	$C_{27}H_{30}O_{14}$	−0.31	577.15588	$[M-H]^-$	flavonoids	[47]
39	–	7.551	laurotetanine	$C_{19}H_{21}NO_4$	0.07	328.15436	$[M+H]^+$	alkaloids	[41]
40	7.557	–	5-(4-Hydroxypentyl)-1,3-benzenediol ★	$C_{11}H_{16}O_3$	−0.11	197.1172	$[M+H]^+$	phenols	
41	–	7.589	Corydine ★	$C_{20}H_{23}NO_4$	−0.21	342.16991	$[M+H]^+$	alkaloids	[43]
42	7.631	–	Trifolin ★	$C_{21}H_{20}O_{11}$	−0.34	447.09298	$[M-H]^-$	flavonoids	[48]
43	7.951	–	Cynaroside	$C_{21}H_{20}O_{11}$	−0.26	447.09299	$[M-H]^-$	flavonoids	[49]
44	–	8.048	Quercitrin	$C_{21}H_{20}O_{11}$	−0.36	447.09312	$[M-H]^-$	flavonoids	[41]
45	8.246	–	Cassythicin	$C_{19}H_{19}NO_4$	0.33	326.13879	$[M+H]^+$	alkaloids	[50]
46	–	8.349	Diosmin ★	$C_{28}H_{32}O_{15}$	−0.77	607.16638	$[M-H]^-$	flavonoids	[51]
47	–	8.503	Neohesperidin ★	$C_{28}H_{34}O_{15}$	−0.78	609.18202	$[M-H]^-$	flavonoids	[52]
48	–	8.644	Hesperetin	$C_{16}H_{14}O_6$	0.57	303.08649	$[M+H]^+$	flavonoids	[53]
49	–	8.648	Hesperidin	$C_{28}H_{34}O_{15}$	0.65	611.19739	$[M+H]^+$	flavonoids	[54]
50	9.196	–	Afzelin	$C_{21}H_{20}O_{10}$	−0.63	431.0981	$[M-H]^-$	flavonoids	[55]
51	9.443	–	Kaempferol ★	$C_{15}H_{10}O_6$	0.05	287.05503	$[M+H]^+$	flavonoids	[56]
52	–	9.930	N-p-Coumaroyltyramine	$C_{17}H_{17}NO_3$	0.32	284.12821	$[M+H]^+$	phenylpropanoids	[57]
53	–	10.391	Crebanine	$C_{20}H_{21}NO_4$	0.3	340.15444	$[M+H]^+$	alkaloids	[58]
54	10.576	10.454	Moupinamide	$C_{18}H_{19}NO_4$	0.24	314.13876	$[M+H]^+$	alkaloids	[59]
55	10.869	–	Tiliroside ★	$C_{30}H_{26}O_{13}$	−0.92	593.12952	$[M-H]^-$	flavonoids	[60]
56	14.447	14.029	15-Hexadecynoic acid ★	$C_{16}H_{28}O_2$	−0.2	253.21616	$[M+H]^+$	organic acids	
57	14.508	–	3-[[6-Deoxy-3,4-bis-O-[(2E)-3-(4-hydroxyphenyl)-1-oxo-2-propen-1-yl]-α-L-mannopyranosyl]oxy]-5,7-dihydroxy-2-(4-hydroxyphenyl)-4H-1-benzopyran-4-one	$C_{39}H_{32}O_{14}$	−0.9	723.17128	$[M-H]^-$	flavonoids	[61]
58	15.609	15.177	Lauryldimethylamine oxide ★	$C_{14}H_{31}NO$	−0.09	230.24782	$[M+H]^+$	alkaloids	[62]
59	–	16.099	Aurantiamide acetate	$C_{27}H_{28}N_2O_4$	0.05	445.21222	$[M+H]^+$	alkaloids	[63]
60	–	16.286	2-Amino-1,3,4-octadecanetriol ★	$C_{18}H_{39}NO_3$	0.55	318.30045	$[M+H]^+$	alcohols	[64]
61	–	16.290	4-Ethylbenzaldehyde	$C_9H_{10}O$	0.59	135.08052	$[M+H]^+$	esters	[65]
62	–	16.297	4-Ethoxy ethylbenzoate	$C_{11}H_{14}O_3$	−0.12	195.10155	$[M+H]^+$	esters	[66]
63	16.529	–	Schinifoline ★	$C_{17}H_{23}NO$	−0.02	258.18524	$[M+H]^+$	alkaloids	[67]

Table 1. *Cont.*

No.	RT/min		Compounds	Molecular Formula	Error/ppm	m/z	Ion Mode	Compound Types	References
	Leaves	Branches							
64	16.882	16.919	1,3:2,4-Di(p-ethylbenzylidene)sorbitol ★	$C_{24}H_{30}O_6$	0.51	415.2117	$[M + H]^+$	alcohols	
65	–	17.097	9-Oxo-ODE	$C_{18}H_{30}O_3$	0.09	295.2268	$[M + H]^+$	organic acids	[68]
66	–	17.368	13(S)-HOTrE	$C_{18}H_{30}O_3$	0.08	293.21224	$[M - H]^-$	organic acids	[69]
67	–	18.395	9-Oxo-10(E),12(E)-octadecadienoic acid	$C_{18}H_{30}O_3$	0.4	295.22687	$[M + H]^+$	organic acids	[70]
68	–	19.147	12-Oxo-10,15(Z)-phytodienoic acid ★	$C_{18}H_{28}O_3$	0.45	293.21124	$[M + H]^+$	organic acids	
69	–	19.440	Linoleoyl ethanolamide ★	$C_{20}H_{37}NO_2$	0.28	324.28979	$[M + H]^+$	alcohols	[71]
70	–	20.267	Sphingosine (d18:1) ★	$C_{18}H_{37}NO_2$	0.6	300.28989	$[M + H]^+$	alcohols	[72]
71	21.806	–	Muscone	$C_{16}H_{30}O$	−0.21	239.23689	$[M + H]^+$	ketones	[73]
72	21.829	–	Pheophorbide A ★	$C_{35}H_{36}N_4O_5$	0.14	593.27594	$[M + H]^+$	alkaloids	

–: not detected, ★: indicates compounds identified for the first time from *L. cubeba*.

2.1.1. Analysis of Non-Volatile Components in Branches

Within the *L. cubeba* branches, a total of 36 non-volatile compounds were identified, encompassing 16 alkaloids (No. 15, 23, 24, 26, 27, 28, 30, 32, 33, 35, 39, 41, 53, 54, 58, and 59). These alkaloids comprised 11 isoquinoline alkaloids (No. 15, 23, 24, 28, 30, 32, 33, 35, 39, 41, and 53), two indole alkaloids (No. 26 and 27), two amide alkaloids (No. 54 and 59), and one other alkaloid (No. 59). Additionally, seven flavonoids (No. 36, 37, 44, 46, 47, 48, and 49), five organic acids (No. 56, 65, 66, 67, and 68), four alcohols (No. 60, 64, 69, and 70), two esters (No. 61 and 62), one ether (No. 14), and one phenylpropanoid (No. 52) were identified. Alkaloids constituted the major component, accounting for nearly 45% of the identified compounds. The sum of flavonoids, organic acids, and alcohol compounds also represented approximately 45% of the total identified compounds in the branches.

2.1.2. Analysis of Non-Volatile Components in Leaves

In *L. cubeba* leaves, a total of 44 non-volatile compounds were identified, including 12 alkaloids (No. 1, 12, 17, 18, 30, 32, 33, 45, 54, 58, 63, and 72). Among the alkaloids, four were isoquinoline alkaloids (No. 30, 32, 33, and 45), two were amide alkaloids (No. 1 and 54), two were pyridine alkaloids (No. 17 and 18), one was a purine alkaloid (No. 12), one was a pyrrolidine alkaloid (No. 72), one was a quinoline alkaloid (63), and one was classified as other (No. 58). Additionally, 10 organic acids (No. 3, 5, 8, 9, 16, 19, 20, 25, 31, and 56), nine flavonoids (No. 34, 36, 38, 42, 43, 50, 51, 55, and 57), five amino acid compounds (No. 6, 10, 11, 21, and 22), three carbohydrates (No. 2, 4, and 7), two phenols (No. 29 and 40), two ketones (No. 29 and 40), and one alcohol were identified. Alkaloids, organic acids, and flavonoids were the major constituents of *L. cubeba* leaves, constituting over 70% of the total identified compounds.

2.2. *Comparative Analysis of Non-Volatile Components in Branches and Leaves*

The comparative analysis of non-volatile components in the methanol extracts of *L. cubeba* branches and leaves revealed substantial differences in their chemical compositions (Figure 1). Out of the 72 identified compounds in *L. cubeba*, only eight (No. 30, 32, 33, 36, 54, 56, 58, and 64) were common to both branches and leaves. Leaves displayed 36 unique compounds (No. 1, 2, 3, 4, 5, 6, 7, 8, 9, 10, 11, 12, 13, 16, 17, 18, 19, 20, 21, 22, 25, 29, 31, 34, 38, 40, 42, 43, 45, 50, 51, 55, 57, 63, 71, and 72), while branches had 28 unique compounds (No. 14, 15, 23, 24, 26, 27, 28, 35, 37, 39, 41, 44, 46, 47, 48, 49, 52, 53, 59, 60, 61, 62, 65, 66, 67, 68, 69, and 70). These distinctive compounds underscore pronounced differences in their chemical profiles.

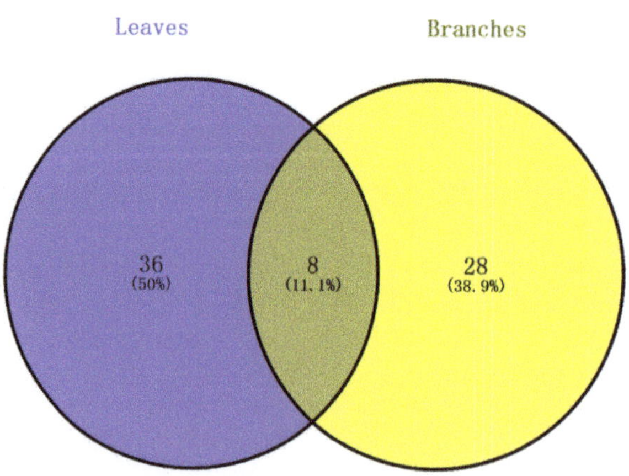

Figure 1. Venn diagram of the non-volatile components of *L. cubeba* branches and leaves.

Alkaloids constituted a major component in both branches and leaves, sharing several compounds such as No. 30, 32, 33, 54, and 58. However, variations exist in the types of alkaloids, with branches primarily featuring isoquinoline alkaloids and leaves encompassing isoquinoline, amide, and other alkaloid categories. Organic acids were prevalent in both branches and leaves, with compound 56 being the sole shared compound (15-Hexadecynoic acid). Nevertheless, other organic acid components exhibited significant differences. Flavonoids, another major class, were identified in both parts, with only Rutin (compound 36) being a shared compound. Other flavonoids were unique to either branches or leaves. Notable distinctions were observed in alcohol and ester content, with branches featuring a higher representation of compounds (No. 60, 64, 69, 70, 61, and 62). Amino acids were exclusively found in leaves (No. 6, 10, 11, 21, and 22). Phenols and ketones were unique to leaves (No. 29 and 40).

In conclusion, while alkaloids, organic acids, and flavonoids were major components in both branches and leaves, the number of shared components was limited. The presence of unique compounds in each part contributed significantly to their distinct chemical profiles, enhancing our understanding of the chemical diversity of *L. cubeba* and the potential biological activities associated with its various components.

2.3. *Antioxidant Activity*

Results of Four In Vitro Antioxidant Activity Tests

The evaluation of in vitro antioxidant activity involves various methods based on different principles, with the most commonly utilized ones being ABTS, DPPH, FRAP, and CUPRAC. ABTS and DPPH assess the antioxidant capacity of samples through measuring absorbance change resulting from the reduction of their respective free radicals under the influence of oxidants. In contrast, FRAP and CUPRAC characterize the activity of antioxidants through reducing metal ions to lower oxidation states and measuring their generation. The comprehensive application of these methods provides a nuanced understanding of antioxidant potential within samples. In this study, we assessed the in vitro antioxidant activity of methanol extracts from both branches and leaves of *L. cubeba* using ABTS, DPPH, FRAP, and CUPRAC methods. For the ABTS, DPPH, and FRAP experiments, antioxidant capacity was expressed as TEAC μmol/g, where higher values signify greater antioxidant capability. For the FRAP method, results were indicated as Fe (II) μmol/g, with higher values reflecting stronger reducing power and thus greater antioxidant potential. The methanol extracts from *L. cubeba* branches exhibited the following results for the four antioxidant assays, as shown in Table 2. These antioxidant activity data indicate that both branches and leaves of *L. cubeba* possess considerable antioxidant capabilities, with a slight predominance in the antioxidant capacity of the branches over the leaves.

Table 2. Antioxidant activity of methanol extracts from branches and leaves of *L. cubeba*.

Parts	ABTS (TEAC μmol/g)	DPPH (TEAC μmol/g)	FRAP (Fe(II) μmol/g)	CUPRAC (TEAC μmol/g)
Branches	42.75 ± 3.94	7.55 ± 0.43	22.21 ± 0.53	42.65 ± 0.35
Leaves	57.78 ± 1.87	9.29 ± 0.39	28.68 ± 0.78	45.89 ± 0.27

3. Discussion

In this investigation, UPLC-HRMS technology facilitated the rapid and precise analysis of non-volatile components within *L. cubeba* branches and leaves. The established analytical method for non-volatile components offered insights into the diverse compounds present in these plant parts, contributing detailed information to enhance our understanding of the plant's chemical characteristics. The identification of 72 compounds, including alkaloids, flavonoids, and organic acids, underscored the chemical diversity of *L. cubeba*. Moreover, methanol extracts from both branches and leaves exhibited noteworthy antioxidant activity in vitro.

While the results align with some previously reported chemical compositions, this study uncovered 24 compounds not documented before, enriching our comprehensive understanding of *L. cubeba* compounds and supporting its chemical taxonomy, development, and utilization [74]. Alkaloids, especially isoquinoline alkaloids, emerged as significant components in the non-volatile fraction of *L. cubeba*, aligning with prior research [74]. Intriguingly, a higher abundance of isoquinoline alkaloids in branches compared to leaves was observed. Further analysis of alkaloid differences identified eight shared compounds, five of which belonged to the alkaloid category (compounds 30, 32, 33, 54, and 58). The predominance of isoquinoline alkaloids in branches, and the greater diversity of alkaloid types in leaves, suggest potential variations in pharmacological activities. Known for their diverse biological activities, especially in pharmaceutical research, the abundance of isoquinoline alkaloids in *L. cubeba* implies their essential role in its medicinal effects.

Flavonoids, renowned for their antioxidant properties, were identified as major components in both branches and leaves of *L. cubeba*. The presence of the shared compound rutin (compound 36) suggests common antioxidant capabilities. However, unique flavonoid compositions in each part may contribute to subtle differences in antioxidant activity. The study also confirmed the presence of organic acids, a less explored aspect of *L. cubeba* chemistry. The only shared organic acid between the branches and leaves was 15-hexadecynoic acid (compound 56), indicating potential variations in their health-promoting properties. Beyond the primary compound categories, differences in alcohols, esters, amino acids, and phenols between the branches and leaves add layers to the plant's chemical diversity, potentially influencing related biological activities and the potential medicinal value of *L. cubeba*.

The assessment of antioxidant potential using ABTS, DPPH, FRAP, and CUPRAC assays demonstrated significant antioxidant capabilities in both the branch and leaf extracts, with a slightly higher antioxidant capacity observed in the branches. In comparison with antioxidant capacities of traditional medicinal plants, such as *Angelica dahurica*, *Fritillaria cirrhosa*, and *Perilla frutescens*, *L. cubeba* branches and leaves exhibited superior or comparable antioxidant abilities [75]. The plant's rich content of alkaloids, flavonoids, and organic acids, known for their antioxidant properties, likely contributes to its robust antioxidant activity, emphasizing the potential health benefits of *L. cubeba* in traditional herbal applications.

In summary, this comparative analysis highlights the diverse chemical characteristics and antioxidant capabilities of *L. cubeba* branches and leaves. As a botanical resource, *L. cubeba* exhibits unique features in terms of chemical composition and antioxidant activity, providing a theoretical foundation for its applications in medicine and the food industry. Future research could delve deeper into the biological activities and pharmacological effects of *L. cubeba* compounds to explore its potential health benefits. This study offers valuable information for the development and utilization of *L. cubeba*, laying a scientific foundation for its diverse applications.

4. Materials and Methods

4.1. Plant Material and Extraction

4.1.1. Plant Material

L. cubeba was sourced from Yunfu, China, in April 2023, and Dr. Xinger Ye, affiliated with the College of Traditional Chinese Medicine Resources at Guangdong Pharmaceutical University, authenticated the plant materials.

4.1.2. Preparation of Liquid-Sample Solution for Mass Spectrometry

The dried leaves and stems of *L. cubeba* were individually pulverized using the DFY-300C Swing Crusher from Wenling Linda Machinery Co., Ltd, Wenling, China. Approximately 1.0 g of each sample powder was precisely weighed into a 100 mL conical flask. Analytical methanol (50 mL) was added accurately, and the mixture was re-weighed. The Q-500DE ultrasound equipment (Dongguan Keqiao Ultrasonic Equipment Co., Ltd., Dongguan, China) was used for ultrasonic extraction at 50 °C with 500 W power and 40 kHz frequency for 30 min. After cooling, the sample was re-weighed, and any weight loss was compensated by adding methanol. Ten milliliters of the upper clear liquid were transferred to a centrifuge tube, and centrifuged at 2200× *g* for 15 min using a high-speed centrifuge. Two hundred microliters of the supernatant were extracted, mixed with 800 μL of chromatographic methanol, diluted to 1 mL, thoroughly mixed, and then filtered through a 0.22 μm microporous membrane. The resultant filtered solution served as the liquid–sample solution for mass spectrometry.

4.1.3. Preparation of Samples for Antioxidant Activity Testing

For antioxidant activity testing, 1.0 g of *L. cubeba* leaves and branches powder was precisely weighed and combined with 40 mL of methanol. Ultrasonic extraction was conducted at 50 °C using an ultrasonic power of 500 W (frequency, 40 kHz) for 50 min, followed by filtration and rotary evaporation to obtain the respective extracts. The yield was 117.7 mg for leaf extract and 61.4 mg for branch extract. The extracts were dissolved in 15 mL of methanol. Based on preliminary experiments, the leaf methanol extract was diluted 10 times, and the branch methanol extract was diluted 5 times to produce the test solutions.

4.2. *The Main Chemicals and Reagents*

Analytical grade methanol from Da Mao Chemical Reagent Co., Ltd., Tianjin, China; chromatography-grade acetonitrile from Honeywell Trading (Shanghai) Co., Ltd., Shanghai, China; and distilled water from Watsons, Hong Kong, China. The total antioxidant capacity assay kits (ABTS, DPPH, FRAP methods) were obtained from Shanghai Macklin Biochemical Technology Co., Ltd., Shanghai, China, and the liquid sample total antioxidant capacity assay kit (Cu^{2+} method) was sourced from Beijing Applygen Technology Co., Ltd., Beijing, China.

4.3. *UPLC-HRMS Analysis*

4.3.1. Instrumentation and Conditions

The analysis employed the Vanquish Flex UPLC system, coupled with the Orbitrap Exploris 120 quadrupole electrostatic field orbital well high-resolution mass spectrometer for UPLC-Q-Orbitrap HRMS, sourced from Thermo Fisher Scientific (Waltham, MA, USA). A Hypersil GOLD C_{18} column (100 mm × 2.1 mm, 1.9 μm) was used for chromatographic analysis with a flow rate of 0.3 mL·min^{-1}, maintaining the column temperature at 35 °C. A 2.00 μL sample was injected into the system. The mobile phase comprised acetonitrile (A) and a 0.1% formic acid solution (B). The gradient elution profile was programmed as follows: starting at 95% B for 5 min, gradually decreasing to 80% B from 5 to 8 min, further decreasing to 75% B from 8 to 20 min, reducing to 5% B from 20 to 22 min, holding at 5% B from 22 to 22.001 min, and finally increasing to 95% B from 22.001 to 25 min.

The mass spectrometry analysis utilized positive and negative ion switching scan modes (Full scan/dd-MS^2). H-ESI ionization was employed with an electrospray voltage of 3.5 kV (+)/2.8 kV (−). The ion transfer tube temperature was set at 325 °C, and the auxiliary gas temperature was maintained at 350 °C, RF Lens at 70%. Nitrogen served as nebulizing gas, auxiliary gas, and sheath gas. The flow rates for sheath gas, auxiliary gas, and sheath gas were 50 Arb, 8 Arb, and 1 Arb, respectively. Primary and secondary resolutions were set at 60,000 (MS) and 15,000 (MS^2), respectively. The ion scan range (m/z) was 100–1500, and the collision energy was normalized. The gradient for collision energy was set at 20%, 40%, and 60%.

4.3.2. Data Analysis and Identification of Compounds

The original data files were processed using Compound Discoverer 3.3 software provided by Thermo Fisher Scientific (Waltham, MA, USA), employing a compound identification method template. This involved peak area extraction, alignment, and matching secondary fragment spectra against the mzCloud network database and the local database mzVault. Filtering criteria included mass deviation control, optimal scores, and comparison with compound information in the compound library. Subsequent analysis of compounds included cross-referencing with literature and online databases (PubChem, CNKI, PubMed) for enhanced understanding.

4.4. Antioxidant Activity

4.4.1. ABTS Radical Scavenging Assay

The ABTS assay followed the Total Antioxidant Capacity Assay Kit. ABTS solution was combined with an oxidizing agent, and the resulting mixture served as the working solution. After 12–16 h of dark storage at room temperature, the ABTS working solution underwent dilution with 80% ethanol, and the absorbance at 734 nm was measured using an Agilent Synergy H1 microplate reader (Agilent Technologies, Inc., VT, USA) until reaching 0.7 ± 0.05 absorbance units. Test and standard solutions were mixed with the ABTS working solution in a 96-well plate, and absorbance at 734 nm was recorded after incubation. Trolox served as the standard, and a series of Trolox standard solutions (0.15, 0.3, 0.6, 0.9, 1.2, 1.5 mM) were prepared. The total antioxidant capacity of each sample was expressed as μmol Trolox/g of herbal medicine dry weight [76].

4.4.2. DPPH Radical Scavenging Assay

The DPPH assay followed the Total Antioxidant Capacity Assay Kit. Test and standard solutions were mixed with the reagent, and after a 20-min dark reaction at room temperature, absorbance was measured at 515 nm using a microplate reader. Trolox served as the standard, and a series of Trolox standard solutions (0.18, 0.15, 0.12, 0.09, 0.06, 0.03 mM) were prepared. The total antioxidant capacity of each sample was expressed as μmol Trolox/g of herbal medicine dry weight [77].

4.4.3. Ferric Reducing Ability of Plasma (FRAP) Assay

The FRAP assay followed the Total Antioxidant Capacity Assay Kit. The FRAP working solution was prepared by mixing TPTZ (2,4,6-tris(2-pyridyl)-s-triazine) diluent, TPTZ solution, and detection buffer solution at a ratio of 10:1:1 ($v/v/v$). After incubation at 37 °C and using within 1–2 h, test and standard solutions were mixed with the FRAP working solution in a 96-well plate and incubated at 37 °C for 3–5 min. After cooling to room temperature, the absorbance of the mixture was recorded at 593 nm using a microplate reader. $FeSO_4$ served as the standard, and a series of $FeSO_4$ standard solutions (0.15, 0.3, 0.6, 0.9, 1.2, 1.5 mM) were prepared. The total antioxidant capacity of each sample was expressed as μmol Fe(II)/g of herbal medicine dry weight [78].

4.4.4. Cupric Reducing Antioxidant Capacity (CUPRAC) Assay

The CUPRAC assay followed the Total Antioxidant Capacity Assay Kit (Cu^{2+} method). The Cu^{2+} working solution was prepared by mixing Cu^{2+} chelating agent solution and Cu^{2+} solution at a ratio of 50:1 (v/v). Test and standard solutions were mixed with the Cu^{2+} working solution in a 96-well plate, incubated at room temperature for 30 min, and absorbance was measured at 570 nm using a microplate reader. Trolox served as the standard, and a series of Trolox standard solutions (1, 0.5, 0.25, 0.125, 0.062, 0.031 mM) were prepared. The total antioxidant capacity of each sample was expressed as μmol Trolox/g of herbal medicine dry weight [79].

4.4.5. Construction of Standard Curves

In this study, standard curves were constructed for the ABTS, DPPH, FRAP, and CUPRAC assays. The ABTS assay's standard curve correlated absorbance values with known Trolox (6-hydroxy-2,5,7,8-etramethylchroman-2-carboxylic acid) concentrations, facilitating the calculation of Trolox Equivalent Antioxidant Capacity (TEAC) using a linear regression equation. Similarly, the DPPH assay utilized absorbance values correlated with various Trolox concentrations to generate a standard curve, enabling the conversion of experimental sample absorbance readings to TEAC values through a linear equation. For the FRAP assay, we created a standard curve by plotting absorbance against different concentrations of Fe(II). The resulting linear regression equation was then applied to compute the FRAP of the tested samples. Likewise, the CUPRAC assay employed a standard curve established with known Trolox concentrations, utilizing the linear equation to quantify the CUPRAC of the samples. These standard curves not only formed the foundation for quantification and data analysis but also enhanced the accuracy and reliability of antioxidant activity assessments. Refer to Figure 2 for the standard curves, and Table 3 for the corresponding equations. The R^2 values, ranging from 0.99133 to 0.99987, indicate excellent linearity, meeting the required standards.

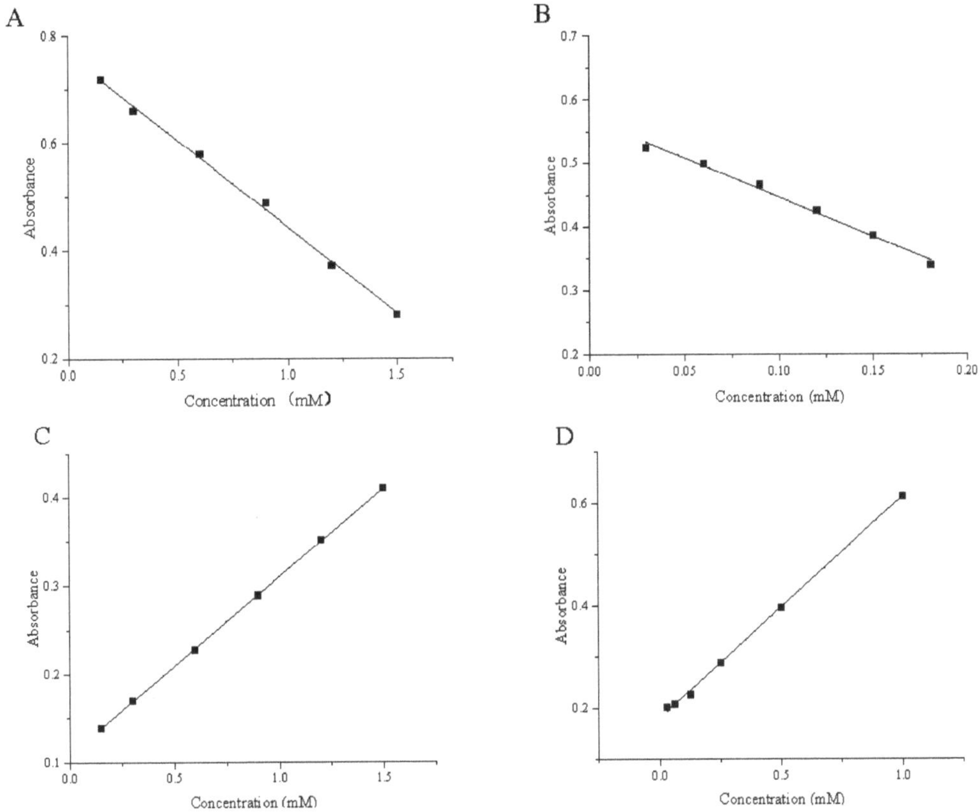

Figure 2. Standard curves for four antioxidant activity methods. ((**A**) Standard curve for Trolox in the ABTS method; (**B**) Standard curve for Trolox in the DPPH method; (**C**) Standard curve for Fe (II) in the FRAP method; (**D**) Standard curve for Trolox in the CUPRAC method).

Table 3. Standard curve equations for four antioxidant activity methods.

Method	Equation	R^2
ABTS	y = −0.32338x + 0.76745	0.99755
DPPH	y = −1.23810x + 0.57000	0.99133
FRAP	y = 0.20124x + 0.10870	0.99987
CUPRAC	y = 0.43161x + 0.18027	0.99903

4.4.6. Statistical Analysis

The experiments were conducted in triplicate, and the results were reported as the mean ± standard deviation.

5. Conclusions

Through a comparative analysis of the non-volatile components and antioxidant activity in the branches and leaves of the traditional medicinal plant *L. cubeba*, we unveiled its diverse chemical composition, encompassing alkaloids, flavonoids, and organic acids across various categories. This underscores its potential as a valuable resource in traditional herbal medicine and the food industry. The distinct variations in alkaloids, organic acids, and flavonoids between the branches and leaves suggest potential differences in their suitability for various applications. Supporting our observations, UPLC-HRMS technology identified 72 constituents, unveiling significant chemical heterogeneity between the branches and leaves, with only eight components shared. This comprehensive characterization contributes to our understanding of *L. cubeba*'s chemical diversity. Regarding antioxidant activity, both the branches and leaves exhibited significant capabilities, with the branches demonstrating slightly higher efficacy. Consistent support from ABTS, DPPH, FRAP, and CUPRAC methods underscores the robust antioxidant potential within *L. cubeba*. This suggests *L. cubeba*'s promising role as a natural antioxidant with implications for health and therapeutic interventions. In summary, *L. cubeba* stands out as a botanical resource with unique chemical composition and potent antioxidant properties, providing theoretical support for its applications in medicine and the food industry. The identified chemical diversity and robust antioxidant activity lay a solid scientific foundation for further exploration. Future research endeavors could delve deeper into the biological activities and pharmacological effects of *L. cubeba* compounds, enhancing our understanding of its potential health benefits. This study contributes valuable insights for the ongoing exploration and utilization of *L. cubeba* in various fields.

Supplementary Materials: The following supporting information can be downloaded at: https://www.mdpi.com/article/10.3390/molecules29040788/s1, Figures S1–S4: UPLC-Q-Orbitrap HRMS chromatograms of *Litsea cubeba*.

Author Contributions: Conceptualization, W.D., Q.W. and G.Q.; methodology, L.D. and Q.W.; software, Y.T. and B.L.; validation, W.D. and Y.T.; formal analysis, L.Z. and Y.X.; investigation, Y.T. and L.Z.; resources, W.D.; data curation, Y.T. and L.Z.; writing—original draft preparation, W.D. and B.L.; writing—review and editing, G.Q. and Q.W.; funding acquisition, W.D. and G.Q. All authors have read and agreed to the published version of the manuscript.

Funding: This research was funded by the following: Guangzhou Basic Research Program Fund Project (No. 202102020630); Scientific research project of Guangdong Provincial Administration of Traditional Chinese Medicine (No. 20231208); Guangdong Medical Research Fund (No. B2021324).

Institutional Review Board Statement: Not applicable.

Informed Consent Statement: Not applicable.

Data Availability Statement: Data are contained within the article and supplementary materials.

Conflicts of Interest: The authors declare no conflicts of interest.

References

1. Editorial Committee of Flora of China, Chinese Academy of Science. *Flora of China*, 1st ed.; Science Press: Beijing, China, 1993; Volume 31, pp. 271–272.
2. Ru, H.; Liu, M.; Liao, T.; Zhu, J.J. Analysis on technological innovation ability and competitive situation of *Litsea cubeba* industry from the perspective of patent, Hunan. *For. Sci. Tec.* **2022**, *49*, 89–94.
3. Yu, L.Y.; Jia, D.; Shen, H.; Sun, X.L.; Qin, L.P.; Han, T. Anti-inflammatory study on 9,9′-O-di-(E)-feruloyl-meso-5,5′-dimethoxysecoisolariciresinol (LCA), an active ingredient in *Litsea cubeba* (Lour.) Pers. *J. Pha. Pra.* **2020**, *38*, 216–220.
4. Zhang, L.; Chen, X.S.; Fan, G.R.; Liao, S.L.; Wang, Z.D. Research progress in application and functions of *Litsea cubeba* essential oil components. *Agric. Univ. Jiangxiensis* **2021**, *43*, 355–363.

5. Li, X.Y.; Gou, Y.H.; Shen, H.J.; Li, Y.H.; Wang, T.; Yin, L.Z. Antibacterial mechanism of *Litsea cubeba* essential oil on Salmonella. *J. Sci. Agric. Uni.* **2021**, *39*, 385–390.
6. Liu, T.; Yang, T.S. Antimicrobial impact of the components of essential oil of *Litsea cubeba* from Taiwan and antimicrobial activity of the oil in food systems. *Int. J. Food. Mic.* **2012**, *156*, 68–75. [CrossRef]
7. Xiang, Y.J.; Wang, H.H.; Sun, Y.D. Advances in the application of *Litsea cubeba* oil. *Chin. J. Cer.* **2020**, *35*, 186–195.
8. Zhang, S.Y.; Guo, Q.; Gao, X.L.; Guo, Z.Q.; Zhao, Y.F.; Chai, X.Y.; Tu, O.F. A phytochemical and pharmacological advance on medicinal plant *Litsea cubeba* (Lauraceae). *Chin. Herb. Med.* **2014**, *39*, 769–776.
9. Feng, T.; Xu, Y.; Cai, X.H.; Du, Z.Z.; Luo, X.D. Antimicrobially Active Isoquinoline Alkaloids from *Litsea cubeba*. *Planta Med.* **2009**, *75*, 76–79. [CrossRef]
10. Guo, Q.; Bai, R.F.; Su, G.Z.; Zhu, Z.X.; Zeng, K.W.; Tu, P.F.; Chai, X.Y. Chemical Constituents from the Roots and Stems of *Litsea cubeba*. *J. Asian Nat. Prod. Res.* **2016**, *18*, 51–58. [CrossRef]
11. Lee, S.S.; Chen, C.K.; Huang, F.M.; Chen, C.H. Two dibenzopyrrocoline alkaloids from *Litsea cubeba*. *J. Nat. Prod.* **1996**, *59*, 80–82. [CrossRef]
12. Zhang, S.S.; Tan, Q.W.; Guan, L.P. Antioxidant, anti-inflammatory, antibacterial, and analgesic activities and mechanisms of quinolines, indoles and related derivatives. *Mini Rev. Med. Chem.* **2021**, *21*, 2261–2275. [CrossRef] [PubMed]
13. Diniz Vilela, D.; Gomes Peixoto, L.; Teixeira, R.R.; Belele Baptista, N.; Carvalho Caixeta, D.; de Souza, A.V.; Machado, H.L.; Pereira, M.N.; Sabino-Silva, R.; Espindola, F.S. The Role of Metformin in Controlling Oxidative Stress in Muscle of Diabetic Rats. *Oxid. Med. Cell Longev.* **2016**, *2016*, 6978625. [CrossRef] [PubMed]
14. Liu, S.; Zhao, C.; Cao, Y.; Li, Y.; Zhang, Z.; Nie, D.; Tang, W.; Li, Y. Comparison of Chemical Compositions and Antioxidant Activity of Essential Oils from *Litsea cubeba*, Cinnamon, Anise, and Eucalyptus. *Molecules* **2023**, *28*, 5051. [CrossRef] [PubMed]
15. She, Q.H.; Li, W.S.; Jiang, Y.Y.; Wu, Y.C.; Zhou, Y.H.; Zhang, L. Chemical Composition, Antimicrobial Activity, and Antioxidant Activity of *Litsea cubeba* Essential Oils in Different Months. *Nat. Prod. Res.* **2020**, *34*, 3285–3288. [CrossRef]
16. Hwang, J.K.; Choi, E.M.; Lee, J.H. Antioxidant activity of *Litsea cubeba*. *Fitoterapia* **2005**, *76*, 684–686. [CrossRef]
17. Zhang, Y.; Fang, H.; Zhang, Y. Study on formation of acrylamide in asparagine-sugar microwave heating systems using UPLC–MS/MS analytical method. *Food Chem.* **2008**, *108*, 542–550. [CrossRef]
18. Zhang, L.; Wang, X.Y.; Guo, J.Z.; Xia, Q.L.; Zhao, G.; Zhou, H.N.; Xie, F.W. Metabolic profiling of Chinese *tobacco* leaf of different geographical origins by GC–MS. *J. Agric. Food Chem.* **2013**, *61*, 2597–2605. [CrossRef]
19. Shen, Q.Y.; Yang, R.J.; Hua, X.; Ye, F.Y.; Wang, H.; Zhao, W.; Wang, K. Enzymatic synthesis and identification of oligosaccharides obtained by transgalactosylation of lactose in the presence of fructose using β-galactosidase from *Kluyveromyces lactis*. *Food Chem.* **2012**, *135*, 1547–1554. [CrossRef]
20. Clifford, M.N.; Knight, S.; Kuhnert, N. Discriminating between the six isomers of dicaffeoylquinic acid by LC-MSn. *J. Agric. Food Chem.* **2005**, *53*, 3821–3832. [CrossRef]
21. Gale, T.V.; Schieffelin, J.S.; Branco, L.M.; Garry, R.F.; Grant, D.S. Elevated L-threonine is a biomarker for Lassa fever and Ebola. *Virol. J.* **2020**, *17*, 188. [CrossRef]
22. Song, M.; Hang, T.J.; Wang, C.; Yang, L.; Wen, A.D. Precolumn derivatization LC-MS/MS method for the determination and pharmacokinetic study of glucosamine in human plasma and urine. *J. Pharm. Anal.* **2012**, *2*, 19–28. [CrossRef] [PubMed]
23. Ma, J.S.; Xu, R.Y.; Wang, B.K.; Qi, Q.; Zhang, C.N. Metabolomics analysis reveals the protective effect of fructooligosaccharide on abnormal metabolism of liver in *Megalobrama amblycephala* induced by *Aeromonas hydrophila*. *Aquacult. Int.* **2023**, *2023*, 1–18. [CrossRef]
24. Fernandez-Fernandez, R.; Lopez-Martinez, J.C.; Romero-Gonzalez, R.; Martinez-Vidal, J.L.; Flores, M.I.A.; Garrido Frenich, A. Simple LC–MS determination of citric and malic acids in fruits and vegetables. *Chromatographia* **2010**, *72*, 55–62. [CrossRef]
25. Moussa, S.; Van Horn, M.R.; Shah, A.; Pollegioni, L.; Thibodeaux, C.J.; Ruthazer, E.S.; Mauzeroll, J. Editors' choice—A miniaturized enzymatic biosensor for detection of sensory–evoked D–serine release in the brain. *J. Electrochem. Soc.* **2021**, *168*, 025502. [CrossRef]
26. Klupczynska, A.; Misiura, M.; Miltyk, W.; Oscilowska, I.; Palka, J.; Kokot, Z.; Matysiak, J. Development of an LC-MS targeted metabolomics methodology to study proline metabolism in mammalian cell cultures. *Molecules* **2020**, *25*, 4639. [CrossRef] [PubMed]
27. Barry, C.G.; Day, C.S.; Bierbach, U. Duplex–Promoted Platination of Adenine–N3 in the Minor Groove of DNA: Challenging a Longstanding Bioinorganic Paradigm. *J. Am. Chem. Soc.* **2005**, *127*, 1160–1169. [CrossRef]
28. Zhang, J.; Shi, L.y.; Ding, L.P.; Liu, Y.; Liang, H.; Tu, P.F.; Li, L.; Zhang, Q.Y. Condensation derivatives of 4-isopropylbenzaldehyde with acetophenone from the *red alga* Laurencia tristicha. *Phytochemistry.* **2021**, *192*, 112960. [CrossRef]
29. Wang, R.; Xiong, X.P.; Yang, M.; He, S.R.; Xu, X.P. A pharmacokinetics study of orally administered higenamine in rats using LC–MS/MS for doping control analysis. *Drug Test Anal.* **2020**, *12*, 485–495. [CrossRef]
30. Larsen, J.; Cornett, C.; Jaroszewski, J.W.; Hansen, S.H. Reaction between drug substances and pharmaceutical excipients: Formation of citric acid esters and amides of carvedilol in the solid state. *J. Pharmaceut. Biomed.* **2009**, *49*, 11–17. [CrossRef]
31. Liu, M.; Zhang, D.; Wang, X.L.; Zhang, L.N.; Han, J.; Yang, M.; Xiao, X.; Zhang, Y.N.; Liu, H.C. Simultaneous quantification of niacin and its three main metabolites in human plasma by LC–MS/MS. *J. Chromatogr. B* **2012**, *904*, 107–114. [CrossRef]
32. Sadilkova, K.; Gospe, S.M.; Hahn, S.H. Simultaneous determination of alpha–aminoadipic semialdehyde, piperideine-6-carboxylate and pipecolic acid by LC–MS/MS for pyridoxine–dependent seizures and folinic acid–responsive seizures. *J. Neurosci.* **2009**, *184*, 136–141. [CrossRef] [PubMed]

33. Magera, M.J.; Helgeson, J.K.; Matern, D.; Rinaldo, P. Methylmalonic acid measured in plasma and urine by stable-isotope dilution and electrospray tandem mass spectrometry. *Clin. Chem.* **2000**, *46*, 1804–1810. [CrossRef] [PubMed]
34. Rostami–Yazdi, M.; Clement, B.; Schmidt, T.J.; Schinor, D.; Mrowietz, U. Detection of Metabolites of Fumaric Acid Esters in Human Urine: Implications for Their Mode of Action. *J. Invest. Dermatol.* **2009**, *129*, 231–234. [CrossRef] [PubMed]
35. Xiao, Y.S.; Vecchi, M.M.; Wen, D.Y. Distinguishing between Leucine and Isoleucine by Integrated LC–MS Analysis Using an Orbitrap Fusion Mass Spectrometer. *Anal. Chem.* **2016**, *88*, 10757–10766. [CrossRef] [PubMed]
36. Liu, J.L.; Eris, T.; Lauren, S.L.; Stearns, G.W.; Westcott, K.R.; Lu, H. Use of LC/MS peptide mapping for characterization of isoforms in 14N–labeled recombinant human leptin. *Tech. Protein Chem.* **1996**, *8*, 155–163.
37. Chen, Q.F.; Zhang, B.C.; Hicks, L.M.; Wang, S.P.; Jez, J.M. A liquid chromatography–tandem mass spectrometry-based assay for indole–3–acetic acid–amido synthetase. *Anal. Chem.* **2009**, *390*, 149–154. [CrossRef]
38. Reed, J.D.; Krueger, C.G.; Vestling, M.M. MALDI-TOF mass spectrometry of oligomeric food polyphenols. *Phytochemistry* **2005**, *66*, 2248–2263. [CrossRef] [PubMed]
39. Xu, F.F.; Qi, R.; Jiang, S.W.; Wang, W.; Chen, Z.Q.; Guo, D.A.; Liu, B. Simultaneous determination of ten compounds in Xiangbin Fang by LC-MRM-MS. *Zhongguo Zhong Yao Za Zhi* **2017**, *32*, 2226–2229.
40. Pan, H.F.; Lundgren, L.N. Phenolic extractives from root bark of *Picea abies*. *Phytochemistry* **1995**, *39*, 1423–1428. [CrossRef]
41. Mollataghi, A.; Hadi, A.H.A.; Awang, K.; Mohamad, J.; Litaudon, M.; Mukhtar, M. (+)–Kunstlerone, a new antioxidant neolignan from the leaves of *Beilschmiedia kunstleri* Gamble. *Molecules* **2011**, *16*, 6582–6590. [CrossRef]
42. Chiwocha, S.D.S.; Abrams, S.R.; Ambrose, S.J.; Cutler, A.J.; Loewen, M.; Ross, A.R.S.; Kermode, A.R. A method for profiling classes of plant hormones and their metabolites using liquid chromatography-electrospray ionization tandem mass spectrometry: An analysis of hormone regulation of thermodormancy of *lettuce* (*Lactuca sativa* L.) seeds. *Plant Physiol.* **2003**, *35*, 405–417. [CrossRef]
43. Husna, H.; Muhammad, H.; Sivasothy, Y.; Khaw, K.; Nafiah, M.A.; Hazni, H.; Litaudon, M.; Wan, R.; Wan, A.; Liew, S.Y. N-Methyl Costaricine and Costaricine, Two Potent Butyrylcholinesterase Inhibitors from *Alseodaphne pendulifolia* Gamb. *Int. J. Mol. Sci.* **2023**, *24*, 10699. [CrossRef]
44. Takemura, T.; Takatsu, Y.; Kasumi, M.; Marubashi, W.; Iwashina, T.H. Flavonoids and their distribution patterns in the flowers of *Gladiolus cultivars*. *Acta Hortic.* **2005**, *673*, 487–493. [CrossRef]
45. Choi, S.J.; Kim, J.K.; Jang, J.M.; Shin, K.H.; Lim, S.S. Rapid identification of the α–glucosidase inhibitory compounds from *Thunberg's Geranium* (*Geranium thunbergii Sieb. et Zucc.*). *Food Sci. Biotechnol.* **2012**, *21*, 987–996. [CrossRef]
46. Li, Y.Q.; Zhou, F.C.; Gao, F.; Bian, J.S.; Shan, F. Comparative Evaluation of Quercetin, Isoquercetin and Rutin as Inhibitors of α-Glucosidase. *J. Agric. Food Chem.* **2009**, *57*, 11463–11468. [CrossRef] [PubMed]
47. Jorge, A.P.; Horst, H.; Sousa, E.; Pizzolatti, M.G.; Silva, F.R.M.B. Insulinomimetic effects of kaempferitrin on glycemia and on 14C–glucose uptake in rat soleus muscle. *Chem. Biol. Interact.* **2004**, *149*, 89–96. [CrossRef] [PubMed]
48. Li, S.Y.; Zhang, Z.Z.; Cain, A.; Wang, B.; Long, M.; Taylor, J. Antifungal Activity of Camptothecin, Trifolin, and Hyperoside Isolated from *Camptotheca acuminata*. *J. Agric. Food Chem.* **2005**, *53*, 32–37. [CrossRef]
49. Yin, R.; Han, F.; Tang, Z.; Liu, R.; Zhao, X.; Chen, X.H.; Bi, K.S. UFLC–MS/MS method for simultaneous determination of luteolin-7-O-gentiobioside, luteolin-7-O-β-D-glucoside and luteolin-7-O-β-D-glucuronide in beagle dog plasma and its application to a pharmacokinetic study after administration of traditional Chinese medicinal preparation: Kudiezi injection. *J. Pharmaceut. Biomed.* **2013**, *72*, 127–133.
50. Uppugundla, N.; Engelberth, A.; Vandhana, R.S.; Clausen, E.C.; Lay, J.O.; Gidden, J.; Carrier, D.J. Switchgrass Water Extracts: Extraction, Separation and Biological Activity of Rutin and Quercitrin. *J. Agric. Food Chem.* **2009**, *57*, 7763–7770. [CrossRef] [PubMed]
51. Cova, D.; De, A.L.; Giavarini, F.; Palladini, G.; Perego, R. Pharmacokinetics and metabolism of oral diosmin in healthy volunteers. *Int J. Clin Pharm Ther.* **1992**, *30*, 29–33.
52. Zhang, J.K.; Sun, C.D.; Yan, Y.Y.; Chen, Q.J.; Luo, F.L.; Zhu, X.Y.; Li, X.; Chen, K.S. Purification of naringin and neohesperidin from Huyou (*Citrus changshanensis*) fruit and their effects on glucose consumption in human HepG2 cells. *Food Chem.* **2012**, *135*, 1471–1478. [CrossRef]
53. Takumi, H.; Nakamura, H.; Simizu, T.; Harada, R.; Kometani, T.; Nadamoto, T.; Mukai, R.; Murota, K.; Kawai, Y.; Terao, J. Bioavailability of orally administered water-dispersible hesperetin and its effect on peripheral vasodilatation in human subjects: Implication of endothelial functions of plasma conjugated metabolites. *Food Funct.* **2012**, *3*, 389–398. [CrossRef] [PubMed]
54. Nectoux, A.M.; Abe, C.; Huang, S.W.; Ohno, N.; Tabata, J.; Miyata, Y.; Tanaka, K.; Tanaka, T.; Yamamura, H.; Matsui, T. Absorption and Metabolic Behavior of Hesperidin (Rutinosylated Hesperetin) after Single Oral Administration to Sprague–Dawley Rats. *J. Agric. Food Chem.* **2019**, *67*, 9812–9819. [CrossRef] [PubMed]
55. Yang, J.H.; Kondratyuk, T.P.; Marler, L.E.; Qiu, X.; Choi, Y.; Cao, H.m.; Yu, R.; Sturdy, M.; Pegan, S.; Liu, Y. Isolation and evaluation of kaempferol glycosides from *the fern Neocheiropteris palmatopedata*. *Phytochemistry* **2010**, *71*, 641–647. [CrossRef] [PubMed]
56. Imran, M.; Salehi, B.; Sharifi-Rad, J.; Gondal, T.A.; Saeed, F.; Imran, A.; Shahbaz, M.; Fokou, P.V.T.; Arshad, M.U.; Khan, H. Kaempferol: A key emphasis to its anticancer potential. *Molecules* **2019**, *24*, 2277. [CrossRef]
57. Nishioka, T.; Watanabe, J.; Kawabata, J.; Niki, R. Isolation and activity of N-p-coumaroyltyramine, an α-glucosidase inhibitor in Welsh onion (*Allium fistulosum*). *Biosci. Biotech. Biochem.* **1997**, *61*, 1138–1141. [CrossRef]

58. Le, P.M.; Srivastava, V.; Nguyen, T.T.; Pradines, B.; Madamet, M.; Mosnier, J.; Trinh, T.T.; Lee, H. Stephanine from *Stephania venosa* (Blume) Spreng Showed Effective Antiplasmodial and Anticancer Activities, the Latter by Inducing Apoptosis through the Reverse of Mitotic Exit. *Phytother Res.* **2017**, *31*, 1357–1368. [CrossRef]
59. Li, J.; Wang, Z.; Fan, M.X.; Hu, G.W.; Guo, M.Q. Potential Antioxidative and Anti-Hyperuricemic Components Targeting Superoxide Dismutase and Xanthine Oxidase Explored from *Polygonatum Sibiricum Red. Antioxidants* **2022**, *11*, 1651. [CrossRef]
60. Qin, N.; Li, C.B.; Jin, M.N.; Shi, L.H.; Duan, H.Q.; Niu, W.Y. Synthesis and biological activity of novel tiliroside derivatives. *Eur. J. Med. Chem.* **2011**, *46*, 5189–5195. [CrossRef] [PubMed]
61. Fiorini, C.; David, B.; Fouraste, I.; Vercauteren, J. Acylated kaempferol glycosides from *Laurus nobilis* leaves. *Phytochemistry* **1998**, *47*, 821–824. [CrossRef]
62. Lotscher, H.R.; DeJong, C.; Capaldi, R.A. Interconversion of high and low ATPase activity forms of ECF1 by the detergent lauryldimethylamine oxide. *Biochemistry* **1984**, *23*, 4140–4143. [CrossRef]
63. Cank, K.B.; Henkin, J.M.; Cook, A.G.; Oberlies, N.H. Droplet probe: A non–destructive residue analysis of Wari ceramics from the imperial heartland. *J. Archaeol. Sci.* **2021**, *134*, 105468. [CrossRef]
64. Hu, Y.W.; Wu, Q.; Qiao, Y.; Zhang, P.; Dai, W.T.; Tao, H.Y.; Chen, S. Disturbances in Metabolic Pathways and the Identification of a Potential Biomarker Panel for Early Cartilage Degeneration in a Rabbit Anterior Cruciate Ligament Transection Model. *Cartilage* **2021**, *13*, 1376–1387. [CrossRef]
65. Caviglioli, G.; Valeria, P.; Brunella, P.; Sergio, C.; Attilia, A.; Gaetano, B. Identification of degradation products of Ibuprofen arising from oxidative and thermal treatments. *J. Pharm. Biomed.* **2002**, *30*, 499–509. [CrossRef] [PubMed]
66. Valente, J.J.; Peddicord, M.B.; Rinaldi, F.A.; Kelly, K.A.; Bolgar, M.S. Identification of leachables observed in the size exclusion chromatograms of a low concentration product stored in prefilled syringes. *J. Pharmceut. Biomed.* **2017**, *139*, 133–142. [CrossRef]
67. Su, C.H.; Cheng, Y.C.; Chang, Y.C.; Kung, T.H.; Chen, Y.L.; Lai, K.H.; Hsieh, H.L.; Chen, C.Y.; Hwang, T.L.; Yang, Y.L. Untargeted LC-MS/MS-Based Multi-Informative Molecular Networking for Targeting the Antiproliferative Ingredients in *Tetradium ruticarpum* Fruit. *Molecules* **2022**, *27*, 4462. [CrossRef] [PubMed]
68. Hu, H.; Wang, Y.Y.; Zhu, H.Q.; Dong, J.; Qiao, J.T.; Kong, L.J.; Zhang, H.C. Two novel markers to discriminate poplar–type propolis from *poplar bud* extracts: 9-oxo-ODE and 9-oxo-ODA. *J. Food Compos. Anal.* **2022**, *105*, 104196. [CrossRef]
69. Kato, T.; Yamaguchi, Y.; Hirano, T.; Yokoyama, T.; Uyehara, T.; Namai, T.; Yamanaka, S.; Harada, N. Unsaturated hydroxy fatty acids, the self defensive substances in rice plant against rice blast disease. *Chem. Lett.* **1984**, *3*, 409–412. [CrossRef]
70. Zhao, B.; Tomoda, Y.; Mizukami, H.; Makino, T. 9-Oxo-(10E,12E)-octadecadienoic acid, a cytotoxic fatty acid ketodiene isolated from eggplant calyx, induces apoptosis in human ovarian cancer (HRA) cells. *J. Nat. Med. Tokyo* **2015**, *69*, 296–302. [CrossRef] [PubMed]
71. Li, Z.X.; Dong, F.; Sun, Y.Z.; Sun, Z.H.; Song, X.Y.; Dong, Y.G.; Huang, X.C.; Zhong, J.Y.; Zhang, R.; Wang, M.Q. Qualitative and quantitative analysis of six fatty acid amides in 11 edible vegetable oils using liquid chromatography-masss pectrometry. *Front Nutr.* **2022**, *9*, 857858. [CrossRef] [PubMed]
72. Colsch, B.; Afonso, C.; Popa, I.; Portoukalian, J.; Fournier, F.; Tabet, J.; Baumann, N. Characterization of the ceramide moieties of sphingoglycolipids from mouse brain by ESI–MS/MS: Identification of ceramides containing sphingadienine. *J. Lipid Res.* **2004**, *45*, 281–286. [CrossRef] [PubMed]
73. Lin, D.D.; Chang, H.C.; Huang, S.H. Characterization of allegedly musk-containing medicinal products in Taiwan. *J. Forensic Sci.* **2004**, *49*, 1187–1193. [CrossRef]
74. Zhang, Y.; Pan, Z.; Wu, K.; Yan, G.; Xu, H.; Gong, Q.; Ni, L. Research Progress on the Chemical Constituents and Pharmacological Activity of *Litsea cubeba* (Lour) Pers. *Rec. Nat. Prod.* **2023**, *17*, 577–594.
75. Song, F.L.; Gan, R.Y.; Zhang, Y.; Xiao, Q.; Kuang, L.; Li, H.B. Total Phenolic Contents and Antioxidant Capacities of Selected Chinese Medicinal Plants. *Int. J. Mol. Sci.* **2010**, *11*, 2362–2372. [CrossRef] [PubMed]
76. Zhu, H.L.; Zhang, J.C.; Li, C.F.; Liu, S.X.; Wang, L. *Morinda citrifolia* L. leaves extracts obtained by traditional and eco–friendly extraction solvents: Relation between phenolic compositions and biological properties by multivariate analysis. *Ind. Crop. Prod.* **2020**, *153*, 112586. [CrossRef]
77. Qin, Y.; Wang, L.; Liu, Y.; Zhang, Q.; Li, Y.; Wu, Z.Q. Release of phenolics compounds from *Rubus idaeus* L. dried fruits and seeds during simulated in vitro digestion and their bio-activities. *J. Funct. Foods* **2018**, *46*, 57–65. [CrossRef]
78. Xia, Q.; Wang, L.P.; Xu, C.C.; Mei, J.; Li, Y.F. Effects of germination and high hydrostatic pressure processing on mineral elements, amino acids and antioxidants in vitro bioaccessibility, as well as starch digestibility in brown rice (*Oryza sativa* L.). *Food Chem.* **2017**, *214*, 533–542. [CrossRef]
79. Saravanakumar, K.; Sarikurkcu, C.; Sarikurkcu, R.T.; Wang, M.H. A comparative study on the phenolic composition, antioxidant and enzyme inhibition activities of two Endemic *Onosma* species. *Ind. Crop. Prod.* **2019**, *142*, 111878. [CrossRef]

molecules

MDPI

Article

Evaluation of the Antibacterial Activity of Gentamicin in Combination with Essential Oils Isolated from Different Cultivars and Morphological Parts of Lavender (*Lavandula angustifolia* Mill.) against Selected Bacterial Strains

Michalina Adaszyńska-Skwirzyńska [1,*], Sławomir Zych [2], Mateusz Bucław [1], Danuta Majewska [1], Małgorzata Dzięcioł [3] and Danuta Szczerbińska [1]

[1] Department of Monogastric Animal Sciences, Faculty of Biotechnology and Animal Husbandry, West Pomeranian University of Technology in Szczecin, Janickiego Str. 29, 71-270 Szczecin, Poland; mateusz.buclaw@zut.edu.pl (M.B.); danuta.majewska@zut.edu.pl (D.M.); danuta.szczerbinska@zut.edu.pl (D.S.)

[2] Laboratory of Chromatography and Mass Spectrometry, Faculty of Biotechnology and Animal Husbandry, West Pomeranian University of Technology in Szczecin, Janickiego Str. 29, 71-270 Szczecin, Poland; slawomir.zych@zut.edu.pl

[3] Department of Chemical Organic Technology and Polymeric Materials, Faculty of Chemical Technology and Engineering, West Pomeranian University of Technology in Szczecin, Piastów Ave. 42, 71-065 Szczecin, Poland; malgorzata.dzieciol@zut.edu.pl

* Correspondence: madaszynska@zut.edu.pl

Abstract: The aim of the study was to investigate the antibacterial effects of essential oils isolated from different cultivars and morphological parts of lavender (*Lavandula angustifolia* Mill.) in combination with the aminoglycoside antibiotic gentamicin. This in vitro study analyzed the effectiveness of the combinations of gentamicin and lavender essential oils against the following strains: *Staphylococcus aureus* ATCC 25923, *Staphylococcus aureus* MRSA and *Pseudomonas aeruginosa* ATCC 9027. The effect of the combination of lavender oils with gentamicin was tested using the checkerboard method. A synergistic effect against *S. aureus* strain ATCC 25923 was found when gentamicin was combined with lavender essential oils isolated from flowers and leafy stalks (flowers: 'Blue River' FICI—0.192; 'Ellagance Purple' FICI—0.288; leafy stalks: 'Blue River' FICI—0.192; 'Ellagance Purple' FICI—0.320). A synergistic effect was also observed for the combination of gentamicin with lavender essential oils from flowers against the resistant strain of *S. aureus* (MRSA) ('Blue River' FICI—0,191; 'Ellagance Purple' FICI—0.263), as well as for the essential oils from leafy stalks ('Blue River' FICI—0.076; 'Ellagance Purple' FICI—0.089). No interaction was observed for the combination of studied essential oils with gentamicin against *P. aeruginosa* strain ATCC 9027 (FICI = 1.083–1.300).

Keywords: lavender essential oil; gentamicin; antibacterial activity; synergism; *Staphylococcus aureus*; *Pseudomonas aeruginosa*

1. Introduction

Considering the exhausting possibilities of classical therapies in the treatment of bacterial infections, new solutions are constantly being sought. For this purpose, the use of substances of natural origin is increasingly often considered, particularly combination therapies involving concurrent administration of biologically active substances of plant origin, e.g., essential oils, with synthetic antibiotics [1–6]. Combination therapy increases the efficacy of antimicrobials agents and prevents strains from acquiring resistance to antibiotics. Importantly, because of the multi-target action of most natural antimicrobial products, there is a negligible risk of generating resistance mechanisms in pathogens [3,7]. There are also other arguments supporting the therapeutic use of natural bioactive substances such as essential oils. Their advantage is demonstrated by a therapeutic effect with a broad spectrum of biological activity [1,5,7]. Lavender (*Lavandula angustifolia* Mill.) essential oils are characterized by antibacterial, antifungal, antioxidant, sedative, analgesic, anti-inflammatory and immunomodulatory properties [4,7–24]. Analyses of the antibacterial properties of lavender essential oils have been carried out by a number of researchers. The obtained results indicate that lavender essential oils show a particularly strong action against various Gram-positive bacteria: *Bacillus cereus, Bacillus subtilis, Listeria monocytogenes, Staphylococcus aureus, Staphylococcus epidermidis, Enterococcus faecalis* or *Streptococcus pyogenes* [4,6,7,11–14,16–22]. It has been demonstrated that lavender essential oils also act against Gram-negative bacteria, such as *Campylobacter jejuni, Escherichia coli, Pseudomonas aeruginosa, Salmonella* Typhimurium, *Salmonella* Enteritidis, *Salmonella* Pullorum or *Klebsiella* sp. [4,6,7,11,12,21,23,24]. As a plant with repellent properties, lavender has evolved mechanisms to defend against microbial attacks by producing protective substances, typically originating from secondary metabolism. These mechanisms involve the synthesis of two main types of substances: prohibitins, which are produced to prevent microbial attacks, and phytoalexins, which are synthesized to repair damage of the plant tissues. The compounds with strong bactericidal activity are mostly classified as phytoalexins, which include components of the essential oils. The increase in antimicrobial resistance has a significant impact on public health, global development, and even the world economy [15,25,26]. The incorrect application and overuse of antibiotics without identifying the etiological factor are the driving factors behind increasing drug resistance [25,26]. Therefore, the search for synergism between synthetic antibiotics and antimicrobial agents, including natural substances such as essential oils, present an excellent research direction, being in agreement with ideas surrounding sustainable development. The great advantage is that synergism allows the dose of a drug to be reduced below the threshold of its toxicity [1,4]. Aminoglycoside antibiotics, which include gentamicin, are an important group of chemotherapeutics used to treat severe infections caused by Gram-negative bacteria, both aerobic and anaerobic [26,27]. The use of gentamicin has become a turning point in the treatment of pruritic infections, mainly caused by β-lactam-resistant *Staphylococcus aureus* (MRSA) and *Pseudomonas aeruginosa* strains. Since the 1980s, it has not been possible to obtain new aminoglycosides that offer high efficacy with relatively low toxicity [28]. This has hindered further research on new antibiotics from this group, and current studies mainly focus on mechanisms of drug resistance. Due to the increasing resistance of bacteria and frequent failure of antibiotic therapies, it seems necessary to search for unconventional methods to improve treatment effectiveness. Therefore, the aim of this study was to investigate the effect of the interaction between lavender essential oils obtained from two lavender (*L. angustifolia*) cultivars and their various morphological parts (flowers and leafy stalks) with gentamicin on selected bacterial strains.

2. Results

The chemical composition of lavender essential oils was presented in our previous publication [29]. The main chemical components detected in the essential oils from the flowers of *L. angustifolia* were linalyl acetate (17.8–31.0%) and linalool (28.5–33.0%), while lavandulol acetate, borneol and caryophyllene oxide were present in lower concentrations (<5%). The essential oils from the leafy stalks of *L. angustifolia* were dominated by borneol (13.0–19.7%) and caryophyllene oxide (7.95–10.0%). Chromatographic analysis showed that the relative percentage content of specific compound classes in the flower essential oils was as follows (%): monoterpene hydrocarbons (4.3–4.8), oxygenated monoterpenes (81.6–82.6), sesquiterpene hydrocarbons (6.8–7.7), and oxygenated sesquiterpenes (3.1–3.7). The following compounds were identified in the oils from leafy stalks (%): monoterpene hydrocarbons (7.6–7.7), oxygenated monoterpenes (51.2–53.8), sesquiterpene hydrocarbons (13.0–14.2) and oxygenated sesquiterpenes (8.0–9.0). The essential oils isolated in the study were characterized by varying antimicrobial activity, with *S. aureus* strains being more sensitive to oils from *L. angustifolia*. The growth of bacterial strains was inhibited by the essential oils as follows (MIC % v/v): *S. aureus* ATCC25922 (0.125–0.5), *S. aureus*

MRSA (0.25–1.25), *P. aeruginosa* ATCC 9027 (0.75–2.5). Table 1 presents the results of the interaction between the essential oils isolated from the flowers of *L. angustifolia* in combination with gentamicin, determined using the checkerboard method. Individual interactions of lavender flower essential oils in combination with gentamicin were found be synergistic against *S. aureus* strains (*S. aureus* ATCC 25923: 'Blue River' FICI—0.192; 'Ellagance Purple FICI—0.288; *S. aureus* MRSA: 'Blue River' FICI—0.191; 'Ellagance Purple' FICI—0.263). A neutral effect was found for the tested combinations against *P. aeruginosa* strain ATCC 9027 ('Blue River' FICI—1.083; 'Ellagance Purple' FICI—1.25). Similarly, in the case of oils isolated from leafy stalks (Table 2), a synergistic effect was found for *Staphylococcus* strains (*S. aureus* ATCC 25923: 'Blue River' FICI—0.192; 'Ellagance Purple' FICI—0.320; *S. aureus* MRSA: 'Blue River' FICI—0.076; 'Ellagance Purple' FICI—0.089). A neutral effect was once again demonstrated for the combination of gentamicin with leafy stalks essential oils against *P. aeruginosa* strain ATCC 9027 ('Blue River' FICI—1.166; 'Ellagance Purple' FICI—1.300).

Table 1. Activity of lavender essential oils from flowers in combination with gentamicin against selected bacterial strains.

Antibacterial Agent	Blue River				Ellagance Purple				Type of Interaction
	MIC_0	MIC_c	FIC	FICI	MIC_0	MIC_c	FIC	FICI	
Staphylococcus aureus ATCC 25923									
Essential oil (% *v*/*v*)	0.125	0.016	0.128	0.192	0.250	0.008	0.032	0.288	synergistic
Gentamicin (µg/mL)	0.250	0.016	0.064		0.125	0.032	0.256		
Staphylococcus aureus MRSA									
Essential oil (% *v*/*v*)	0.250	0.032	0.128	0.191	1.250	0.016	0.013	0.263	synergistic
Gentamicin (µg/mL)	16.0	1.0	0.063		16.0	4.0	0.250		
Pseudomonas aeruginosa ATCC 9027									
Essential oil (% *v*/*v*)	0.750	0.625	0.833	1.083	2.0	1.500	0.750	1.250	no interaction
Gentamicin (µg/mL)	2.0	0.500	0.250		2.0	1.0	0.5		

Explanations: MIC—minimal inhibitory concentration; FIC—fractional inhibitory concentration; FICI—fractional inhibitory concentration index; MIC_0 = MIC of an individual sample alone; MIC_c = MIC of an individual sample of the most effective combination; FIC of essential oil = MIC of essential oil in combination with gentamicin/MIC of essential oil alone; FIC of gentamicin = MIC of gentamicin in combination with essential oil /MIC of gentamicin alone; FICI = FIC of essential oil + FIC of gentamicin. Interpretation: FICI $\leq$ 0.5, synergistic; FICI > 0.5–1.0, additive; FICI > 1.0–4.0, no interaction; FICI > 4.0, antagonistic [30].

Table 2. Activity of lavender essential oils from leafy stalks in combination with gentamicin against selected bacterial strains.

Antibacterial Agent	Blue River				Ellagance Purple				Type of Interaction
	MIC_0	MIC_c	FIC	FICI	MIC_0	MIC_c	FIC	FICI	
Staphylococcus aureus ATCC 25923									
Essential oil (% *v*/*v*)	0.500	0.032	0.164	0.192	0.250	0.016	0.064	0.320	synergistic
Gentamicin (µg/mL)	0.125	0.016	0.128		0.125	0.032	0.256		
Staphylococcus aureus MRSA									
Essential oil (% *v*/*v*)	1.250	0.016	0.013	0.076	1.250	0.032	0.026	0.089	synergistic
Gentamicin (µg/mL)	32.0	2.0	0.063		32.0	2.0	0.063		
Pseudomonas aeruginosa ATCC 9027									
Essential oil (% *v*/*v*)	1.50	1.0	0.666	1.166	2.5	2.0	0.80	1.300	no interaction
Gentamicin (µg/mL)	2.0	1.0	0.500		2.0	1.0	0.50		

Explanations: MIC—minimal inhibitory concentration; FIC—fractional inhibitory concentration; FICI—fractional inhibitory concentration index; MIC_0 = MIC of an individual sample alone; MIC_c = MIC of an individual sample of the most effective combination; FIC of essential oil = MIC of essential oil in combination with gentamicin/MIC of essential oil alone; FIC of gentamicin = MIC of gentamicin in combination with essential oil/MIC of gentamicin alone; FICI = FIC of essential oil + FIC of gentamicin. Interpretation: FICI $\leq$ 0.5, synergistic; FICI > 0.5–1.0, additive; FICI > 1.0–4.0, no interaction; FICI > 4.0, antagonistic [30].

3. Discussion

Aminoglycoside antibiotics belong to the group of chemotherapeutics that inhibit bacterial protein biosynthesis, and include antibiotics of natural origin, such as gentamicin and tobramycin, as well as semi-synthetic antibiotics like amikacin [26]. Aminoglycosides exert a strong effect on aerobic bacteria, mainly Gram-negative, but also certain Gram-positive bacteria. They exhibit particularly strong antibacterial activity against strains belonging to genera *Escherichia*, *Klebsiella*, *Enterobacter*, *Pseudomonas*, *Hemophilus*, and *Staphylococcus*. Aminoglycosides are substances that contain tri- or tetrasaccharide structures, with streptamine or its derivatives being their common component. The mechanism of action of aminoglycoside antibiotics involves irreversible binding to the 30S ribosomal subunit, which hinders the attachment of aminoacyl-tRNA and causes the misreading of genetic information. This in turn leads to the incorporation of false amino acids, disruption of enzymatic and structural protein synthesis, which initiates irreversible damage to bacterial cell membranes [25,31,32]. Resistance to aminoglycoside antibiotics can develop very rapidly. It involves the formation of enzymes that inactivate aminoglycoside antibiotics. The genetic information of these enzymes is stored in plasmids. Another possible mechanism of microbial resistance to aminoglycoside antibiotics is an alteration in the amino acid sequence of certain ribosomal proteins, which prevents the binding of the antibiotic to the 30S ribosomal subunit. The ability of bacteria to develop antibiotic resistance depends on their adaptability to selective pressure. One of the mechanisms relates to the presence of efflux pumps in bacteria, which allow the antibiotic to be expelled from the cell. Another mechanism involves changes in the composition and function of the cell membrane, which result in its reduced permeability. The next pathway is antibiotic inactivation by extracellular and intracellular enzymes. Bacterial cell adaptation to antibiotic action can involve the reduction of the substrate targeted by the antibiotic or bacterial mutations [31,32]. Generally, two types of antibiotic resistance can be distinguished. The first is natural antibiotic resistance, resulting from the cell's biology, structural or functional characteristics [32]. The second type is acquired antibiotic resistance. It can occur, for instance, due to chromosomal mutations or through the transfer of genetic material from another bacterium via plasmids [32]. The transfer of genes through plasmids occurs through conjugation, transduction, and transformation, or is facilitated by proteinaceous filaments termed fimbriae or pili [33]. In the transduction process, genes encoding resistance are passed from a resistant bacterial cell to a susceptible one. Antibiotic-sensitive cells can take up genetic material that has been released through autolysis of resistant cells—a process known as transformation [33,34]. The antibiotic resistance profile of *Staphylococcus* strains continues to evolve, contributing to the spread of new bacterial clones [35–37].

Most of the essential oils contain one main chemical component that is responsible for their biological and pharmacological properties [7,38,39]. The chemical composition of essential oil may vary significantly creating their unique chemotypes within plant species with the same morphological features. Additionally, the composition depends on many factors, such as the country of origin, the part of the plant and the production method [40]. For example, cinnamon essential oil contains 50–75% of trans-cinnamaldehyde when extracted from the bark of the true cinnamon tree (*Cinnamomum zeylanicum*). However, the oil produced from the leaves of this tree contains 50–75% of eugenol and only a trace amount of cinnamaldehyde, making it similar in composition, activity, and scent to clove essential oil [41]. Camphor is derived from the wood, bark, and leaves of *Cinnamomum camphora* (as "camphor brown" oil). However, the first distillation fraction is referred to as "camphor white" mainly containing 1,8-cineole (30–60%; similar to eucalyptus oil) [42]. In contrast, essential oil distilled from *C. camphora* var. *linaloolifera* (also known as Ho wood) typically contains more than 90% of linalool [43]. Each of these main components has demonstrated a broad range of highly antimicrobial activities against different pathogens [40]. Information available in the literature indicates that linalool is the chemical compound responsible for the antibacterial activity of the essential oil from *L. angustifolia*. However, it should be emphasized that essential oils derived from leafy stalks are characterized by low content of linalool, yet they still exhibit antibacterial activity. The overall concept of antimicrobial synergy is based on the principle that the combination of two or more antimicrobial agents (even in lower amounts) may enhance their efficacy. This is manifested, for example, due to their hydrophobicity, by reaction with lipids present in the bacterial cell membrane (e.g., destroying cell structures or increasing the permeability of the main component), a reduction in the required dose of the active substance or reduced antimicrobial resistance [44]. The biosynthesis of secondary metabolites and their proportion in essential oils vary due to environmental factors, such as seasonal variation, light availability, vegetation stage, presence of additional commensal microorganisms as well as nature of soil (e.g., pH) [42]. Moreover, Gram-positive bacteria seem to be much more susceptible to essential oil than Gram-negative [4]. All tested lavender essential oils exhibited more effective antibacterial activity against *S. aureus* strains (MIC % v/v: 0.125–1.25) compared to *P. aeruginosa* strains (MIC % v/v: 0.75–2.50). This suggests that lavender oils may show weaker activity against Gram-negative bacteria in general, particularly the genus *Pseudomonas*, which naturally occurs only in soil and water. *Pseudomonas* has developed a range of cellular defense mechanisms through adaptation to adverse environmental conditions, which may explain the observed lower susceptibility to lavender essential oils compared to *S. aureus*. Different antibacterial activity of essential oils can be possibly related to its chemical composition and content of some other compounds with synergistic activity. Available literature indicates the large variability in antimicrobial properties of essential oils isolated from *L. angustifolia* flowers. Strong antimicrobial activity against the reference strains of *S. aureus* CECT 4459 with an MIC level of 0.0025% w/v was demonstrated by Djenane et al. [45], while weak activity was reported by Thosar et al. with an MIC value of 0.003% w/v against *S. aureus* ATCC 25923 [46]. In turn, according to De Martino et al. *L. angustifolia* essential oil did not show any activity against strains of *S. aureus* and *P. aeruginosa* [12]. In studies performed by de Rapper et al., the value of lavender essential oil MIC against *S. aureus* MRSA and *P. aeruginosa* ATCC 11093 was 0.2% w/v, regardless of whether *Staphylococcus*, MRSA or gentamicin-resistant MRSA was tested (strain analogous to that tested in our study) [47].

In our studies, after analyzing individual combinations of gentamicin with lavender essential oils, it was observed that their effects on tested microorganisms varied. Some combinations indicated synergism (*S. aureus* ATCC 25923 FICI: 0.192–0.32; *S. aureus* MRSA FICI: 0.076–0.263), while others showed lack of interaction (*P. aeruginosa* ATCC 9027 FICI: 1.08–1.30). It should be emphasized that an antagonistic interaction was not recorded in any case. No data were found in the literature on the effect of essential oils from different cultivars and morphological parts of lavender in combination with gentamicin. The conducted research indicates that their biological activity slightly varied among two studied lavender cultivars and was also affected by the part of the plant used for the isolation of essential oil.

Importantly, a synergistic interaction between gentamicin and lavender essential oils was obtained against the resistant isolate (*S. aureus* MRSA), which was included in the list of pathogens urgently requiring development of new antibiotics by the World Health Organization (WHO) in 2017 [48]. A very interesting observation is that essential oils isolated from the leafy stalks of both studied lavender cultivars are very effective enhancers of gentamicin activity against this resistant strain. Upon comparing the obtained FICI values, it can be noticed that the ability to enhance the gentamicin activity was significantly higher in the case of both 'Blue River' and 'Ellagance Purple' cultivars in comparison to essential oils obtained from their flowers. These results indicate that the essential oil from the leafy stalks of lavender, despite the lower content of linalool, can also be a valuable natural bioactive product with potential practical application. It also confirms that the antimicrobial activity of lavender essential oils is the result of more than linalool content alone, and further research for the possible explanation of this fact is required. For this purpose, the biological activity of other major and minor components of lavender essential oils should be tested in analogous conditions to identify the remaining active compounds.

Some authors have shown synergistic effects with gentamicin for other essential oils against Gram-positive and Gram-negative bacteria [1,44,49–51]. This was confirmed in our previous study on commercial lavender essential oil [7] and the currently studied oils isolated from different cultivars and morphological parts of lavender, whose combinations with gentamicin have not yet been examined. The obtained results demonstrate synergy between the tested essential oils and gentamicin and are thus very promising. Further research is necessary to confirm the effectiveness of these combinations through in vivo studies.

4. Materials and Methods

4.1. Isolation of Essential Oils

Plant raw material comprised dried flowers and leafy stalks of two cultivars of *Lavandula angustifolia*: 'Blue River' and 'Ellagance Purple'. Directly before isolation of essential oils, plant material was pounded in a mortar and weighed sample (20.00 g) was placed in a 1000 mL round-bottomed flask, immersed in 400 mL distilled water, and connected to Deryng apparatus. Hydrodistillation process was performed for 3 h and the obtained oils were dried over anhydrous sodium sulfate. For this purpose, 1.0 mL of methylene chloride and desiccant were added to the vial with essential oil. After storage in the refrigerator for 24 h, the drying agent was removed by filtration and the solvent was evaporated to obtain a pure essential oil. All isolated essential oils were analyzed using gas chromatography with mass selective detector (GC-MS), what was described previously [29]. (See Supplementary Materials for details).

4.2. Microdilution Checkerboard Method

Two bacterial strains of the American Type Culture Collection (*S. aureus* ATCC 25923, *P. aeruginosa* ATCC 9027, KwikStik™, Microbiologics, St. Cloud, MS, USA) and one isolate from purulent skin lesions in a horse (*S. aureus* MRSA—bacteria from the culture collection of the Labo-Wet Laboratory, Szczecin, Poland) were used for the study. *S. aureus* and *P. aeruginosa* are versatile bacterial pathogens and common etiological agents in polymicrobial infections. Both *S. aureus* and *P. aeruginosa* exhibit intrinsic and acquired antibiotic resistance, making infections by these pathogens increasingly difficult to treat. Microbial communities containing both pathogens are shaped by interactions ranging from parasitic to mutualistic, with the net impact of these interactions in many cases resulting in enhanced virulence. Moreover, synergism between *S. aureus* and *P. aeruginosa* has been observed in multiple models of infection, including wounds and chronic lung infection. The disc-diffusion method was used to determine the preliminary classification of the tested strains for susceptibility to gentamicin (commercial disc 10 μg, OXOID, Argenta, Poznan, Poland). Interpretive criteria of zone diameter (mm) were used according to CLSI VET01S 5th edition (*Staphylococci* and *P. aeruginosa* isolated from humans and most animal species: $\leq$12 (R) resistant, 13–14 (I) intermediate, $\geq$15 (S) susceptible) [52]. Gentamicin (256 mg/mL; Oxoid Limited, Hampshire, England) diluted in pure deionised water was used for microdilution testing as the active agent, and isolated lavender oils. Dimethylsulfoxide—DMSO (POCH, Gliwice, Poland) was used as an organic solvent to dilute only the oil. In order to determine the susceptibility of the tested microorganisms to the analysed antimicrobial agents, the determination of minimum inhibitory concentration (MIC). All identifications were made on individually packed, sterile, divided, 96-well polystyrene titration plates with flat bottoms. Again, interpretive criteria of MIC (μg/mL) were used according to CLSI VET01S 5th edition ($\geq$16 (R), 8 (I), $\leq$4 (S) for *Staphylococci* and *P. aeruginosa* isolated from humans and most animals' species [52]. The Clinical and Laboratory Standard Institute (CLSI) recommendations were followed [52,53]. Each test was repeated three times. The medium was used as a ready-to-use cation-adjusted Mueller–Hinton broth (CAMHB) (Graso, Starogard Gdański, Poland). The final volume of broth in each well was 100 μL. For gentamicin, a series of two-fold dilutions were made in the range of 0.002 $\div$ 256 mg/mL, and for essential oils, a concentration gradient was prepared in the range of was 0.008 $\div$ 5% v/v. To avoid the toxicity of DMSO, the final concentration of DMSO in the well did not exceed 5% v/v for *P. aeruginosa* and 10% v/v for both *Staphylococci*. Colonies of each strain were selected from 18- to 24-h nonselective blood agar plates. The inoculum of 1–2 $\times$ 10^8 CFU/mL, corresponding to 0.5 McFarland standard measured in a DEN-1 densitometer (BioSan, Józefów, Poland) were employed in the tests (according to CLSI, the final concentration in each well was approximately 5 $\times$ 10^5 CFU/mL). The microtiter plate was incubated in an incubator at +35.0 $\pm$ 2 °C for 18 $\pm$ 2 h. Due to natural clouding of the medium at high concentrations of the essential oil and DMSO, the result was read macroscopically, and taken into account accordingly. Both antimicrobial agents were considered inefficient when clouding characteristic only for bacteria growth was present. The study of the effect of gentamicin in combination with lavender oils was carried out using the checkerboard method, according to the methodology described in the previous article [7]. MIC data of the gentamicin and lavender essential oils were converted into Fractional Inhibitory Concentration (FIC) and defined as the antimicrobial concentration in an inhibitory concentration with a second compound to the concentration of the antimicrobial by itself [30]. In the combination assays, the checkerboard procedure described by Rosato et al. [49] was followed to evaluate the synergistic action of the lavender essential oils with gentamicin. In our experimental protocol, the substance combinations were analysed by calculating the FIC index (FICI) using the following formulas:

$$\text{FIC of essential oil} = \frac{\text{MIC value of essential oil combined with gentamicin}}{\text{MIC value of essential oil alone}} \quad (1)$$

$$\text{FIC of gentamicin} = \frac{\text{MIC value of gentamicin combined with essential oil}}{\text{MIC value of gentamicin alone}} \quad (2)$$

$$\text{FICI} = \text{FIC value of essential oil} + \text{FIC value of gentamicin} \quad (3)$$

Generally, the FICI value was interpreted as: synergistic when $\leq$0.5; additive when >0.5 and $\leq$1; noninteractive (>1 but $\leq$4) and antagonistic when >4 [30].

5. Conclusions

New therapeutic solutions are currently being sought as the problem of drug resistance continues to increase. One of the strategies includes searching for combined treatment options using natural biologically active products with known drugs. For the tested combinations of lavender essential oils with gentamicin against *P. aeruginosa* ATCC 9027 strain, no interaction was found. However, the conducted analyses demonstrated the possibility of using lavender essential oils to enhance the antibacterial activity of gentamicin against *S. aureus* ATCC 25923 and MRSA strains. Despite some differences between the essential oils obtained from the two tested lavender cultivars ('Blue River' and 'Ellagance Purple'), their flowers and leafy stalks, synergistic effects with gentamicin were found in all cases. The obtained results are very promising and important, especially in the context of searching for new possibilities of treating infections in both humans and animals regarding antibiotic-resistant strains. Further, the presented findings encourage and justify further research to verify the results in vivo, aimed at developing antibiotic formulations with biologically active natural substances, characterized by increased effectiveness and lower toxicity.

Supplementary Materials: The following supporting information can be downloaded at: https://www.mdpi.com/article/10.3390/molecules28155781/s1, GC-MS data: Table S1. Retention parameters of compounds identified in essential oils from flowers and leafy stalks of *Lavandula angustifolia* cultivars: 'Blue River' and 'Ellagance Purple', obtained by GC-MS method; Figure S1. Chromatogram of essential oil from flowers of 'Blue River' cultivar of *Lavandula angustifolia*; Figure S2. Chromatogram of essential oil from flowers of 'Ellagance Purple' cultivar of *Lavandula angustifolia*; Figure S3. Chromatogram of essential oil from leafy stalks of 'Blue River' cultivar of *Lavandula angustifolia*; Figure S4. Chromatogram of essential oil from leafy stalks of 'Ellagance Purple' cultivar of *Lavandula angustifolia*; Figure S5. Mass spectrum of eucalyptol present in *Lavandula angustifolia* essential oils, compared with eucalyptol standard mass spectrum from NIST 02 library; Figure S6. Mass spectrum of linalool present in *Lavandula angustifolia* essential oils, compared with linalool standard mass spectrum from NIST 02 library; Figure S7. Mass spectrum of borneol present in *Lavandula angustifolia* essential oils, compared with borneol standard mass spectrum from NIST 02 library; Figure S8. Mass spectrum of linalool acetate present in *Lavandula angustifolia* essential oils, compared with linalool acetate standard mass spectrum from NIST 02 library; Figure S9. Mass spectrum of lavandulol acetate present in *Lavandula angustifolia* essential oils, compared with lavandulol acetate standard mass spectrum from NIST 02 library; Figure S10. Mass spectrum of caryophyllene present in *Lavandula angustifolia* essential oils, compared with caryophyllene standard mass spectrum from NIST 02 library; Figure S11. Mass spectrum of caryophyllene oxide present in *Lavandula angustifolia* essential oils, compared with caryophyllene oxide standard mass spectrum from NIST 02 library; Figure S12. Chromatogram of linalool standard; Figure S13. Mass spectrum of linalool, compared with linalool standard mass spectrum from NIST 02 library.

Author Contributions: Conceptualization, M.A.-S., M.D. and D.S.; methodology, M.A.-S.; formal analysis, M.A.-S. and S.Z.; investigation, M.A.-S., S.Z. and D.S.; resources, M.A.-S., M.D. and D.S.; data curation, M.A.-S., M.B., D.M., S.Z. and M.D.; writing—original draft, M.A.-S.; writing—review and editing, M.A.-S. and M.D.; visualization, M.A.-S., M.B., D.M. and D.S.; supervision, M.A.-S. and M.D. All authors listed have made a substantial, direct and intellectual contribution to the work, and approved it for publication. All authors have read and agreed to the published version of the manuscript.

Funding: This research received no external funding.

Institutional Review Board Statement: Not applicable.

Informed Consent Statement: Not applicable.

Data Availability Statement: Not applicable.

Acknowledgments: The authors thank the Labo-Wet Laboratory, Szczecin, Poland.

Conflicts of Interest: The authors declare no conflict of interest.

Sample Availability: Samples of essential oils are available from the authors.

References

1. Yap, P.S.; Yiap, B.C.; Ping, H.C.; Lim, S.H. Essential oils, a new horizon in combating bacterial antibiotic resistance. *Open Microbiol. J.* **2014**, *8*, 6–14. [CrossRef]
2. Alam, M.; Bano, N.; Ahmad, T.; Sharangi, A.B.; Upadhyay, T.K.; Alraey, Y.; Alabdallah, N.M.; Rauf, M.A.; Saeed, M. Synergistic Role of Plant Extracts and Essential Oils against Multidrug Resistance and Gram-Negative Bacterial Strains Producing Extended-Spectrum β-Lactamases. *Antibiotics* **2022**, *11*, 855. [CrossRef]
3. Jia, J.; Feng, Z.; Xiaohua, M.; Zhiwei, W.C.; Yixue, X.L.; Yu, Z.C. Mechanisms of drug combinations: Interaction and network perspectives. *Nat. Rev. Drug Discov.* **2009**, *8*, 111–128. [CrossRef]
4. Wińska, K.; Mączka, W.; Łyczko, J.; Grabarczyk, M.; Czubaszek, A.; Szumny, A. Essential Oils as Antimicrobial Agents-Myth or Real Alternative? *Molecules* **2019**, *11*, 2130. [CrossRef]
5. Mahmoud, A.M.; El-Baky, R.M.A.; Ahmed, A.B.F.; Gad, G.F.M. Antibacterial Activity of Essential Oils and in Combination with Some Standard Antimicrobials against Different Pathogens Isolated from Some Clinical Specimens. *Am. J. Microbiol. Res.* **2016**, *1*, 16–25.
6. Aljaafari, M.N.; AlAli, A.O.; Baqais, L.; Alqubaisy, M.; AlAli, M.; Molouki, A.; Ong-Abdullah, J.; Abushelaibi, A.; Lai, K.S.; Lim, S.E. An Overview of the Potential Therapeutic Applications of Essential Oils. *Molecules* **2021**, *3*, 628. [CrossRef]

7. Adaszyńska-Skwirzyńska, M.; Szczerbińska, D.; Zych, S. Antibacterial activity of lavender essential oil and linalool combined with gentamicin on selected bacterial strains. *Med. Wet.* **2020**, *176*, 15–118. [CrossRef]
8. Bakkali, F.; Averbeck, S.; Averbeck, D.; Idaomar, M. Biological effects of essential oils—A review. *Food Chem. Toxicol.* **2008**, *46*, 446–475. [CrossRef]
9. Nazzaro, F.; Fratianni, F.; De Martino, L.; Coppola, R.; De Feo, V. Effect of Essential Oils on Pathogenic Bacteria. *Pharmaceuticals* **2013**, *6*, 1451–1474. [CrossRef]
10. Sienkiewicz, M.; Denys, P.; Kowalczyk, E. Antibacterial and immunostimulatory effect of essential oils. *Int. Rev. Allergol. Clin. Immunol.* **2011**, *17*, 40–44.
11. Tardugno, R.; Serio, A.; Pellati, F.; D'Amato, S.; Chaves López, C.; Bellardi, M.G.; Di Vito, M.; Savini, V.; Paparella, A.; Benvenuti, S. *Lavandula x intermedia* and *Lavandula angustifolia* essential oils: Phytochemical composition and antimicrobial activity against foodborne pathogens. *Nat. Prod. Res.* **2019**, *22*, 3330–3335. [CrossRef]
12. De Martino, L.; De Feo, V.; Nazzaro, F. Chemical composition and in vitro antimicrobial and mutagenic activities of seven Lamiaceae essential oils. *Molecules* **2009**, *14*, 4213–4230. [CrossRef]
13. Roller, S.; Ernest, N.; Buckle, J. The antimicrobial activity of high-necrodane and other lavender oils on methicillin-sensitive and -resistant *Staphylococcus aureus* (MSSA and MRSA). *J. Altern. Complement. Med.* **2009**, *15*, 275–279. [CrossRef]
14. Kwiatkowski, P.; Łopusiewicz, Ł.; Kostek, M.; Drozłowska, E.; Pruss, A.; Wojciuk, B.; Sienkiewicz, M.; Zielińska-Bliźniewska, H.; Dołęgowska, B. The Antibacterial Activity of Lavender Essential Oil Alone and in Combination with Octenidine Dihydrochloride against MRSA Strains. *Molecules* **2019**, *1*, 95. [CrossRef]
15. Padiyara, P.; Inoue, H.; Sprenger, M. Global Governance Mechanisms to Address Antimicrobial Resistance. *Infect. Dis.* **2018**, *11*, 1178633718767887. [CrossRef]
16. Todorova, D.; Yavorov, N.; Lasheva, V.; Damyanova, S.; Kostova, I. Lavender Essential Oil as Antibacterial Treatment for Packaging Paper. *Coatings* **2023**, *13*, 32. [CrossRef]
17. Tkachenko, H.; Opryshko, M.; Gyrenko, O.; Maryniuk, M.; Buyun, L.; Kurhaluk, N. Antibacterial Properties of Commercial Lavender Essential Oil against Some Gram-Positive and Gram-Negative Bacteria. *Agrobiodiversity Improv. Nutr. Health Life Qual.* **2022**, *6*, 2. [CrossRef]
18. Batiha, G.E.S.; Teibo, J.O.; Wasef, L.; Shaheen, H.M.; Akomolafe, A.P.; Teibo, T.K.A.; Al.-kuraishy, H.M.; Al.-Garbeeb, A.I.; Alexiou, A. A review of the bioactive components and pharmacological properties of *Lavandula* species. *Naunyn-Schmiedeberg's Arch. Pharmacol.* **2023**, *396*, 877–900. [CrossRef]
19. Walasek-Janusz, M.; Grzegorczyk, A.; Zalewski, D.; Malm, A.; Gajcy, S.; Gruszecki, R. Variation in the Antimicrobial Activity of Essential Oils from Cultivars of *Lavandula angustifolia* and *L. × intermedia*. *Agronomy* **2022**, *12*, 2955. [CrossRef]
20. Han, X.; Chen, Q.; Zhang, X.; Peng, J.; Zhang, M.; Zhong, Q. The elimination effects of lavender essential oil on *Listeria monocytogenes* biofilms developed at different temperatures and the induction of VBNC state. *Lett. Appl. Microbiol.* **2022**, *74*, 1016–1026. [CrossRef]
21. Cavanagh, H.; Wilkinson, J. Biological activities of lavender essential oil. *Phytother. Res.* **2002**, *16*, 301–308. [CrossRef]
22. Altun, M.; Yapici, B.M. Determination of chemical compositions and antibacterial effects of selected essential oils against human pathogenic strains. *An. Acad. Bras. Cienc.* **2022**, *94*, e20210074. [CrossRef]
23. Hossain, S.; Heo, H.; De Silva, B.C.J.; Wimalasena, S.H.M.P.; Pathirana, H.N.K.S.; Heo, G.-J. Antibacterial activity of essential oil from lavender (*Lavandula angustifolia*) against pet turtle-borne pathogenic bacteria. *Lab. Anim. Res.* **2017**, *33*, 195–201. [CrossRef]
24. Adaszyńska-Skwirzyńska, M.; Zych, S.; Szczerbińska, D. In Vitro antibacterial effect of enrofloxacin combined with lavender essential oil on selected *Salmonella* serotypes isolated most commonly in poultry. *Med. Wet.* **2023**, *79*, 182–185. [CrossRef]
25. Llor, C.; Bjerrum, L. Antimicrobial resistance: Risk associated with antibiotic overuse and initiatives to reduce the problem. *Ther. Adv. Drug Saf.* **2014**, *6*, 229–241. [CrossRef]
26. Krause, K.M.; Serio, A.W.; Kane, T.R.; Connolly, L.E. Aminoglycosides: An Overview. *Cold Spring Harb. Perspect. Med.* **2016**, *6*, a027029. [CrossRef]
27. Garneau-Tsodikova, S.; Labby, K.J. Mechanisms of Resistance to Aminoglycoside Antibiotics: Overview and Perspectives. *Medchemcomm* **2016**, *1*, 11–27. [CrossRef]
28. Becker, B.; Cooper, M.A. Aminoglycoside antibiotics in the 21st century. *ACS Chem. Biol.* **2013**, *1*, 105–115. [CrossRef]
29. Adaszyńska-Skwirzyńska, M.; Dzięcioł, M.; Szczerbińska, D. *Lavandula angustifolia* Essential Oils as Effective Enhancers of Fluconazole Antifungal Activity against *Candida albicans*. *Molecules* **2023**, *28*, 1176. [CrossRef]
30. van Vuuren, S.; Viljoen, A. Plant-based antimicrobial studies-methods and approaches to study the interaction between natural products. *Planta Med.* **2011**, *11*, 1168–1182. [CrossRef]
31. Larsson, D.G.J.; Flach, C.F. Antibiotic resistance in the environment. *Nat. Rev. Microbiol.* **2022**, *20*, 257–269. [CrossRef]
32. Zhang, F.; Cheng, W. The Mechanism of Bacterial Resistance and Potential Bacteriostatic Strategies. *Antibiotics* **2022**, *11*, 1215. [CrossRef]
33. Li, B.; Webster, T.J. Bacteria antibiotic resistance: New challenges and opportunities for implant-associated orthopedic infections. *J. Orthop. Res.* **2018**, *1*, 22–32. [CrossRef]
34. Chellat, M.F.; Raguž, L.; Riedl, R. Targeting Antibiotic Resistance. *Angew. Chem. Int. Ed. Engl.* **2016**, *23*, 6600–6626. [CrossRef]
35. Hershberg, R. Antibiotic-Independent Adaptive Effects of Antibiotic Resistance Mutations. *Trends Genet.* **2017**, *8*, 521–528. [CrossRef]

36. Munita, J.M.; Arias, C.A. Mechanisms of Antibiotic Resistance. *Microbiol. Spectr.* **2016**, *4*, 464–473. [CrossRef]
37. Polyzou, A.; Slavakis, A.; Pournaras, S.; Maniatis, A.N.; Sofianou, D.; Tsakris, A. Predominance of a methicillin-resistant *Staphylococcus aureus* clone susceptible to erythromycin and several other non-β-lactam antibiotics in a greek hospital. *J. Antimicrob. Chemother.* **2001**, *48*, 231–234. [CrossRef]
38. Guimarães, A.C.; Meireles, L.M.; Lemos, M.F.; Guimarães, M.C.C.; Endringer, D.C.; Fronza, M.; Scherer, R. Antibacterial Activity of Terpenes and Terpenoids Present in Essential Oils. *Molecules* **2019**, *13*, 2471. [CrossRef]
39. Kalemba, D.; Kunicka, A. Antibacterial and antifungal properties of essential oils. *Curr. Med. Chem.* **2003**, *10*, 813–829. [CrossRef]
40. de Groot, A.C.; Schmidt, E. Tea tree oil: Contact allergy and chemical composition. *Contact Dermat.* **2016**, *75*, 129–143. [CrossRef]
41. Liu, Q.; Meng, X.; Li, Y.; Zhao, C.N.; Tang, G.Y.; Li, H.B. Antibacterial and Antifungal Activities of Spices. *Int. J. Mol. Sci.* **2017**, *18*, 1283. [CrossRef]
42. Lee, S.H.; Kim, D.S.; Park, S.H.; Park, H. Phytochemistry and Applications of *Cinnamomum camphora* Essential Oils. *Molecules* **2022**, *27*, 2695. [CrossRef]
43. Zhang, T.; Zheng, Y.; Fu, C.; Yang, H.; Liu, X.; Qiu, F.; Wang, X.; Wang, Z. Chemical Variation and Environmental Influence on Essential Oil of *Cinnamomum camphora*. *Molecules* **2023**, *28*, 973. [CrossRef]
44. Szewczuk, M.A.; Zych, S.; Oster, N.; Karakulska, J. Activity of Patchouli and Tea Tree Essential Oils against *Staphylococci* Isolated from Pyoderma in Dogs and Their Synergistic Potential with Gentamicin and Enrofloxacin. *Animals* **2023**, *13*, 1279. [CrossRef]
45. Djenane, D.; Yanguela, J.; Roncales, P.; Aider, M. Use of essential oils as natural food preservatives: Effect on the growth of *Salmonella enteritidis* in liquid whole eggs stored underabuse refrigerated conditions. *J. Food Res.* **2013**, *2*, 65–78. [CrossRef]
46. Thosar, N.; Basak, S.; Bahadure, R.N.; Rajurkar, M. Antimicrobial efficacy of five essential oils against oral pathogens: An in vitro study. *Eur. J. Dent.* **2013**, *7*, 71–77. [CrossRef]
47. De Rapper, S.; Kamatou, G.; Viljoen, A.; van Vuuren, S. The in vitro antimicrobial activity of *Lavandula angustifolia* essential oil in combination with other aroma-therapeutic oils. *J. Evid. Based Complement. Altern. Med.* **2013**, *2013*, 852049.
48. Tacconelli, E.; Carrara, E.; Savoldi, A.; Harbarth, S.; Mendelson, M.; Monnet, D.L.; Pulcini, C.; Kahlmeter, G.; Kluytmans, J.; Carmeli, Y.; et al. Discovery, research, and development of new antibiotics: The WHO priority list of antibiotic-resistant bacteria and tuberculosis. *Lancet Infect. Dis.* **2018**, *3*, 318–327. [CrossRef]
49. Rosato, A.; Piarulli, M.; Corbo, F.; Muraglia, M.; Carone, A.; Vitali, M.E.; Vitali, C. In Vitro synergistic action of certain combinations of gentamicin and essential oils. *Curr. Med. Chem.* **2010**, *17*, 3289–3295. [CrossRef]
50. Moussaoui, F.; Alaoui, F. Evaluation of antibacterial activity and synergistic effect between antibiotic and the essential oils of some medicinal plants. *Asian Pac. J. Trop. Biomed.* **2016**, *6*, 32–37. [CrossRef]
51. Ismail, M.; Kemegne, G.A.; Njayou, F.N.; Penlap, V.; Mbacham, W.F.; Kamdem, S.L.S. Chemical composition, antibiotic promotion and in vivo toxicity of *Piper nigrum* and *Syzygium aromaticum* essential oil. *Afri. J. Biochem. Res.* **2017**, *11*, 58–71.
52. Clinical and Laboratory Standards Institute (CLSI). *Performance Standards for Antimicrobial Disk and Dilution Susceptibility Tests for Bacteria Isolated from Animals*, 5th ed.; CLSI supplement VET01S: Wayne, PA, USA, 2020.
53. European Committee for Antimicrobial Susceptibility Testing (EUCAST). Terminology Relating to Methods for the Determination of Susceptibility of Bacteria to Antimicrobial Agents. In *Eucast Definitive Document E.Def. 1.2.*; European Society of Clinical Microbiology and Infectious Diseases (ESCMID): Basel, Switzerland, 2002; Volume 6, pp. 503–508.

molecules

MDPI

Article

Comparison of Chemical Compositions and Antioxidant Activity of Essential Oils from Litsea Cubeba, Cinnamon, Anise, and Eucalyptus

Shutian Liu, Chen Zhao, Yuwei Cao, Yan Li, Zhuo Zhang, Dechao Nie, Weixuan Tang and Yanling Li *

Animal Science and Technology College, Beijing University of Agriculture, No. 7 Beinong Road, Changping, Beijing 102206, China; liushutian622@163.com (S.L.); zhaochenunique@163.com (C.Z.); cyw2222021@126.com (Y.C.); liyan06122022@163.com (Y.L.); zzhuo0126@163.com (Z.Z.); niedechao0403@163.com (D.N.); winsometang@163.com (W.T.)

* Correspondence: yanl_li@163.com or 20137302@bua.edu.cn

Abstract: The purpose of this study was to compare the antioxidant activity of litsea cubeba oil (LCO), cinnamon oil (CO), anise oil (AO), and eucalyptus oil (EUC) in vitro. The chemical compositions of the essential oils (EOs) were analyzed using gas chromatography-mass spectrometry (GC-MS). The antioxidant activity of the four EOs was evaluated through scavenging DPPH free radicals, chelating Fe^{2+}, scavenging hydroxyl free radicals, and inhibiting yolk lipid peroxidation. The results showed that the major compounds found in LCO, CO, AO, and EUC are citral (64.29%), cinnamaldehyde (84.25%), anethole (78.51%), and 1,8-cineole (81.78%), respectively. The four EOs all had certain antioxidant activity. The ability to scavenge DPPH radical was ranked in the order of LCO > CO > AO > EUC. The hydroxyl radical scavenging ability was ranked in the order of EUC > CO > LCO > AO. The chelating Fe^{2+} capacity was ranked in the order of EUC > AO > CO > LCO. The yolk lipid peroxidation inhibition ability was ranked in the order of CO > AO > EUC > LCO. In different antioxidant activity assays, the antioxidant activity of the EOs was different. It was speculated that the total antioxidant activity of an EO may be the result of the joint action of different antioxidant capacities.

Keywords: litsea cubeba oil; cinnamon oil; eucalyptus oil; anise oil; antioxidant activity

1. Introduction

In livestock production, intensive farming patterns and harmful environmental factors (e.g., bacteria) can lead to oxidative stress in animals. The overproduction of reactive oxygen species and an imbalance of antioxidant systems can cause oxidative stress [1]. Oxidative stress can destroy a variety of cellular components via DNA hydroxylation, protein denaturation, lipid peroxidation, and membrane rupture, which results in cell apoptosis and other cell death patterns [2,3]. Oxidative stress causes oxidative damage to the digestive tract, which, in turn, induces an inflammatory response in the organism. This ultimately leads to stunted growth, reduced immunity, and even death in the animal, which can seriously affect economic efficiency [4]. Eliminating and slowing down oxidative stress is a key step in protecting animals from injury. Some synthetic antioxidants, such as butylhydroxytoluene (BHT) and butylhydroxyanisole (BHA), may have carcinogenic potential and pose a risk to animal health and product quality. Therefore, it is important to find natural green antioxidants to reduce oxidative stress in animals.

Essential oils (EOs) are aromatic and volatile mixtures composed of dozens to hundreds of compounds, among which monoterpenes, sesquiterpenes, and their oxygen-containing derivatives are the main components [2,3,5]. The antioxidative and antibacterial activities of EOs are derived from these components. The toxicity and side effects of EOs are low, meaning they can be widely used in animal husbandry [6]. As a natural antioxidant,

EOs have been used in livestock and poultry production. Previous studies have reported that EOs reduce fat oxidation and improve the shelf-life of meat quality [7]. EOs can alleviate oxidative damage and inhibit the activation of NF-κB signaling pathways, thereby alleviating the damage of immune functions caused by oxidative stress [8,9]. Other studies have reported that EO supplementation increased the activity of antioxidant enzymes in the body and improved the growth performance and immune functions of animals [10]. Therefore, the antioxidant activity of EOs has important biological significance [11]. Some studies have indicated that *Litsea cubeba* (Lour.) Pers. oil (LCO), *Cinnamomum cassia* (L.) D. Don oil (CO), *Pimpinella anisum* L. oil (AO), and *Eucalyptus* spp. oil (EUC) have antibacterial, anti-inflammatory, and antioxidant activities, and these four EOs are widely used in the pharmaceutical and food industries in China [12–15]. Thus, the purpose of this study was to evaluate the chemical compositions of LCO, CO, AO, and EUC and compare their antioxidant activity via a DPPH radical scavenging assay, Fe^{2+} chelating assay, hydroxyl radical scavenging assay, and yolk lipid peroxidation assay. This study provides a theoretical basis for the application of EOs as a natural antioxidant in animal husbandry.

2. Results

2.1. Chemical Compositions of Essential Oils

The chemical compositions of the four EOs are shown in Table 1. There were 29, 20, 19, and 13 different active components that were detected in LCO, CO, AO, and EUC, respectively. The major components of LCO were citral (64.29%), d-limonene (12.39%), 4,5-epoxycarene (2.62%), β-caryophyllene (2.37%), and others (17.97%). CO contained cinnamaldehyde (84.25%), o-coumaric acid (6.43%), 3-(2-Methoxyphenyl)-2-propen (1.76%), cinnamyl acetate (1.46%), and others (6.1%). The major components of AO were anethole (78.51%), estragole (6.60%), 1-(3-methyl-2-butenyloxy)-4-(1-propenyl)benzene (3.47%), and d-limonene (2.0%). EUC contained 1,8-cineole (81.78%), 4-carene (5.35%), β-lauricene (4.58%), β-pinene (3.53%) and others (4.76%).

Table 1. Chemical constituents and contents of the four essential oils.

No.	Retention Indices	Retention Time RT/min	Compounds	Composition (% of Total)			
				LCO	CO	AO	EUC
1	847	2.015	Hydroperoxide, 1-methylhexyl	-	-	-	0.03
2	948	6.71	α-Pinene	1.46	-	0.98	-
3	943	7.251	Camphene	0.35	-	-	0.16
4	982	7.75	Benzaldehyde	-	1.06	-	-
5	897	8.075	Sabinene hydrate	1.08	-	-	-
6	943	8.194	β-Pinene	1.13	-	-	3.53
7	938	8.57	6-Methyl-5-hepten-2-one	1.80	-	-	-
8	958	8.695	β-Myrcene	0.71	-	-	4.58
9	969	9.162	α-Phellandrene	-	-	0.48	1.97
10	976	9.236	trans-β-Ocimene	-	-	0.37	0.30
11	919	9.53	4-Carene	-	-	-	5.35
12	1042	9.825	1-methyl-3-(1-methylethyl)-benzen	-	-	-	1.81
13	1018	9.95	D-Limonene	12.39	-	2.00	-
14	1059	10.092	1,8-cineole	-	-	0.7	81.79
15	998	10.818	Pinene	-	-	-	0.19
16	1082	12.229	3,7-Dimethyl-1,6-octadiene 3-ol	2.08	-	1.41	-
17	1174	13.294	3,3,5-Trimer-1,4-hexadiene	0.26	-	-	-
18	868	13.33	1,3-Hexadiene	-	-	-	0.25
19	1125	13.535	Citronellal	2.47	-	-	-

Table 1. *Cont.*

No.	Retention Indices	Retention Time RT/min	Compounds	Composition (% of Total)			
				LCO	CO	AO	EUC
20	1163	13.791	1,2,3,6-Tetrahydrobenzaldehyde	1.32	-	-	-
21	1181	13.793	Phenylpropyl aldehyde	-	0.74	-	-
22	1138	14.201	(1S)-endo)-(-)-borneol	0.10	-	-	-
23	1163	14.292	4,5-Epoxycarene	2.62	-	-	-
24	1137	14.303	4-Terpinenol	-	-	0.30	-
25	1172	14.746	Estragole	-	-	6.60	-
26	1143	14.767	α-Pinoresinol	0.78	-	-	0.05
27	1189	15.29	trans-Cinnamaldehyde	-	0.39	-	-
28	1174	15.891	β-Citral	28.71	-	-	-
29	1158	16.18	3-Methyl-2-cyclohexen-1-one	0.13	-	-	-
30	1171	16.256	4-Methoxybenzaldehyde	-	-	1.06	-
31	1228	16.322	Geraniol	1.93	-	-	-
32	1174	16.659	α-Citral	35.58	-	-	-
33	1189	16.884	Cinnamaldehyde	-	83.86	-	-
34	1031	17.086	7-Oxabicyclo [4.1.0] heptan-2-one	0.32	-	-	-
35	1190	17.16	Anethole	-	-	78.51	-
36	1199	18.101	2,7-Dimethyl-2,7-diol	0.24	-	-	-
37	1203	18.704	2,4,4,7-Tetramethyl-5,7-octadiene 3-ol	0.21	-	-	-
38	869	18.92	6-Hepten-3-ol	0.39	-	-	-
39	1221	18.961	α-cobalene	-	0.57	-	-
40	1424	19.094	2-methyl-epoxide	-	-	0.32	-
41	1398	19.284	β-Elemiene	0.33	-	-	-
42	1430	19.794	trans-α-bergamot	-	-	1.09	-
43	1494	19.925	Isoeugenol	-	0.18	-	-
44	1494	19.938	β-Caryophyllene	2.37	-	0.80	-
45	1430	20.221	trans-Bergamottin	-	0.12	-	-
46	1374	20.38	O-coumaric acid	-	6.43	-	-
47	1367	20.522	Cinnamyl acetate	-	1.46	-	-
48	1386	20.793	Balsamene	-	0.19	-	-
49	1435	21.111	γ-Ylang-ylangolene	-	0.16	-	-
50	1431	21.536	1,5-Dimethyl-8-(1-methylethylidene)-1,5-cyclododecene	-	-	0.24	-
51	1440	21.608	4,7-Dimethyl-1-(1-methylethyl)	-	0.4	-	-
52	1500	21.797	β-Red myrcene	-	0.38	0.2	-
53	1216	21.904	β-cobalene	-	0.17	-	-
54	1430	22.183	4,8,11,11-Tetramethyl-tricyclo[7.2.0.0(3,8)]undecylene-4-ene	-	0.16	-	-
55	1378	22.267	3-(2-Methoxyphenyl)-2-propenal	-	1.76	-	-
56	1564	22.924	trans-Nerolidol	-	0.34	0.24	-
57	1507	23.301	Graphene oxide	0.56	0.35	-	-
58	1580	24.757	alpha-Dauerol	-	-	0.23	-
59	1572	25.133	1-(3-Methyl-2-butenyloxy)-4-(1-propenyl)benzene	-	-	3.47	-
60	1490	30.762	β-Serinene	-	0.15	-	-
61	2192	31.513	trans-Geraniol	0.10	-	-	-
62	1281	31.632	Isododecane epoxide	0.2	-	-	-
63	1342	32.762	(2Z)-3,7-Dimethyl-2,6-octadienoic acid	0.22	-	-	-
64	1454	32.892	1-(2,2,5α-Trimethylperhydro-1-benzothiophen-1-yl)-2-buten-1-one	0.16	-	-	-
			Others	2.00	1.13	1.00	0.27
			Total	100	100	100	100

Note: "-" indicates that EO does not contain this component. LCO: litsea cubeba oil, CO: cinnamon oil, AO: anise oil, EUC: eucalyptus oil.

2.2. *The Antioxidant Activity of Essential Oils*

2.2.1. Effect of EOs on DPPH Radical Scavenging Rates

Figure 1 shows the effects of the EO type and the EO concentration on the scavenging rates of DPPH radicals. EO type (E) and EO concentration (C) had significant effects on DPPH radical scavenging rates ($p_E < 0.01$, $p_C < 0.01$), and the interactions between EO type and concentration (E × C) were significant ($p_E \times p_C < 0.01$). The DPPH radical scavenging rate quadratically increased ($p_Q < 0.01$) with an increase in the concentration of LCO, CO, AO, and EUC. In comparing rates among EOs, the DPPH radical scavenging rate differed ($p < 0.05$) at a concentration of 2.5 mg/mL (CO > LCO > AO, EUC), at a concentration of 10 and 20 mg/mL (CO, LCO > AO > EUC), at a concentration of 40 mg/mL (LCO > CO > AO > EUC), and at a concentration of 80 mg/mL (LCO > CO > AO > EUC). The BHA had consistently greater ($p < 0.05$) hydroxyl radical scavenging rates compared to all EOs, except there was no significant difference ($p > 0.05$) in DPPH radical scavenging between LCO and BHA at the concentration of 80 mg/mL.

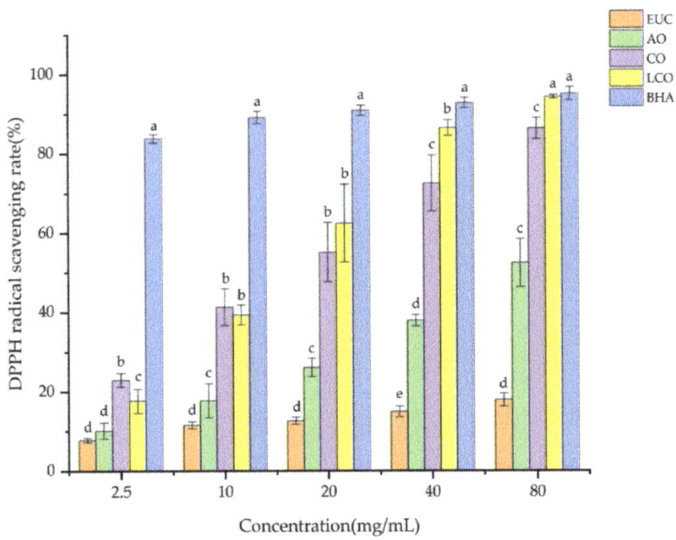

Figure 1. Effects of different concentrations of EOs on DPPH radical scavenging rates. EOs (E) and their different concentrations (C) had significant effects on DPPH radical scavenging rates ($p_E < 0.01$, $p_C < 0.01$), and their interaction (E × C) was significant ($p_E \times p_C < 0.01$). Different letters show differences ($p < 0.05$) among EOs. LCO: litsea cubeba oil, CO: cinnamon oil, AO: anise oil, EUC: eucalyptus oil; BHA: butylated hydroxyanisole.

2.2.2. Effect of EOs on Fe^{2+} Chelating Ability

Figure 2 shows the effects of the EO type and the EO concentration on Fe^{2+} chelating capacity. EO type (E) and EO concentration (C) had significant effects on the Fe^{2+} chelating ability ($p_E < 0.01$, $p_C < 0.01$), and the interactions between EO type and concentration (E × C) were significant ($p_E \times p_C < 0.01$). The Fe^{2+} chelating capacity quadratically increased ($p_Q < 0.01$) with an increase in the concentration of LCO, and linearly increased ($p_L < 0.01$) with an increase in the concentration of CO, AO, and EUC. In comparing capacity among EOs, the Fe^{2+} chelating capacity differed ($p < 0.05$) at five different EO concentration levels (2, 6, 8, 10, and 12 mg/mL) (EUC > AO > CO > LCO). The VC had a consistently greater ($p < 0.05$) Fe^{2+} chelating capacity compared to all EOs at all of the concentrations. At the concentration of 12 mg/mL, the chelation rate of VC to Fe^{2+} was 82.59%, and the chelation rates of AO and EUC to Fe^{2+} were 70.15% and 75.39%, respectively, reaching 84.94% and 91.28% of VC.

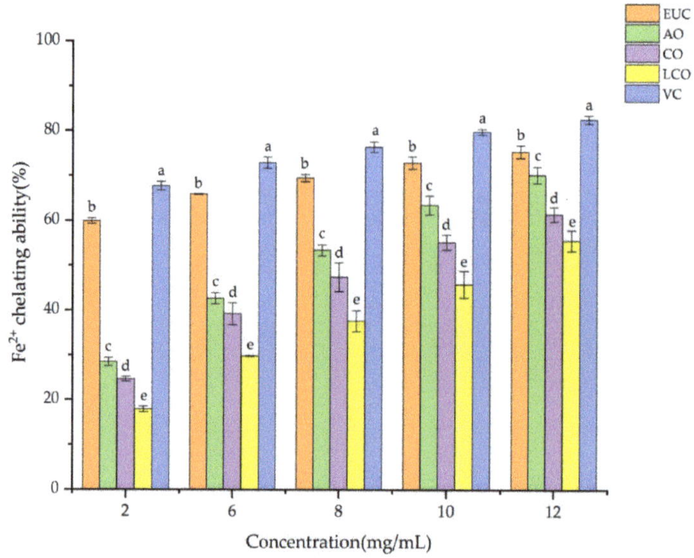

Figure 2. Effects of different concentrations of EOs on Fe^{2+} chelating ability. EOs (E) and their different concentrations (C) had significant effects on Fe^{2+} chelating capacity ($p_E < 0.01$, $p_C < 0.01$), and their interaction (E × C) was significant ($p_E \times p_C < 0.01$). Different letters show differences ($p < 0.05$) among EOs. LCO: litsea cubeba oil, CO: cinnamon oil, AO: anise oil, EUC: eucalyptus oil; VC: Vitamin C.

2.2.3. Effect of EOs on Hydroxyl Radical Scavenging Rates

The effects of the EO type and the EO concentration on the scavenging rates of hydroxyl radicals are shown in Figure 3. EO type (E) and EO concentration (C) had significant effects on the hydroxyl radical scavenging rate ($p_E < 0.01$, $p_C < 0.01$), and the interactions between EO type and concentration (E × C) were significant ($p_E \times p_C < 0.01$). The hydroxyl radical scavenging rate quadratically increased ($p_Q < 0.01$) with an increase in the concentration of LCO, CO, AO, and EUC. In comparing rates among EOs, the hydroxyl radical scavenging rate differed ($p < 0.05$) at five different EO concentration levels (1, 4, 8, 16, and 32 mg/mL) (EUC > CO > LCO > AO). The VC had a consistently greater ($p < 0.05$) hydroxyl radical scavenging rate compared to all EOs at all of the concentrations. At the concentration of 32 mg/mL, the hydroxyl radical scavenging rate of VC was 85.66%, and the hydroxyl radical scavenging rate of EUC was 75.05%, which reached more than 80% of the level of VC.

2.2.4. Effects of EOs on the Inhibition of Yolk Lipid Peroxidation

Figure 4 shows the effect of the EO type and the EO concentration on the lipid peroxidation inhibition rate of yolk. EO type (E) and EO concentration (C) had significant effects on the lipid peroxidation inhibition rate of yolk ($p_E < 0.01$, $p_C < 0.01$), and the interactions of EO type and concentration (E × C) were significant ($p_E \times p_C < 0.01$). The lipid peroxidation inhibition rate of yolk quadratically increased ($p_Q < 0.01$) with increasing the concentration of LCO, CO, AO and EUC. In comparing among EOs, the lipid peroxidation inhibition rate of yolk differed ($p < 0.05$) at a concentration of 1.25, 5, 10, 20 mg/mL (PG > CO > AO > EUC > LCO) and at the concentration of 4 mg/mL (CO > AO, EUC > LCO). At the concentration of 2.5 mg/mL, the inhibition rate of PG on yolk lipid peroxidation was 90.41%, and that of CO was 86.42%, reaching 95.59% of PG.

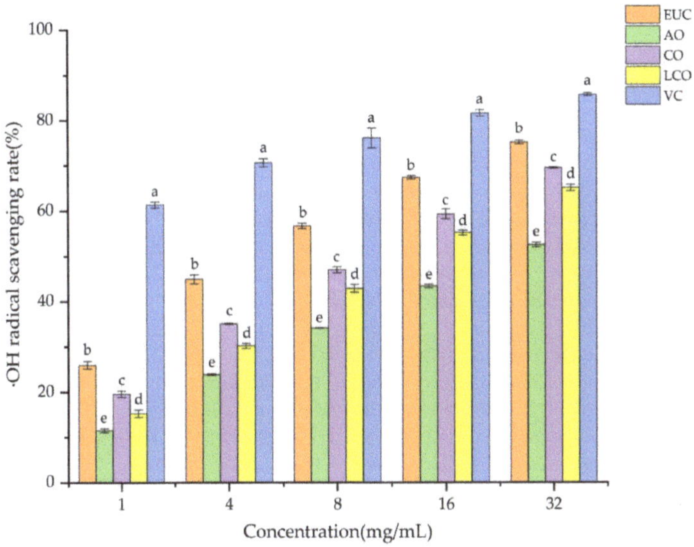

Figure 3. Effects of different concentrations of EOs on ·OH radical scavenging rates. EOs (E) and their different concentrations (C) had significant effects on ·OH radical scavenging rates ($p_E < 0.01$, $p_C < 0.01$), and their interaction (E × C) was significant ($p_E \times p_C < 0.01$). Different letters show differences ($p < 0.05$) among EOs. LCO: litsea cubeba oil, CO: cinnamon oil, AO: anise oil, EUC: eucalyptus oil; VC: Vitamin C.

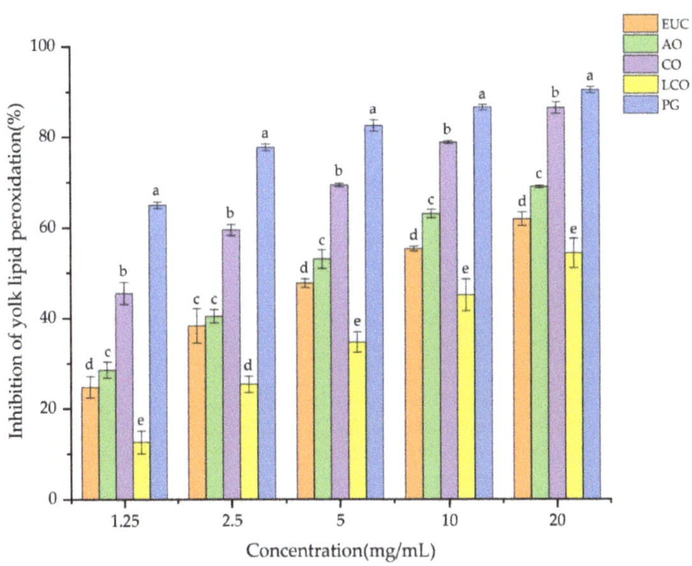

Figure 4. Effect of different concentrations of EOs on yolk lipid peroxidation inhibition. EOs (E) and their different concentrations (C) had significant effects on yolk lipid peroxidation inhibition ($p_E < 0.01$, $p_C < 0.01$), and their interaction (E × C) was significant ($p_E \times p_C < 0.01$). Different letters show differences ($p < 0.05$) among EOs. LCO: litsea cubeba oil, CO: cinnamon oil, AO: anise oil, EUC: eucalyptus oil; PG: propyl gallate.

3. Discussion

A reduction in antioxidant defense mechanisms and the production of free radicals can lead to oxidative stress, which damages proteins, lipids, and enzymes [16]. Free radicals exist in the body widely, and they are the main cause of lipid peroxidation and the root of oxidative damage to macromolecular substances [17]. Some studies have shown that oxidative stress can cause inflammation and other diseases by producing excess free radicals to mediate oxidative damage to cells [18]. Antioxidants can scavenge free radicals and stop free radical reactions. As a result of the carcinogenicity and hepatotoxicity of synthetic antioxidants (such as BHA and BHT), EOs have attracted increasing attention as green natural antioxidants. Some studies have found that EOs can prevent free radical chain reactions and delay the lipid peroxidation process [6,19,20].

EOs are complex mixtures of different volatile and non-volatile components [21]. Different EOs have different chemical compositions. In our study, it was found that the active components of the four studied EOs were very complex and varied greatly. Citral, the main component of LCO, and cinnamic aldehyde, the main component of CO, are aldehydes. Anisole, the main component of AO, and 1, 8-eudinolein, the main component of EUC, are terpenoid compounds. The reasons for the differences in EO active components may be related to variety, heredity, maturity stage, culture conditions, etc. [22].

It has been reported that EOs can reduce or eliminate free radicals, block free radical chain reactions, and delay lipid peroxidation [23]. In our study, the antioxidant activity of four EOs was evaluated through scavenging DPPH free radicals, chelating Fe^{2+}, scavenging hydroxyl free radicals, and inhibiting yolk lipid peroxidation. Our study found that the antioxidant activity of EOs is related to the EO concentration and EO type. The DPPH and hydroxyl radical scavenging rate, the Fe^{2+} chelating ability, and the inhibition rate of the lipid peroxidation of yolk were dose-dependent, and they linearly or quadratically increased with an increase in EO concentration, which suggests that the antioxidant activity of EOs varies with concentration. Similarly, El amrani et al. [24] found that the DPPH radical inhibition percentages of cinnamon and clove essential oils presented a dose dependent effect. Other studies have found that the scavenging effect of AO was stronger than BHA and BHT and increased with the increase of concentration [25]. In DPPH radical scavenging experiments, the position of different EOs changes at different concentrations (cross effect). Similar results have been observed in our previous study, where it was found that the antioxidant activity of five citrus EOs increased with an increase in concentration. Additionally, the scavenging effect of bergamot EO was higher than that of lemon EO at low concentrations of 16–80 mg/mL, but the results were the opposite at higher concentrations of 112–144 mg/mL [26]. This is due to the interaction between the type of EO and its concentration. In addition, different EOs had different antioxidant activity. Wei et al. [27] measured the antioxidant activity of 25 EOs and found that cinnamon leaf oil, clove leaf oil, and thyme oil had good antioxidant activity, while sandalwood oil showed poor antioxidant activity. Similarly, Ghazghazi et al. [28] found significant differences in the antioxidant activity of two EOs (*Eucalyptus marginata* L. and *Eucalyptus pauciflora* L. EOs). Another study analyzed the antioxidant activity of LCO extracted in different months, and the results showed that LCO extracted in July had a better hydroxyl radical scavenging rate, and LCO extracted in August had a better DPPH scavenging activity and ferric reducing antioxidant power [29]. In this study, at the same concentration, EUC and CO had good radical hydroxyl scavenging ability, while AO and LCO had poor scavenging ability. This difference may be due to the different chemical compositions of different EOs, and the compositions and contents of EOs may affect their overall antioxidant activity [30].

In addition, the antioxidant activity of EOs is related to their chemical compositions [31]. It has been reported that phenols contribute greatly to the antioxidant capacity of EOs [32]. The phenolic hydroxyl can release hydrogen ions to bind with free radicals and block the oxidative chain reaction [33], and the antioxidant activity of EOs is significantly positively correlated with the phenol content [34]. Mechergui et al. [35] reported that the antioxidant activity of oregano oil mainly depended on the carvall and thymol contents.

In addition, fatty acids, esters, ketones, alcohols, and terpenoids have previously been reported to have antioxidant activity [36]. Adefegha et al. [37] showed that the free radical scavenging ability and metal chelating ability of Masson pine EO may be attributed to phenolic monoterpenes and oxygenated monoterpenes in EOs. Some studies have shown that the antioxidant activity of different antioxidants mainly depends on their stability after absorbing lone pair electrons, and phenols > aldehydes > alcohols [38]. The four EOs showed different antioxidant activity, which may have been caused by the different chemical components of different EOs. The active components of EOs are complex and diverse, and whether the antioxidant activity of different active components are based on synergistic, antagonistic, or additive effects needs to be further studied.

Various antioxidant activity assays have been used to evaluate the antioxidant capacity of EOs in vitro, and EOs showed different antioxidant activity using different assays. In our study, we evaluated the antioxidant activity of EOs using four methods: scavenging DPPH radical, chelating Fe^{2+}, scavenging hydroxyl radical, and inhibiting yolk lipid peroxidation. DPPH free radical is a stable radical that is widely used as a tool to evaluate the free radical scavenging activity of EOs [39]. The ability of EOs to scavenge DPPH free radicals may be related to their ability to provide hydrogen atoms. EOs can provide hydrogen atoms to DPPH radicals to form stable end products (DPPH-H), which will not further trigger or aggravate lipid oxidation [40]. It has been found that monoterpenes, such as citral, carvone, laurene, and γ-terpinene, have strong DPPH radical scavenging activity [41]. The scavenging ability of EOs against DPPH free radicals is related to their content of unsaturated hydrocarbon. LCO had the strongest scavenging ability against DPPH free radicals among the four EOs, which may be due to the effects of citral, the main component of LCO. The accumulation of Fe^{2+} in cells can induce the production of free radicals and malondialdehyde [37,42]. EOs can chelate with metal ions to form stable complexes that inhibit the formation of metal-induced free radicals. Some phenols in EOs can effectively chelate ferrous ions [43]. Singh et al. [44] found that the chelating activity of EOs of *Zanthoxylum armatum* DC was significantly higher than that of BHA and BHT, which may be attributed to the phenolic compounds contained in EOs that can chelate metal ions. In our study, EUC showed a good Fe^{2+} chelating ability and increased in a dose-dependent manner, which may be due to the large number of compounds in the oil and their possible affinity for Fe^{2+}. Hydroxyl free radical is a kind of highly active oxidant that can directly damage various biofilms and lead to many diseases [45]. Hydroxyl free radicals can extract electrons from polyunsaturated fatty acids and produce lipid radicals, which can trigger lipid peroxidation. In addition, hydroxyl free radicals are highly reactive products produced via the decomposition of hydrogen peroxide in the presence of Fe^{2+} and other metals, which can aggravate oxidative stress in the body, lead to immune system dysfunction, and affect the digestion, absorption, and transformation of nutrients [46]. Thus, a reduction in hydroxyl radicals can reduce lipid peroxidation and protect the immune system. In our study, all four EOs could remove hydroxyl radicals, among which EUC has the best effect. The scavenging effects of EOs on hydroxyl free radicals can not only act on the non-chain process before the oxidation reaction chain to remove the hydroxyl radicals, starting the chain reaction, but also remove the free radicals in the chain extension process, producing a dual-antioxidant effect. Lipid peroxidation is considered to be an important mechanism of cell damage under oxidative stress and is involved in the pathological processes of many diseases [47]. Previous studies have shown that EOs can effectively inhibit lipid peroxidation. Gargouri et al. [48] found that Henna EO showed very high potential for scavenging free radicals and inhibiting lipid peroxidation, which could be used to combat the oxidative stress generated by Raji cells. Alizadeh et al. [49] speculated that the EO of *Zeilan cinnamomum* L. had a strong free radical scavenging ability and the potential to inhibit lipid oxidation reactions, which was consistent with the results of our experiment. In our study, CO showed the best inhibition of lipid peroxidation of yolk, which may be attributed to the fact that its main component, 1,8 eucalyptol, is a monoterpenoid. It has been found that monoterpene hydrocarbon, γ-terpinene, retards the peroxidation of linoleic acid because its chaincarrying peroxyls are HOO• radicals, which react rapidly with linoleylperoxyl radicals [50]. In our study, the four EOs showed different antioxidant activity in different antioxidant tests. EUC showed good hydroxyl radical scavenging ability and Fe^{2+} chelating ability, but poor DPPH radical scavenging ability and yolk lipid peroxidation inhibition. Similarly, Bi et al. [51] found that the EOs from Nandina domestica fruits exhibited significant scavenging activity against DPPH free radical and ATBS free radical, moderate scavenging activity against superoxide anion free radical, and low activity against metal chelating power. This difference may be due to the fact that the total antioxidant activity of EOs is the result of a combination of one or several pathways. In our study, EUC had the best hydroxyl radical scavenging ability and chelating Fe^{2+} ability, and CO had better yolk lipid peroxidation inhibition ability and DPPH and hydroxyl radical scavenging ability. Therefore, EUC and CO have good antioxidant activity and have the potential to be used in practical production as a new green antioxidant.

In summary, our results show that the four EOs possessed significant antioxidant activity, but their antioxidant capacity varied with EO type and concentration. In addition, the different antioxidant abilities of EOs may be due to the different chemical compositions of EOs. Combined with the results of the four antioxidant experiments, it is speculated that the total antioxidant activity of EOs may comprise different activities including scavenging free radicals, chelating Fe^{2+}, and inhibiting lipid peroxidation etc.

4. Materials and Methods

4.1. Chemicals and Reagents

Butylated hydroxyanisole was purchased from Beijing Solarbio Science and Technology Co., Ltd. (Beijing, China). DPPH was purchased from Sigma–Aldrich (Shanghai, China) and Sigma–Aldrich (St. Louis, MO, USA). Propyl gallat, vitamin C, Acido salicilico, and 2-thiobarbituric acid (TBA) were purchased from Sinopharm Chemical Reagent Co., Ltd. (Shanghai, China).

4.2. Essential Oils

LCO (purity 80%), CO (purity 80%), AO (purity 87%), and EUC (purity 80%) were purchased from Nanjing Vincero International Trade Co., Ltd. (Nanjing, China).

4.3. Gas Chromatography-Mass Spectrometry (GC-MS) Analysis

The EO samples were diluted 1:100 with hexane and then injected into an Rxi-5Sil MS (Restek, Bellefonte, Newcastle, PA, USA, 30 m × 0.25 mm × 0.25 μm) column via the GC-MS injection system. The column temperature was initially set at 50 °C and held for 5 min, then increased up to 320 °C at a rate of 6 °C/min for 5 min and solvent delay for 3 min. Helium was used as a carrier with a shunt ratio of 10:1 and a flow rate of 1 mL/min. Total ion flow chromatography (TIC) was obtained by analyzing the samples. The data were collected using the GC-MS solution 2.6 software and screened and matched with NIST and other dedicated standard spectrum libraries to identify each component of the EOs. Finally, the relative content was calculated using area normalization.

4.4. Antioxidant Activity

4.4.1. Experimental Design

The antioxidant activity of the four EOs at different concentrations was evaluated by measuring DPPH free radical scavenging ability, Fe^{2+} chelating ability, hydroxyl radical scavenging ability, and yolk lipid peroxidation inhibition. The experiment was a completed randomized design with 4 EOs (LCO, CO, AO, and EUC) × 5 concentrations of factorial arrangements of treatments. The concentration of each EO was 2.5, 10, 20, 40, and 80 mg/mL in the DPPH measurements; 2, 6, 8, 10, and 12 mg/mL in the Fe^{2+} chelating ability assay; 1, 4, 8, 16, and 32 mg/mL in the hydroxyl radical scavenging ability assay; and 1.25, 2.5, 5, 10, and 20 mg/mL in the yolk lipid peroxidation inhibition assay. Butylated hydroxyanisole (BHA), propyl gallate (PG), and vitamin C (VC), as strong antioxidants, were used as controls, respectively.

4.4.2. DPPH Radical Scavenging Ability Assay

The DPPH free radical scavenging activity was determined according to a previously described method [52]. LCO, CO, AO, EUC, and BHA were diluted with anhydrous ethanol to 2.5, 10, 20, 40, and 80 mg/mL, respectively. A 2 mL EOs diluent and 2 mL 0.2 mmol/L DPPH ethanol solution were taken to prepare 4 mL of the tested solution in a tube. After shaking, the solution was kept away from light at room temperature for 30 min. Next, 200 μL of the tested solution was added to a 96-well microtiter plate. The absorbance was measured using an automatic microplate reader at 517 nm, and the clearance rate was calculated. There were 3 parallel groups in each group. The DPPH free radical scavenging rate was calculated according to Formula (1). A_1 is the absorbance of the ethanol solution of DPPH mixed with the diluent of plant EOs, A_0 is the absorbance of the DPPH ethanol solution mixed with anhydrous ethanol, and A_2 is the absorbance of the plant EOs diluent mixed with absolute ethanol.

$$\text{DPPH radical scavenging rate} = [A_0 - (A_1 - A_2)]/A_0 \times 100\% \quad (1)$$

4.4.3. Fe^{2+} Chelating Ability Assay

The Fe^{2+} chelating ability was determined as described by Oboh et al. [53]. LCO, CO, AO, EUC, and strong antioxidant (VC) were diluted with anhydrous ethanol to 2, 6, 8, 10, and 12 mg/mL, respectively. A total of 1 mL of the diluted sample solution was taken, and 0.1 mL of 2 mmol/L $FeCl_2$ and 0.3 mL of 5 mmol/L phenanthrazine were successively added to the clean test tube. Then, 2.6 mL of distilled water was added to prepare 4 mL of the tested solution, and the solution was left at room temperature for 20 min. A total of 200 μL of the tested solution was added to a 96-well microtiter plate. The absorbance was measured using an automatic microplate reader at 517 nm, and the clearance rate was calculated. There were 3 parallel groups in each group. The chelating capacity of Fe^{2+} was calculated according to Formula (2). A_1 is the absorbance of the tested solution added to EOs, A_0 is the absorbance of absolute ethanol sample solution without EOs, and A_2 is the absorbance of distilled water without phenanthrazine.

$$Fe^{2+} \text{ chelating capacity } (\%) = [A_0 - (A_1 - A_2)/A_0] \times 100\% \quad (2)$$

4.4.4. Hydroxyl Radical Scavenging Ability Assay

The hydroxyl radical scavenging ability was measured according to the method of Radünz [54] with some modifications. LCO, CO, AO, EUC, and strong antioxidant (VC) were diluted with anhydrous ethanol to 1, 4, 8, 16, and 32 mg/mL, respectively. A total of 1 mL of essential oil diluent was taken from each, and 1 mL of a 2 mmol/L $FeSO_4$, 1 mL of a 6 mmol/L salicylic acid, and 1 mL of a 2 mmol/L H_2O_2 were added to prepare 4 mL of the tested sample solution. The solution was mixed well and left for 30 min at room temperature. A total of 200 μL of the tested solution was added to a 96-well microtiter plate. The absorbance was measured using an automatic microplate reader at 510 nm and the clearance rate was calculated. There were 3 parallel groups in each group. The hydroxyl radical scavenging rate was calculated according to Formula (3). A_1 is the absorbance of the tested solution added to EOs; A_0 is the absorbance of absolute ethanol sample solution without EOs; A_2 is the absorbance of distilled water without H_2O_2.

$$\text{The hydroxyl radical scavenging rate } (\%) = [A_0 - (A_1 - A_2)]/A_0 \times 100\% \quad (3)$$

4.4.5. Yolk Lipid Peroxidation Inhibition Assay

The yolk lipid peroxidation inhibition rate was determined according to a previously described method [55]. The yolk of fresh eggs was put into a 50 mL beaker, the same volume of phosphate buffer was added, the sealing film was fastened, and the solution was stored at −4 °C. Four EOs and PG were diluted with absolute ethanol to 1.25, 2.5, 5, 10, and 20 mg/mL sample dilutions. A total of 0.5 mL of egg yolk stock solution was taken and 12 mL of phosphate buffer was added to prepare a 1:25 egg yolk suspension. A total of 200 μL of the yolk suspension was taken, a 100 μL EO sample diluent was added, and then 200 μL of a 25 mmol/L $FeSO_4$ was added and supplemented to 1 mL with phosphate buffer. After shaking at 37 °C for 30 min, 250 μL of a 20% trichloroacetic acid was added, 3500 r/min centrifugation was performed for 10 min until clarification, the supernatant was absorbed, and 250 μL of a 0.8% TBA was added. A total of 1.5 mL of the sample solution was prepared to be tested and reacted in a boiling water bath for 15 min. A total of 200 μL of the tested solution was added to a 96-well microtiter plate. The absorbance was measured using an automatic microplate reader at 510 nm, and the clearance rate was calculated. There were 3 parallel groups in each group. The yolk lipid peroxidation inhibition rate was calculated according to Formula (4). A_1 is the absorbance of the tested solution added to EOs; A_0 is the absorbance of absolute ethanol sample solution without EOs; A_2 is the absorbance of the tested solution without yolk.

$$\text{The yolk lipid peroxidation inhibition rate (\%)} = [A_0 - (A_1 - A_2)/A_0] \times 100\% \quad (4)$$

5. Statistical Analysis

Data for antioxidant activity were analyzed using the SAS 9.4 mixing procedure with a model including EO type, EO concentration, and their interactions as fixed effects and three replications of the experiment as random effects. The effects of increasing the EO concentration were examined through linear and quadratic orthogonal contrasts using the CONTRAST statement of SAS. Differences were declared significant at $p \leq 0.05$. The graphs were drawn using the Origin 2021 software (Northampton, MA, USA).

6. Conclusions

The major compounds found in LCO, CO, AO, and EUC are citral, cinnamaldehyde, anethole, and 1,8-cineole, respectively. The four EOs effectively scavenged DPPH, chelated Fe^{2+}, scavenged hydroxyl radicals, and inhibited lipid peroxidation in a dose-dependent manner. Compared with that of the other EOs, the DPPH radical scavenging ability of LCO was the strongest; EUC had the greatest activity in its Fe^{2+} chelating ability and hydroxyl radical scavenging rate; and CO had the highest yolk lipid peroxidation ability. It is speculated that the total antioxidant activity of EOs might be the result of the joint actions of different antioxidant capacities.

Author Contributions: Y.L. (Yanling Li) covered the project. S.L., C.Z. and Y.C. designed and performed the experiments and analyzed the raw data. Z.Z., D.N., Y.L. (Yan Li) and W.T. assisted with the experiments. Y.L. (Yanling Li) supervised the project. All authors have read and agreed to the published version of the manuscript.

Funding: This work was supported by Beijing Natural Science Foundation (6222006).

Institutional Review Board Statement: Not applicable.

Informed Consent Statement: Not applicable.

Data Availability Statement: Data present in this study are available on request from the corresponding author.

Acknowledgments: Thanks for the experimental environment provided by the Animal Nutrition Laboratory of the Beijing University of Agriculture.

Conflicts of Interest: The authors declare no conflict of interest.

Sample Availability: Samples of the compounds are available from the authors.

References

1. Zahra, K.F.; Lefter, R.; Ali, A.; Abdellah, E.C.; Trus, C.; Ciobica, A.; Timofte, D. The Involvement of the Oxidative Stress Status in Cancer Pathology: A Double View on the Role of the Antioxidants. *Oxid. Med. Cell Longev.* **2021**, *2021*, 9965916. [CrossRef]
2. Li, G.; Xiang, S.; Pan, Y.; Long, X.; Cheng, Y.; Han, L.; Zhao, X. Effects of Cold-Pressing and Hydrodistillation on the Active Non-volatile Components in Lemon Essential Oil and the Effects of the Resulting Oils on Aging-Related Oxidative Stress in Mice. *Front. Nutr.* **2021**, *8*, 689094. [CrossRef]
3. Gonzalez-Mas, M.C.; Rambla, J.L.; Lopez-Gresa, M.P.; Blazquez, M.A.; Granell, A. Volatile Compounds in Citrus Essential Oils: A Comprehensive Review. *Front. Plant Sci.* **2019**, *10*, 12. [CrossRef]
4. Zeng, Z.; Zhang, S.; Wang, H.; Piao, X. Essential oil and aromatic plants as feed additives in non-ruminant nutrition: A review. *J. Anim. Sci. Biotechnol.* **2015**, *6*, 7. [CrossRef]
5. Diaz-Sanchez, S.; D'Souza, D.; Biswas, D.; Hanning, I. Botanical alternatives to antibiotics for use in organic poultry production. *Poult. Sci.* **2015**, *94*, 1419–1430. [CrossRef]
6. Bączek, K.B.; Kosakowska, O.; Przybył, J.L.; Pióro-Jabrucka, E.; Costa, R.; Mondello, L.; Gniewosz, M.; Synowiec, A.; Węglarz, Z. Antibacterial and antioxidant activity of essential oils and extracts from costmary (*Tanacetum balsamita* L.) and tansy (*Tanacetum vulgare* L.). *Ind. Crops Prod.* **2017**, *102*, 154–163. [CrossRef]
7. Falowo, A.B.; Mukumbo, F.E.; Idamokoro, E.M.; Afolayan, A.J.; Muchenje, V. Phytochemical Constituents and Antioxidant Activity of Sweet Basil (*Ocimum basilicum* L.) Essential Oil on Ground Beef from Boran and Nguni Cattle. *Int. J. Food Sci.* **2019**, *2019*, 2628747. [CrossRef]
8. Younis, N.S.; Abduldaium, M.S.; Mohamed, M.E. Protective Effect of Geraniol on Oxidative, Inflammatory and Apoptotic Alterations in Isoproterenol-Induced Cardiotoxicity: Role of the Keap1/Nrf2/HO-1 and PI3K/Akt/mTOR Pathways. *Antioxidants* **2020**, *9*, 977. [CrossRef]
9. Younis, N.S.; Mohamed, M.E. Protective effects of myrrh essential oil on isoproterenol-induced myocardial infarction in rats through antioxidant, anti-inflammatory, Nrf2/HO-1 and apoptotic pathways. *J. Ethnopharmacol.* **2021**, *270*, 113793. [CrossRef]
10. Elbaz, A.M.; Ashmawy, E.S.; Salama, A.A.; Abdel-Moneim, A.E.; Badri, F.B.; Thabet, H.A. Effects of garlic and lemon essential oils on performance, digestibility, plasma metabolite, and intestinal health in broilers under environmental heat stress. *BMC Vet. Res.* **2022**, *18*, 430. [CrossRef]
11. Simitzis, P.E. Enrichment of Animal Diets with Essential Oils-A Great Perspective on Improving Animal Performance and Quality Characteristics of the Derived Products. *Medicines* **2017**, *4*, 35. [CrossRef]
12. Thielmann, J.; Muranyi, P. Review on the chemical composition of *Litsea cubebaessential* oils and the bioactivity of its major constituents citral and limonene. *J. Essent. Oil Res.* **2019**, *31*, 361–378. [CrossRef]
13. Abd El-Hack, M.E.; Alagawany, M.; Abdel-Moneim, A.E.; Mohammed, N.G.; Khafaga, A.F.; Bin-Jumah, M.; Othman, S.I.; Allam, A.A.; Elnesr, S.S. Cinnamon (*Cinnamomum zeylanicum*) Oil as a Potential Alternative to Antibiotics in Poultry. *Antibiotics* **2020**, *9*, 210. [CrossRef]
14. Adnan, M. Bioactive potential of essential oil extracted from the leaves of Eucalyptus globulus (*Myrtaceae*). *J. Pharmacogn. Phytochem.* **2019**, *8*, 213–216.
15. Koriem, K.M.M.; Fadl, N.N.; El-Zayat, S.R.; Hosny, E.N.; Abbas El-Shamy, K.; Arbid, M.S.; Morsy, F.A.; El-Azma, M.H. Geranium oil and anise oil inhibit brain cerebral cortex and hippocampus inflammation in depressed animal model. *Nutr. Food Sci.* **2020**, *51*, 439–456. [CrossRef]
16. Zhuang, S.; Yu, R.; Zhong, J.; Liu, P.; Liu, Z. Rhein from Rheum rhabarbarum Inhibits Hydrogen-Peroxide-Induced Oxidative Stress in Intestinal Epithelial Cells Partly through PI3K/Akt-Mediated Nrf2/HO-1 Pathways. *J. Agric. Food Chem.* **2019**, *67*, 2519–2529. [CrossRef]
17. Pisoschi, A.M.; Pop, A. The role of antioxidants in the chemistry of oxidative stress: A review. *Eur. J. Med. Chem.* **2015**, *97*, 55–74. [CrossRef]
18. Chatterjee, S. Oxidative stress, inflammation, and disease. In *Oxidative Stress and Biomaterials*; Academic Press: Cambridge, MA, USA, 2016; pp. 35–58.
19. Fancello, F.; Petretto, G.L.; Zara, S.; Sanna, M.L.; Addis, R.; Maldini, M.; Foddai, M.; Rourke, J.P.; Chessa, M.; Pintore, G. Chemical characterization, antioxidant capacity and antimicrobial activity against food related microorganisms of *Citrus limon* var. pompia leaf essential oil. *LWT Food Sci. Technol.* **2016**, *69*, 579–585. [CrossRef]
20. Lin, L.Y.; Chuang, C.H.; Chen, H.C.; Yang, K.M. Lime (*Citrus aurantifolia* (Christm.) Swingle) Essential Oils: Volatile Compounds, Antioxidant Capacity, and Hypolipidemic Effect. *Foods* **2019**, *8*, 398. [CrossRef]
21. Deng, W.; Liu, K.; Cao, S.; Sun, J.; Zhong, B.; Chun, J. Chemical Composition, Antimicrobial, Antioxidant, and Antiproliferative Properties of Grapefruit Essential Oil Prepared by Molecular Distillation. *Molecules* **2020**, *25*, 217. [CrossRef]
22. Lin, X.; Cao, S.; Sun, J.; Lu, D.; Zhong, B.; Chun, J. The Chemical Compositions, and Antibacterial and Antioxidant Activities of Four Types of Citrus Essential Oils. *Molecules* **2021**, *26*, 3412. [CrossRef]
23. Bhavaniramya, S.; Vishnupriya, S.; Al-Aboody, M.S.; Vijayakumar, R.; Baskaran, D. Role of essential oils in food safety: Antimicrobial and antioxidant applications. *Grain Oil Sci. Technol.* **2019**, *2*, 49–55. [CrossRef]
24. Amrania, S.E.; Lalamib, A.E.O.; Zoubic, Y.E.; Moukhafia, K.; Bouslamtia, R.; Lairinia, S. Evaluation of antibacterial and antioxidant effects of cinnamon and clove essential oils from Madagascar. *Sci. Direct* **2019**, *13*, 762–770.

25. Singh, G.; Kapoor, I.P.S.; Singh, P.; Heluani, C.S.d.; Catalan, C.A.N. Chemical composition and antioxidant potential of essential oil and oleoresins from anise seeds (*Pimpinella anisum* L.). *Int. J. Essent. Oil Ther.* **2008**, *2*, 122–130.
26. Li, Y.; Liu, S.; Zhao, C.; Zhang, Z.; Nie, D.; Tang, W.; Li, Y. The Chemical Composition and Antibacterial and Antioxidant Activities of Five Citrus Essential Oils. *Molecules* **2022**, *27*, 7044. [CrossRef]
27. Wei, A.; Shibamoto, T. Antioxidant/lipoxygenase inhibitory activities and chemical compositions of selected essential oils. *J. Agric. Food Chem.* **2010**, *58*, 7218–7225. [CrossRef]
28. Li, H.; Chu, X.; Li, D.; Zeng, Z.H.; Peng, X.X. Construction and immune protection evaluation of recombinant polyvalent OmpAs derived from genetically divergent ompA by DNA shuffling. *Fish Shellfish Immunol.* **2016**, *49*, 230–236. [CrossRef]
29. She, Q.H.; Li, W.S.; Jiang, Y.Y.; Wu, Y.C.; Zhou, Y.H.; Zhang, L. Chemical composition, antimicrobial activity and antioxidant activity of *Litsea cubeba* essential oils in different months. *Nat. Prod. Res.* **2020**, *34*, 3285–3288. [CrossRef]
30. Dhifi, W.; Bellili, S.; Jazi, S.; Bahloul, N.; Mnif, W. Essential Oils' Chemical Characterization and Investigation of Some Biological Activities: A Critical Review. *Medicines* **2016**, *3*, 25. [CrossRef]
31. Peng, B.; Bai, R.F.; Li, P.; Han, X.Y.; Wang, H.; Zhu, C.C.; Zeng, Z.P.; Chai, X.Y. Two new glycosides from *Dryopteris fragrans* with anti-inflammatory activities. *J. Asian Nat. Prod. Res.* **2016**, *18*, 59–64. [CrossRef]
32. Li, Y.; Tan, B.; Cen, Z.; Fu, Y.; Zhu, X.; He, H.; Kong, D.; Wu, H. The variation in essential oils composition, phenolic acids and flavonoids is correlated with changes in antioxidant activity during *Cinnamomum loureirii* bark growth. *Arab. J. Chem.* **2021**, *14*, 3249. [CrossRef]
33. Tohidi, B.; Rahimmalek, M.; Arzani, A. Essential oil composition, total phenolic, flavonoid contents, and antioxidant activity of *Thymus* species collected from different regions of Iran. *Food Chem.* **2017**, *220*, 153–161. [CrossRef]
34. Zhang, Q.A.; Fan, X.H.; Zhang, Z.Q.; Li, T.; Zhu, C.P.; Zhang, X.R.; Song, W. Extraction, antioxidant capacity and identification of Semen Astragali Complanati (*Astragalus complanatus* R. Br.) phenolics. *Food Chem.* **2013**, *141*, 1295–1300. [CrossRef]
35. Mechergui, K.; Coelho, J.A.; Serra, M.C.; Lamine, S.B.; Boukhchina, S.; Khouja, M.L. Essential oils of *Origanum vulgare* L. subsp. *glandulosum* (Desf.) Ietswaart from Tunisia: Chemical composition and antioxidant activity. *J. Sci. Food Agric.* **2010**, *90*, 1745–1749. [CrossRef]
36. Liu, Y.; Sun, L.Y.; Zhu, Z.J.; Lin, W.; Qu, W.; Zeng, Z.G. Measles Virus Infection in Pediatric Liver Transplantation Recipients. *Transplant. Proc.* **2015**, *47*, 2715–2718. [CrossRef]
37. Adefegha, S.A.; Olasehinde, T.A.; Oboh, G. Essential Oil Composition, Antioxidant, Antidiabetic and Antihypertensive Properties of Two Afromomum Species. *J. Oleo Sci.* **2017**, *66*, 51–63. [CrossRef]
38. Gulcin, I. Antioxidants and antioxidant methods: An updated overview. *Arch. Toxicol.* **2020**, *94*, 651–715. [CrossRef]
39. Ma, Y.-L.; Zhu, D.-Y.; Thakur, K.; Wang, C.-H.; Wang, H.; Ren, Y.-F.; Zhang, J.-G.; Wei, Z.-J. Antioxidant and antibacterial evaluation of polysaccharides sequentially extracted from onion (*Allium cepa* L.). *Int. J. Biol. Macromol.* **2018**, *111*, 92–101. [CrossRef]
40. Ray, A.; Jena, S.; Dash, B.; Kar, B.; Halder, T.; Chatterjee, T.; Ghosh, B.; Panda, P.C.; Nayak, S.; Mahapatra, N. Chemical diversity, antioxidant and antimicrobial activities of the essential oils from Indian populations of *Hedychium coronarium* Koen. *Ind. Crops Prod.* **2018**, *112*, 353–362. [CrossRef]
41. Ciesla, L.; Kryszen, J.; Stochmal, A.; Oleszek, W.; Waksmundzka-Hajnos, M. Approach to develop a standardized TLC-DPPH* test for assessing free radical scavenging properties of selected phenolic compounds. *J. Pharm. Biomed. Anal.* **2012**, *70*, 126–135. [CrossRef]
42. Susanne, H.; Erich, F.E. Transition metal ion-catalyzed oxygen activation during pathogenic processes. *FEBS Lett.* **1999**, *443*, 1–7. [CrossRef]
43. Formisano, C.; Oliviero, F.; Rigano, D.; Saab, A.M.; Senatore, F. Chemical composition of essential oils and in vitro antioxidant properties of extracts and essential oils of *Calamintha origanifolia* and *Micromeria myrtifolia*, two Lamiaceae from the Lebanon flora. *Ind. Crops Prod.* **2014**, *62*, 405–411. [CrossRef]
44. Singh, G.; Kapoor, I.P.S.; Singh, P.; de Heluani, C.S.; de Lampasona, M.P.; Catalan, C.A.N. Chemistry and Antioxidant Properties of Essential Oil and Oleoresins Extracted from the Seeds of Tomer (*Zanthoxylum armatum* DC). *Int. J. Food Prop.* **2013**, *16*, 288–300. [CrossRef]
45. Zhang, P.; Yuan, S. Production of hydroxyl radicals from abiotic oxidation of pyrite by oxygen under circumneutral conditions in the presence of low-molecular-weight organic acids. *Geochim. Cosmochim. Acta* **2017**, *218*, 153–166. [CrossRef]
46. Wang, Y.; Jiang, F.; Cheng, H.; Tan, X.; Liu, Y.; Wei, C.; Song, E. Astragaloside IV Protects against Oxidative Stress in Calf Small Intestine Epithelial Cells via NFE2L2-Antioxidant Response Element Signaling. *Int. J. Mol. Sci.* **2019**, *20*, 6131. [CrossRef]
47. Al-Menhali, A.S.; Banu, S.; Angelova, P.R.; Barcaru, A.; Horvatovich, P.; Abramov, A.Y.; Jaganjac, M. Lipid peroxidation is involved in calcium dependent upregulation of mitochondrial metabolism in skeletal muscle. *Biochim. Biophys. Acta Gen. Subj.* **2020**, *1864*, 129487. [CrossRef]
48. Zeng, Z.; Wang, H.; Shang, F.; Zhou, L.; Little, P.J.; Quirion, R.; Zheng, W. Lithium ions attenuate serum-deprivation-induced apoptosis in PC12 cells through regulation of the Akt/FoxO1 signaling pathways. *Psychopharmacology* **2016**, *233*, 785–794. [CrossRef]
49. Alizadeh Behbahani, B.; Falah, F.; Lavi Arab, F.; Vasiee, M.; Tabatabaee Yazdi, F. Chemical Composition and Antioxidant, Antimicrobial, and Antiproliferative Activities of *Cinnamomum zeylanicum* Bark Essential Oil. *Evid. Based Complement Alternat. Med.* **2020**, *2020*, 5190603. [CrossRef]

50. Han, X.; Liu, Z.; Jo, M.C.; Zhang, K.; Li, Y.; Zeng, Z.; Li, N.; Zu, Y.; Qin, L. CRISPR-Cas9 delivery to hard-to-transfect cells via membrane deformation. *Sci. Adv.* **2015**, *1*, e1500454. [CrossRef]
51. Bi, S.F.; Zhu, G.Q.; Wu, J.; Li, Z.K.; Lv, Y.Z.; Fang, L. Chemical composition and antioxidant activities of the essential oil from *Nandina domestica* fruits. *Nat. Prod. Res.* **2016**, *30*, 362–365. [CrossRef]
52. Chen, Z.; Mei, X.; Jin, Y.; Kim, E.H.; Yang, Z.; Tu, Y. Optimisation of supercritical carbon dioxide extraction of essential oil of flowers of tea (*Camellia sinensis* L.) plants and its antioxidative activity. *J. Sci. Food Agric.* **2014**, *94*, 316–321. [CrossRef]
53. Oboh, G.; Akinbola, I.A.; Ademosun, A.O.; Sanni, D.M.; Odubanjo, O.V.; Olasehinde, T.A.; Oyeleye, S.I. Essential Oil from Clove Bud (*Eugenia aromatica* Kuntze) Inhibit Key Enzymes Relevant to the Management of Type-2 Diabetes and Some Pro-oxidant Induced Lipid Peroxidation in Rats Pancreas in vitro. *J. Oleo Sci.* **2015**, *64*, 775–782. [CrossRef]
54. Radünz, M.; Mota Camargo, T.; Santos Hackbart, H.C.d.; Inchauspe Correa Alves, P.; Radünz, A.L.; Avila Gandra, E.; da Rosa Zavareze, E. Chemical composition and in vitro antioxidant and antihyperglycemic activities of clove, thyme, oregano, and sweet orange essential oils. *LWT* **2021**, *138*, 632. [CrossRef]
55. Zeng, W.C.; Zhang, Z.; Gao, H.; Jia, L.R.; He, Q. Chemical composition, antioxidant, and antimicrobial activities of essential oil from pine needle (*Cedrus deodara*). *J. Food Sci.* **2012**, *77*, C824–C829. [CrossRef]

molecules

MDPI

Article

Valorization of *Prunus* Seed Oils: Fatty Acids Composition and Oxidative Stability

Sandra Rodríguez-Blázquez [1,2], Esther Gómez-Mejía [1], Noelia Rosales-Conrado [1], María Eugenia León-González [1,*], Beatriz García-Sánchez [2] and Ruben Miranda [2]

1 Department of Analytical Chemistry, Faculty of Chemistry, Complutense University of Madrid, Complutense Avenue, 28040 Madrid, Spain; sandro08@ucm.es (S.R.-B.); egomez03@ucm.es (E.G.-M.); nrosales@ucm.es (N.R.-C.)

2 Department of Chemical Engineering and Materials, Faculty of Chemistry, Complutense University of Madrid, Complutense Avenue, 28040 Madrid, Spain; beatriga@ucm.es (B.G.-S.); rmiranda@ucm.es (R.M.)

* Correspondence: leongon@ucm.es

Abstract: *Prunus* fruit seeds are one of the main types of agri-food waste generated worldwide during the processing of fruits to produce jams, juices and preserves. To valorize this by-product, the aim of this work was the nutritional analysis of peach, apricot, plum and cherry seeds using the official AOAC methods, together with the extraction and characterization of the lipid profile of seed oils using GC-FID, as well as the measurement of the antioxidant activity and oxidative stability using the 2,2-diphenyl-1-picrylhydrazyl (DPPH) free-radical scavenging method. Chemometric tools were required for data evaluation and the obtained results indicated that the main component of seeds were oils (30–38%, w). All seed oils were rich in oleic (C18:1n9c) and linoleic (C18:2n6c) acids and presented heart-healthy lipid indexes. Oil antioxidant activity was estimated in the range IC_{50} = 20–35 $mg \cdot mL^{-1}$, and high oxidative stability was observed for all evaluated oils during 1–22 storage days, with the plum seed oil being the most antioxidant and stable over time. Oxidative stability was also positively correlated with oleic acid content and negatively correlated with linoleic acid content. Therefore, this research showed that the four *Prunus* seed oils present interesting healthy characteristics for their use and potential application in the cosmetic and nutraceutical industries.

Keywords: *Prunus* seed oils; peach seeds; apricot seeds; plum seeds; cherry seeds; fatty acids; antioxidant activity; oxidative stability; by-product valorization

1. Introduction

Currently, there is a high level of interest in the search for new alternatives for the recovery of waste from the agri-food industry [1,2]. During the industrial processing of fruits, a large amount of waste and by-products such as peels, stones and seeds are generated [1,3,4]. The deposition of these materials in landfill sites has significant negative food-security, economic and environmental impacts [5]. Therefore, to reduce environmental pollution along with economic losses, different research studies have reported that agri-food waste material could be exploited as a source of high-value-added compounds that could be applied in the cosmetic, pharmaceutical and nutraceutical sectors [2,3,6].

The processing of some members of the Rosaceae family in the genus *Prunus*, including peach (*Prunus persica*), apricot (*Prunus armeniaca*), plum (*Prunus domestica*) and sweet cherry (*Prunus avium*), is of great importance worldwide [7]. According to the 2023 campaign for stone fruits [8], 110,692 tons of apricot, 805,368 tons of peach, 164,685 tons of plum and 140,166 tons of cherry were produced in Spain.

All *Prunus* species are highly appreciated by consumers and, thus, they are being studied not only because of their taste, color and sweetness, but also for their nutritional composition and bioactive properties [9,10]. Their entire stone is divided into a central softer part known as the kernel or seed, and an outer hard part named the shell. Depending on the fruit, the seed of the stone accounts for approximately 15–30 wt.% of the entire stone, while the remaining 70–85 wt.% corresponds to the stone's shell [11]. *Prunus* seeds are one of the main components discarded during the production of juices and jams, and in other processing industries. This waste constitutes a huge nutritional loss, since seeds are a good source of unsaturated fatty acids, proteins, dietary fibers, carbohydrates, polyphenols, vitamins and other bioactive compounds [12,13]. The presence of proteins, carbohydrates and dietary fibers is essential for the maintenance of human tissues, the production of neurotransmitters, the generation of energy reserves and the proper functioning of the human intestine, among others [14].

Among the main components of seeds, due to their multiple bioactivities, are the oils [12]. The levels of bioactive compounds in seed oil depends on the extraction method used. Although non-traditional techniques are currently used that reduce the use of solvents, such as cold pressing, supercritical methods, ultrasonic-assisted extraction and microwave-assisted extraction [15], the reference method par excellence is Soxhlet extraction. Due to its simplicity and high extraction yield, it is one of the most widely used techniques for the recovery of fatty acids from oils [16]. The most common solvent used in this extraction technique is *n*-hexane due to its high solubility with oils, low cost, high volatility, low boiling point and easy removal from solids [17].

Prunus seed oils are mainly characterized by triacylglycerides of different chemical natures. The main fatty acids found in *Prunus* seed oils are oleic (52–66%), linoleic (25–35%) and palmitic acids (3–10%) [9,18]. The high content of unsaturated fatty acids (UFA) in the oils reduces the concentration of low-density lipoproteins (LDL) which, when circulating in the body, are deposited in the blood vessels, reducing dysrhythmias, mortality caused by coronary disease and the rate of atherosclerosis, as well as blood pressure [19,20]. In addition, the high content of polyunsaturated fatty acids (PUFA) in seed oils has been related to the development and/or regeneration of cell membranes and a protective effect against dementia and Alzheimer's disease [19,21]. Furthermore, oils are characterized by a low content of saturated fatty acids (SFA), which increase LDL protein levels and the risk of coronary heart disease [22]. A PUFA/SFA ratio below 0.45 in the diet is a risk factor for increased blood cholesterol levels [23].

The health quality of lipids, based on fatty acid composition, is determined using indexes. The desirable fatty acid (DFA) index provides information on the hypocholesterolemic properties (reduction of total cholesterol) of the lipids analyzed [24]. The hypocholesterolemic/hypercholesterolemic (HH) ratio can become an indicator of the cholesterol effect of a fat source. Atherogenicity (AI) and thrombogenicity (TI) indexes are also used to indicate the risk of developing cardiovascular irregularities [25]. The n-6/n-3 PUFA ratio is another important parameter to consider when establishing the nutritional value of oils as it is related to lipid metabolism, neurogenesis and cell apoptosis [12,26,27].

In addition to the importance of knowing the content of fatty acids present in the oils, it is also important to know their antioxidant activity and their stability against lipid oxidation [18]. Oil lipid oxidation is one of the main causes of the loss of quality in color, taste, aroma and nutritional value due to the degradation of essential fatty acids and the production of toxic compounds that can contribute to the development of cancer, atherosclerosis, heart disease and allergic responses [28]. The oxidation process depends mainly on exposure to light, the temperature, the presence of oxygen, the composition of fatty acids and the composition of antioxidant compounds such as polyphenols and tocopherols [29,30]. Bozan et al. [31] found that a high polyunsaturated content of linolenic acid and long-chain fatty acids reduces the oxidative stability of the oils. In addition, Redondo et al. [32] studied the relationship between the lipid composition and oxidative stability of 22 different types of fats and observed that a higher oxidative stability correlates with a lower SFA content.

Commonly used methods to determine the oxidative stability of lipids include the determination of the peroxide value; the oxidative stability index; the determination of the induction time in the Rancimat test; the determination of the amount of aldehydes formed

(TBA method) such as lipid oxidation by-products; and the 2,2-diphenyl-1-picrylhydrazyl (DPPH) free-radical scavenging method [33,34]. In addition, kinetic methods are used in conjunction with these methods to evaluate the degradation process that lipids undergo [35].

Therefore, to study the possible valorization of *Prunus* seeds as functional ingredients, the present work aims to perform a nutritional analysis of the seeds of *P. armeniaca*, *P. persica*, *P. avium* and *P. domestica*, together with the extraction and characterization of the oils obtained from the mentioned seeds in terms of the fatty acid profile, lipid quality indexes and antioxidant activity.

2. Results and Discussion

2.1. Evaluation of the Nutritional Analysis of Prunus Seeds

The characterization of the approximate composition of peach, apricot, plum and cherry seeds is presented in Table 1. It was performed in terms of the moisture, ash, fat, crude fiber, protein and carbohydrates content, which allowed us to estimate the nutritional value and quality of seed by-products and, thus, their potential applicability as functional ingredients.

Table 1. Nutritional analysis of peach, apricot, plum and cherry seeds.

Sample	Seed (%, w)	Moisture (%, w)	Ash (%, w)	Fat (%, w)	Crude Fiber (%, w)	Protein Nitrogen (%, w)	Carbohydrates (%, w)
Peach	2.4 ± 0.3^{a}	7.6 ± 0.4^{a}	6.1 ± 0.1^{a}	30 ± 3^{a}	8.63 ± 0.02^{a}	35 ± 2^{a}	13 ± 3^{a}
Apricot	12.4 ± 0.6^{b}	5.8 ± 0.3^{b}	4.8 ± 0.4^{b}	38 ± 2^{b}	7.49 ± 0.02^{b}	28.7 ± 0.8^{b}	15 ± 3^{b}
Plum	9.5 ± 0.3^{c}	4.7 ± 0.4^{c}	2.16 ± 0.02^{c}	37.4 ± 0.4^{b}	21.4 ± 0.2^{c}	16 ± 2^{c}	18 ± 2^{c}
Cherry	10.3 ± 0.5^{d}	3.6 ± 0.1^{d}	1.43 ± 0.02^{d}	36.0 ± 0.2^{b}	23.9 ± 0.6^{d}	10.3 ± 0.7^{d}	25 ± 1^{d}

Values are expressed as mean ± standard deviation (n = 3), in dry weight. Values followed by a different superscript in a column differ significantly (p-value < 0.05) according to ANOVA and Fisher's LSD test.

As it is presented in Table 1, significant variations (p-value < 0.05) among the samples studied were observed in the seed-to-whole stone ratio, moisture, ash, crude fiber, protein nitrogen and carbohydrates contents. These differences were highly likely due to the plants' genotype, but also to their geographical origin and fruit maturity stages. However, two statistically different groups were observed in the fat content of the seeds: the first group contained peach seeds and the other group contained apricot, plum and cherry seeds.

As can be seen in Table 1, all *Prunus* seeds showed low moisture content, between 3.6 and 7.6% (w), which is beneficial for storage over long periods of time, as they are not susceptible to microorganism attack [36]. In addition, it is noteworthy that every single seed studied was characterized as a suitable source of fat, with percentages between 30 and 38% (w) over the whole seed, followed by protein (10–35%, w), crude fiber (7–24%, w) and carbohydrates (13–25%, w). In line with the results shown in Table 1, kernels are known to be particularly rich in oil [37]. In fact, the seeds with the highest lipid content were apricot (38 ± 2%, w), plum (37.4 ± 0.4%, w) and cherry (36.0 ± 0.2%, w), forming a homogeneous group statistically richer in fat content (p-value < 0.05) compared to peach seeds (30 ± 3%, w). The fact that seeds are rich in oils is highly relevant in the food and cosmetic industries, making it possible to recover this waste [38,39]. On the other hand, the presence of a high protein content is of vital importance for the strengthening and maintenance of the muscles and bones that make up the human body, thus providing a high energy intake [40]. In addition, the high content of crude fiber and carbohydrates in seeds display several benefits, such as the reduction of cholesterol, diabetes, coronary heart disease and even the prevention and/or treatment of obesity [41–43], showing the high quality and the potential of these bio-residues as functional ingredients [37]. The obtained results from the approximate analysis are comparable with the results of other researchers [37,44–48], which found that *Prunus* seeds were characterized by a protein content of 6–20% (w), a crude fiber content of 15–20% (w), an oil content of 11–57% (w), a moisture content of 5–7% (w), an ash content of 1–3% (w) and a carbohydrate content of 18–27% (w).

2.2. Evaluation of the Physico-Chemical Quality Characteristics of Prunus Seed Oils

2.2.1. Density Determination

The oil density is an identifying quality that allows the quality and purity of the oil to be determined [7]. Table 2 shows the density values obtained for peach, apricot, plum and cherry seed oils, which ranged from 0.896 to 0.917 g·mL^{-1}, and were in agreement with those reported by other authors [7,49]. The highest density was exhibited by the cherry seed oil (0.917 ± 0.005 g·mL^{-1}), followed by plum seed oil (0.903 ± 0.002 g·mL^{-1}), apricot seed oil (0.897 ± 0.003 g·mL^{-1}) and peach seed oil (0.896 ± 0.001 g·mL^{-1}). According to the Fisher's LSD test, three homogeneous groups (p-value < 0.05) were observed, determining that peach and apricot oils did not differ significantly from each other at the 95% confidence level, although they diverged significantly from plum and cherry oils. Neagu et al. [50] reported that the density of vegetable oils is conditioned by their fatty acid composition, minor constituents and temperature. Accordingly, the similarity between peach and apricot seed oils can be likely attributed to a similar fatty acid content. Therefore, determining the lipid composition of the oils is necessary.

Table 2. Density values of peach, apricot, plum and cherry seed oils.

Sample	Density (g·mL^{-1})
Peach oil	0.896 ± 0.001 ^{a}
Apricot oil	0.897 ± 0.003 ^{a}
Plum oil	0.903 ± 0.002 ^{b}
Cherry oil	0.917 ± 0.005 ^{c}

Data obtained are expressed as mean ± standard deviation (n = 3). Values with different letters in the same column denote significant differences (p-value < 0.05) among samples according to ANOVA and Fisher's LSD test.

2.2.2. Fatty Acid Composition

The fatty acid profile of *Prunus* seed oils was determined using gas chromatography coupled to a flame ionization detector (GC-FID) with previous derivatization to their corresponding methyl esters following the method proposed by Lee et al. [51]. For the identification of the fatty acids present in peach, apricot, cherry and plum seed oils, the chromatogram of FAME 37 component SUPELCO standard mixture (Figure S1, Supplementary Materials) and PUFA No. 3 Menhaden oil Ref 47085—standard mix (Figure S2, Supplementary Materials) were registered. For quantification purposes, an internal standard calibration was carried out with the response factor (RF) using tridecanoic acid (C13:0) as an internal standard. The internal standard was added directly (1 mg) before methylation to correct the losses that could occur in the process of fatty acid derivatization to methyl esters. According to data from the literature [52], the recovery of fatty acids after derivatization processes ranges from 85.6 to 114.1%. The response factors (RF) for each fatty acid in the internal standard calibration ranged from 1.069 to 1.132. The limit of quantification (LOQ) was established as 0.33 mg·g^{-1} and the limit of detection (LOD) was 0.1089 mg·g^{-1}. As an example, the chromatograms of plum and cherry seed oils can be observed in Figures S3 and S4 (Supplementary Materials), respectively. A total of 10 fatty acids was identified in peach, apricot and plum seed oils: palmitic acid (C16:0), palmitoleic acid (C16:1n7), margaric acid (C17:0), stearic acid (C18:0), cis-vaccenic acid (C18:1n7c), oleic acid (C18:1n9c), linoleic acid (C18:2n6c), α-linolenic acid (C18:3n3), arachidic acid (C20:0) and gondoic acid (C20:1n9). Moreover, two additional saturated fatty acids were identified in the cherry seed oil: behenic acid (C22:0) and lignoceric acid (C24:0). The lipid content was expressed as a percentage (%) considering a response factor (RF) of 1 and the results are indicated in Table 3. As previously reported by Lazos et al. [7], Atik et al. [53] and Perifanova et al. [54], the oils exhibited a high percentage of unsaturated fatty acids (UFA), ranging from 86% (cherry oil) to 92.2% (apricot oil), with oleic (48.6–72.7%) and linoleic acid (16.4–39.3%) being the dominant ones. The content of saturated fatty acids (SFA) present in the oils varied in the range of 7.8% to 14%, with palmitic acid as the main one (5.71–8.1%). Meanwhile, the levels of other fatty acids present in the oils were below 1% (Table 3).

Table 3. Fatty acid composition of peach, apricot, plum and cherry seed oils.

Fatty Acids	Peach Oil (%)	Apricot Oil (%)	Plum Oil (%)	Cherry Oil (%)
Palmitic acid (C16:0)	$(7.95 \pm 0.08)^{a}$	$(6.36 \pm 0.03)^{b}$	$(5.71 \pm 0.03)^{b}$	$(8.1 \pm 0.8)^{a}$
Palmitoleic acid (C16:1n7)	$(0.579 \pm 0.002)^{a}$	$(1.10 \pm 0.03)^{b}$	$(0.81 \pm 0.01)^{c}$	$(0.39 \pm 0.01)^{d}$
Margaric acid (C17:0)	$(0.0612 \pm 0.0008)^{a}$	$(0.051 \pm 0.002)^{b}$	$(0.0529 \pm 0.0001)^{a,b}$	$(0.092 \pm 0.007)^{c}$
Stearic acid (C18:0)	$(1.401 \pm 0.004)^{a}$	$(1.27 \pm 0.05)^{a}$	$(2.86 \pm 0.05)^{b}$	$(3.8 \pm 0.6)^{c}$
Cis-Vaccenic acid (C18:1n7c)	$(1.302 \pm 0.007)^{a}$	$(1.863 \pm 0.024)^{b}$	$(1.185 \pm 0.005)^{c}$	$(0.71 \pm 0.02)^{d}$
Oleic acid (C18:1n9c)	$(52.9 \pm 0.4)^{a}$	$(49.6 \pm 0.5)^{b}$	$(72.7 \pm 0.2)^{c}$	$(48.6 \pm 0.9)^{b}$
Linoleic acid (C18:2n6c)	$(35.4 \pm 0.3)^{a}$	$(39.3 \pm 0.5)^{b}$	$(16.4 \pm 0.2)^{c}$	$(36.1 \pm 0.9)^{a}$
α-Linolenic acid (C18:3n3)	$(0.129 \pm 0.006)^{a}$	$(0.172 \pm 0.008)^{b}$	$(0.081 \pm 0.001)^{c}$	$(0.1063 \pm 0.0003)^{d}$
Arachidic acid (C20:0)	$(0.143 \pm 0.006)^{a}$	$(0.14 \pm 0.01)^{a}$	$(0.1952 \pm 0.0004)^{a}$	$(1.3 \pm 0.3)^{b}$
Gondoic acid (C20:1n9)	$(0.090 \pm 0.002)^{a}$	$(0.104 \pm 0.005)^{b}$	$(0.079 \pm 0.002)^{c}$	$(0.398 \pm 0.001)^{d}$
Behenic acid (C22:0)	ND	ND	ND	(0.23 ± 0.04)
Lignoceric acid (C24:0)	ND	ND	ND	(0.18 ± 0.02)
$\sum$SFA	$(9.55 \pm 0.09)^{a}$	$(7.8 \pm 0.1)^{a}$	$(8.82 \pm 0.02)^{a}$	$(14 \pm 2)^{b}$
$\sum$UFA	$(90.45 \pm 0.09)^{a}$	$(92.2 \pm 0.1)^{a}$	$(91.18 \pm 0.02)^{a}$	$(86 \pm 2)^{b}$
$\sum$MUFA	$(54.9 \pm 0.4)^{a}$	$(52.7 \pm 0.6)^{b}$	$(74.7 \pm 0.2)^{c}$	$(50.1 \pm 0.9)^{d}$
$\sum$PUFA	$(35.5 \pm 0.3)^{a}$	$(39.5 \pm 0.5)^{b}$	$(16.5 \pm 0.2)^{c}$	$(36.2 \pm 0.9)^{a}$
PUFA/SFA ratio	$(3.7198 \pm 0.0001)^{a}$	$(5.046 \pm 0.003)^{b}$	$(1.86 \pm 0.03)^{a}$	$(2.7 \pm 0.4)^{c}$

Results are the mean of two replicates, expressed in percentages with estimates of standard deviation. Values on the same row with different letters denote significant differences (p-value < 0.05) among samples according to ANOVA and Fisher's LSD test. ND: undetectable. SFA: saturated fatty acids. UFA: unsaturated fatty acids. MUFA: monounsaturated fatty acids. PUFA: polyunsaturated fatty acids (unsaturation ≥ 2). PUFA/SFA: ratio between polyunsaturated and saturated fatty acids.

On the other hand, the total saturated fatty acid (SFA) and unsaturated fatty acid (UFA) content of the cherry seed oils differed significantly (p-value < 0.05) with the other oils studied. All *Prunus* seed oils were rich in unsaturated fatty acids, which could have multiple positive health effects. The seed oils had a high content of monounsaturated fatty acids (MUFA), with oleic acid (48.6–72.7%) being the main component of the oils, which could exert beneficial effects on the cardiovascular system and on the proper development and/or functioning of the human brain [55]. Seed oils were also characterized based on their outstanding polyunsaturated fatty acid (PUFA) content (16.5–39.5%), particularly defined by a high content of linoleic acid (16.4–39.3%), which is essential for a healthy diet and for cell membrane development [19]. However, although the saturated fatty acid content represented the minority in all oils, a slight increase was observed in cherry seed oil with a value of 14 ± 2%. In the present study, the PUFA/SFA ratio in the seed oils was especially high (1.86–5.046%), indicating that the oils were healthy, and that they contained an adequate proportion of healthy fatty acids.

To evaluate the fatty acid content relationships with peach, apricot, plum and cherry seed oils, a principal component analysis (PCA) was performed. The results of the PCA analysis are shown in the graph depicted in Figure 1. Two principal components with eigenvalues greater than or equal to 1 accounted for 92.822% of the total data variability. The first principal component (PC1) accounted for 64.540% of the total variability and it was mainly related to margaric acid (C17:0), behenic acid (C22:0), arachidic acid (C20:0), lignoceric acid (C24:0) and gondoic acid (C20:1n9). The second principal component (PC2) explained 28.282% of the total variability and it was defined by the strong correlation with linoleic (C18:2n6c) and α-linolenic acid (C18:3n3). The PCA graph indicated the presence of three homogeneous groups. The first one, formed by peach and apricot seed oils, was characterized by a high content of unsaturated fatty acids such as palmitoleic acid (C16:1n7), cis-vaccenic acid (C18:1n7c) and α-linolenic acid (C18:3n3). The presence of high linolenic acid content in oils can have multiple health benefits, as this essential omega-3 (n-3) polyunsaturated fatty acid plays vital roles in proper brain development and function, cardiovascular health and the anti-inflammatory response [56]. In addition, the presence of high contents of other UFAs such as cis-vaccenic acid and palmitoleic acid has an anti-inflammatory and protective effect against cardiovascular diseases [57,58]. The second group consisted of plum seed oil, which was characterized by a high oleic acid content (C18:1n9c). This type of non-essential fatty acid in the oil can be used in the treatment and prevention of various disorders, such as autoimmune or cardiovascular diseases, metabolic disorders and cancer [55]. The third and last group consisted of cherry seed oil, which is characterized by a high SFA content, especially behenic acid (C22:0), margaric acid (C17:0) and arachidic acid (C20:1n9c).

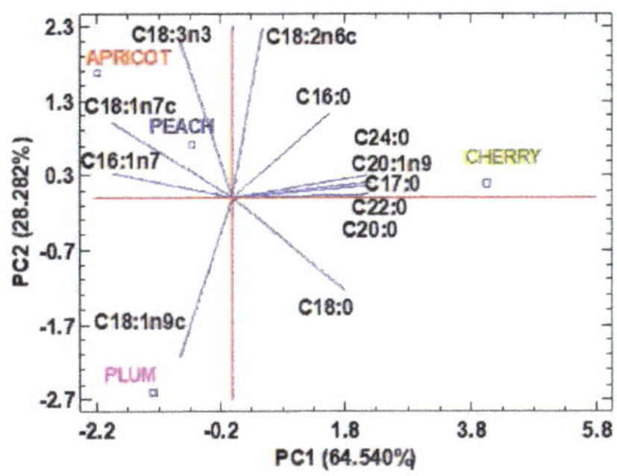

Figure 1. Two−dimensional plot of the principal component analysis (PCA) of the fatty acids present in peach, apricot, plum and cherry seed oils.

Regarding the correlations between the different fatty acids presented in the four different oils (Figure 1), it was observed that the UFA, palmitoleic acid (C16:1n7) and cis-vaccenic acid (C18:1n7c) were highly positively correlated with each other. Palmitoleic acid was correlated negatively with the saturated fatty acids margaric acid (C17:0), behenic acid (C22:0) and arachidic acid (C20:0); and the unsaturated fatty acid gondoic acid (C20:1n9). However, cis-vaccenic fatty acid was negatively correlated with stearic acid (C18:0). A high negative correlation was also observed between the two main components of the oils: linoleic acid (C18:2n6c) and oleic acid (C18:1n9c).

2.2.3. Lipid Health Quality Indexes

The atherogenicity index (AI) showed two homogeneous groups (p-value < 0.05): on the one hand, peach and cherry seed oil were grouped together, and on the other, apricot and plum seed oil were grouped together. All oils showed low values of this index, where the lowest value was found in plum seed oil (0.0626) and the highest in cherry seed oil (0.09). The results corresponding to the thrombogenicity (TI) index showed that peach, apricot and plum seed oils were statistically similar (p-value $\geq$ 0.05), while cherry seed oil differed from them. The lowest value corresponded to the apricot kernel oil (0.166) and the highest to the cherry kernel oil (0.28). According to the literature [23,24,59], low values of both the AI and TI are related to the prevention of coronary heart disease. Thus, the lower these values, the healthier the food, indicating the promising potential of these seed oils.

According to the desirable fatty acid (DFA) index, three statistically homogeneous groups were found (peach and apricot oil, apricot and plum oil and, lastly, cherry oil). High values (90–94) were observed for all four *Prunus* seed oils (Table 4), evidencing their high hypocholesterolaemic properties. The hypocholesterolemic/hypercholesterolemic (H/H) ratio correlates with the DFA index and measures the bioactive properties of oils to lower blood cholesterol levels [60]. In this case, the oils were grouped into two statistically homogeneous groups and showed high values for this nutritional index (11.3–15.83).

Table 4. Indexes of the nutritional quality of peach, apricot, plum and cherry seed oils.

Lipid Indexes	Peach Oil	Apricot Oil	Plum Oil	Cherry Oil
Desirable fatty acid (DFA)	$(91.85 \pm 0.09)^{a}$	$(93.44 \pm 0.5)^{a,b}$	$(94.05 \pm 0.03)^{b}$	$(90 \pm 1)^{c}$
Atherogenicity (AI)	$(0.088 \pm 0.001)^{a}$	$(0.0691 \pm 0.0004)^{b}$	$(0.0626 \pm 0.0003)^{b}$	$(0.09 \pm 0.01)^{a}$
Thrombogenicity (TI)	$(0.207 \pm 0.002)^{a}$	$(0.166 \pm 0.002)^{a}$	$(0.188 \pm 0.001)^{a}$	$(0.28 \pm 0.04)^{b}$
Hypocholesterolemic/ Hypercholesterolemic (H/H)	$(11.3 \pm 0.1)^{a}$	$(14.29 \pm 0.08)^{b}$	$(15.83 \pm 0.06)^{b}$	$(11 \pm 1)^{a}$
n6/n3 fatty acid ratio	$(275 \pm 10)^{a}$	$(228 \pm 8)^{b}$	$(201.5 \pm 0.6)^{c}$	$(339 \pm 9)^{d}$

Values are expressed as mean ± standard deviation (n = 2). Values with different letters in the same row denote significant differences (p-value < 0.05) among samples according to ANOVA and Fisher's LSD test. n-6/n-3: ratio between omega-6 and omega-3 fatty acids.

On the other hand, all seed oils were shown to have a higher proportion of omega-6 fatty acids than omega-3 fatty acids (Table 4). The oils presented significant differences among them (p-value < 0.05), with the lowest value found in plum seed oil (201.5 ± 0.6). Although these values suggest a health risk, the presence of high amounts of linoleic acid is required by the human body for the maintenance of cell membranes, brain function and the transmission of nervous impulses in normal conditions and the correct oxygenation of the blood [61]. Therefore, a balanced omega-6/omega-3 ratio diet is needed.

Considering all the nutritional lipid indexes (AI, TI, H/H, DFA, n6/n3 ratio) used to evaluate the quality of the oils, plum seed oil was the one that presented the best nutritional quality. However, all *Prunus* seed oils could play beneficial roles in human health, particularly in the prevention and/or treatment of coronary and cardiovascular diseases and obesity [62,63]. Due to the interesting nutritional characteristics of *Prunus* seed oils, they could be used in the food and/or nutraceutical industries as natural food supplements or additives [37,39].

2.2.4. Antioxidant Activity

The determination of the oil antioxidant activity is another parameter that is used to evaluate the quality of oils, since this bioactive property correlates with the lipid composition and the presence of natural antioxidants in the oil [64]. Table 5 shows the antioxidant activity of peach, apricot, plum and cherry seed oils (expressed as $mg \cdot mL^{-1}$ of oil). Trolox was used as a standard and its IC_{50} was 0.0025 ± 0.0001 $mg \cdot mL^{-1}$. All studied oils showed high values of IC_{50}, ranging from 20 to 35 $mg \cdot mL^{-1}$, with respect to the Trolox standard. Furthermore, the IC_{50} values obtained for *Prunus* seed oils were higher than those reported by Fratianni et al. [38], indicating the interesting potential of the oils obtained from the agri-food waste. Apricot and plum oils were those with the highest antioxidant capacity (IC_{50} = 20–21 $mg \cdot mL^{-1}$), compared to peach and cherry oils, which were characterized by a significantly lower (p-value < 0.05) antioxidant capacity (IC_{50} = 31–35 $mg \cdot mL^{-1}$).

Table 5. Antioxidant activity determined after 24 h storage of peach, apricot, plum and cherry kernel oils.

Oils	DPPH IC_{50} ($mg \cdot mL^{-1}$ of Oil)
Peach oil	$(31 \pm 3)^{a}$
Apricot oil	$(21.2 \pm 0.9)^{b}$
Plum oil	$(20 \pm 3)^{b}$
Cherry oil	$(35 \pm 4)^{a}$

Values are expressed as mean ± standard deviation (n = 2). Values with different letters denote significant differences (p-value < 0.05) among samples according to ANOVA and Fisher's LSD test. IC_{50} values are the concentration of sample required to scavenge 50% of 2,2-diphenyl-1-picrylhydrazyl (DPPH) free radical.

To establish the possible relationship between the fatty acid composition (Table 3) and the antioxidant capacity of seed oils, a Pearson correlation analysis was carried out

(Figure 2). The correlation coefficients ranges from −1 to +1 to express the linear relationship between the different study factors. The correlation analysis showed that the main fatty acids affecting the oils' antioxidant capacity (IC_{50} value) were palmitic acid (C16:0) and palmitoleic acid (C16:1n7). A high positive correlation was also observed between the content of palmitic acid and the IC_{50} value (r = 0.97). A higher content of palmitic acid in the oil led to an increase in the IC_{50} value and, therefore, a decrease in the antioxidant capacity. Palmitic acid is associated with increasing total cholesterol levels in plasma [38]; however, it was found in low proportions in oils (5.71–8.1%). Conversely, a high negative correlation was observed between the IC_{50} value and the palmitoleic acid (C16:1n7) content (r = −0.89), indicating that the high content of this type of UFA in the oils contributes positively to the antioxidant capacity (lowest IC_{50} value) and acts beneficially in the human body, protecting against oxidative stress [55].

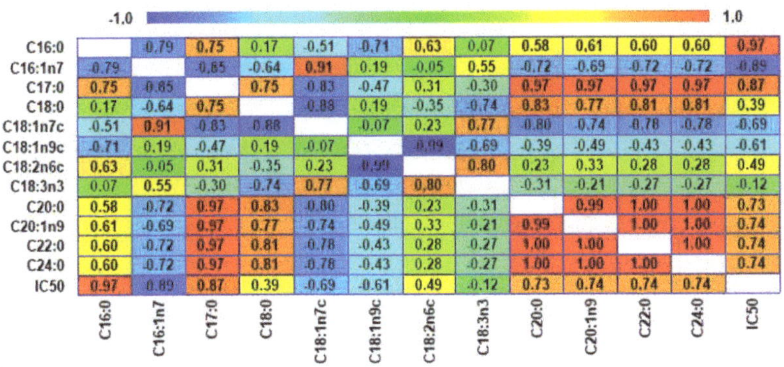

Figure 2. Pearson correlation heat map between fatty acid contents and antioxidant activity of *Prunus* seed oils. IC_{50} values mean the concentration of sample required to scavenge 50% of DPPH free radical.

2.3. Comparative Study of the Oxidative Stability of Seed Oils

Lipid oxidation is one of the biggest problems affecting oil quality. Therefore, the study of the oxidative stability is required.

The oil oxidative stability was measured over a period of 1–22 days using the 2,2-diphenyl-1-picrylhydrazyl (DPPH) free-radical scavenging method. The results obtained are shown in Table 6.

Table 6. Variation in the antioxidant capacity of peach, apricot, plum and cherry seed oils with storage time.

Storage Time (h)	IC_{50} Peach Oil ($mg \cdot mL^{-1}$ of Oil)	IC_{50} Apricot Oil ($mg \cdot mL^{-1}$ of Oil)	IC_{50} Plum Oil ($mg \cdot mL^{-1}$ of Oil)	IC_{50} Cherry Oil ($mg \cdot mL^{-1}$ of Oil)
24 (1 day)	$(31 \pm 3)^{a}$	$(21.2 \pm 0.9)^{a}$	$(20 \pm 3)^{a}$	$(35 \pm 4)^{a}$
48 (2 days)	$(37 \pm 1)^{b}$	n.m.	$(21.9 \pm 0.7)^{a,b}$	n.m.
72 (3 days)	n.m.	$(28.7 \pm 0.5)^{b}$	n.m.	$(41.6 \pm 0.2)^{a,b}$
120 (5 days)	$(37.8 \pm 0.6)^{b}$	n.m.	n.m.	n.m.
168 (7 days)	n.m.	n.m.	$(25 \pm 1)^{b}$	n.m.
240 (10 days)	$(39 \pm 3)^{c}$	$(57 \pm 1)^{c}$	n.m.	$(46 \pm 1)^{b,c}$
360 (15 days)	n.m.	n.m.	$(26 \pm 3)^{b}$	$(51 \pm 4)^{c}$
528 (22 days)	n.m.	n.m.	$(26.2 \pm 0.3)^{b}$	n.m.

Values are expressed as mean ± standard deviation (n = 2). IC_{50} values mean the concentration of sample required to scavenge 50% of DPPH free radical and n.m. signifies not measured on that specific storage time. For each type of oil, values with different letters in the same column denote significant differences (p-value < 0.05) between storage times according to ANOVA and Fisher's LSD test.

To evaluate the trend of the oxidative stability, IC_{50} values were plotted versus storage time (Figure 3). The curves shown in Figure 3 were non-linear and fitted adequately to a logarithmic model (with correlation coefficients (R^2) between 0.8547 and 0.9727). Thus, the variation in antioxidant capacity during storage time followed a logarithmic model of the first-order degradation kinetic reaction [35,65]. In the logarithmic curve of plum oil, an apparently constant trend was observed between the IC_{50} values and the storage times, indicating its high stability against lipid oxidation. However, in apricot, peach and cherry seed oils, an increasing trend of the IC_{50} value was observed at 240 h (22 days) of storage time, which indicated that the lipid oxidation phenomenon had occurred.

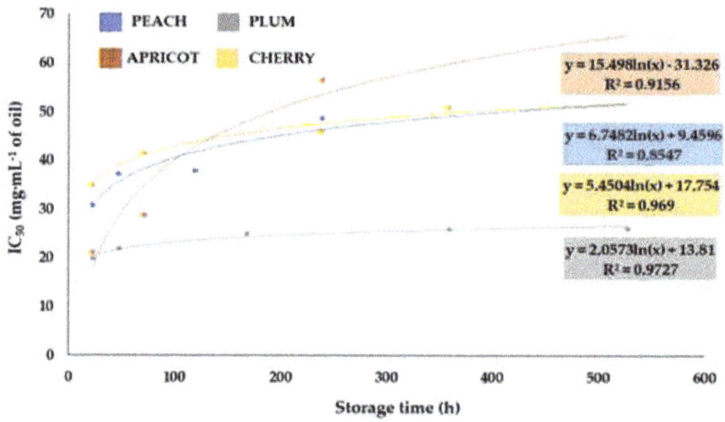

Figure 3. Kinetics curves of logarithmic model of IC_{50} values versus storage time of peach, apricot, plum and cherry seed oils.

To determine the time at which the oil was stable against the oxidation of its fatty acids the $t_{1/2}$ value was estimated, which refers to the time at which the concentration of oil antioxidants is reduced by half. For this purpose, the IC_{100} was calculated as the sample concentration required to remove 100% of the free radical DPPH. From this value, ln(100-IC_{100}) ($\ln_{c.antioxidants}$) was calculated and plotted against storage time, following the first-order linear kinetic equation ($\ln_{c.antioxidants} = \ln_{C0} - kt$). The data related to the linear fit (intercept, slope and correlation coefficient (R^2)) are given in Table 7.

Table 7. Parameters of the linear fit (intercept, slope, correlation coefficient (R^2)) of $\ln_{c.antioxidants}$ versus storage time of peach, apricot, plum and cherry kernel oils.

Prunus Seed Oil	Intercept (mg·mL^{-1})	Slope (h^{-1})	$t_{1/2}$ (h)	R^2
Peach	(−0.012 ± 0.003)	(4.0 ± 0.4)	58 (2 days)	0.90
Apricot	(−0.006 ± 0.001)	(4.2± 0.1)	110 (4 days)	1.00
Plum	(−0.0004 ± 0.0001)	(4.0 ± 0.3)	1732 (72 days)	0.78
Cherry	(−0.0057 ± 0.0001)	(3.4 ± 0.2)	121 (5 days)	0.94

The intercept refers to the logarithm of the initial concentration of antioxidant compounds ($\ln_{C0}$) and the slope to the first-order constant (k). A linear trend in the data was observed in all oils.

It was observed that the oxidative stability of all oils conformed to first-order kinetics with high correlation factors (R^2) ranging from 0.78 to 1.00. The times at which the antioxidant concentration halved were different for each oil. On the one hand, the longest time and, thus, the highest stability against lipid oxidation, was observed for the plum oil ($t_{1/2}$ = 1732 h (72 days)). On the other hand, peach oil showed the shortest stability time ($t_{1/2}$ = 58 h (2 days)). Apricot kernel oil and cherry oil showed $t_{1/2}$ values of 110 and 121 h (4 and 5 days), respectively.

The results obtained according to literature data [32,61] evidenced that the oil composition strongly affects its antioxidant activity and oxidative stability. Consequently, the effect of fatty acids on oil oxidative stability was studied using principal component analysis based on the stability time data reported in Table 7 and the data concerning fatty acid composition (Table 3). Two principal components, with eigenvalues greater than or equal to 1, were extracted. They accounted for 93.213% of the total data variability (Figure 4).

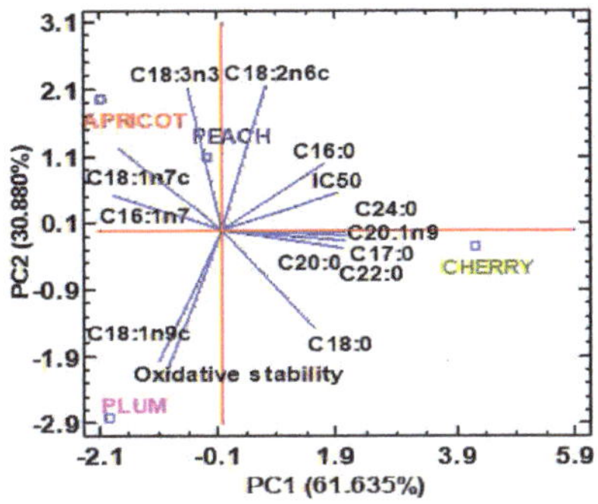

Figure 4. Two-dimensional principal component analysis (PCA) plot of fatty acid content, antioxidant activity (IC_{50}) and oxidative stability of peach, apricot, plum and cherry seed oils.

The first principal component (PC1) represented 60.401% of the total data variability and it was mainly related to margaric acid (C17:0), behenic acid (C22:0), arachidic acid (C20:0), lignoceric acid (C24:0) and gondoic acid (C20:1n9). The second principal component (PC2) explained 32.813% of the total data variability and it was defined by the strong correlation with both linoleic (C18:2n6c) and α-linolenic acids (C18:3n3). In the PCA graph depicted in Figure 4, a high positive correlation was also observed between the oxidative stability and the oleic acid content. On the contrary, the maximum negative correlation was observed between the oxidative stability and the content of linoleic acid. Similarly, Nederal et al. [66] observed that the oxidative stability of cold-pressed pumpkin oils was positively correlated with the oleic acid content and negatively correlated with the linoleic and α-linolenic acid contents. This fact could be explained by the presence of consecutive double bonds, which are more susceptible to attack by the oxygen present in the environment. Furthermore, it was observed that plum seed oil had the greatest stability against the oxidation of fatty acids due to its high content of oleic monounsaturated fatty acid.

The adequate antioxidant activity and oxidative stability of *Prunus* seed oils opens new fields of application in the cosmetic industry for their use as active ingredients in antioxidant cosmetics [39].

3. Materials and Methods

3.1. Reagents and Solvents

Analytical grade reagents were required in the procedures. *n*-Hexane (96%) and methanol (MeOH, ≥99%) for HPLC gradient quality were supplied by Scharlab (Barcelona, Spain). Sodium hydroxide pellets (NaOH) (98%), sulphuric acid (H_2SO_4, 98%), boric acid (≥99%) and methylene blue (82%) were obtained from Panreac (Barcelona, Spain). Dimethyl sulfoxide (DMSO, ≥99.9%) and 2,2-diphenyl-1-picrylhydrazyl (DPPH, ≥99.9%) were provided by Sigma-Aldrich (St. Louis, MO, USA). Methyl red, Kjeldahl catalyst tables and distilled water system were purchased from Merck (Madrid, Spain). Fatty acid standards FAME 37 component SUPELCO Ref CRM47885, PUFA No. 3 Menhaden oil Ref 47085-U and tridecanoic acid (C13:0, ≥ 99%) were purchased from Sigma-Aldrich (Barcelona, Spain). The standard Trolox was provided by Sigma-Aldrich (Burghasen, Germany).

3.2. *Sample Preparation*

Plum (*Prunus domestica*) and cherry (*Prunus avium*) pits were purchased from The Jerte Valley Cooperatives Group (Cáceres, Spain). Peach pits (*Prunus persica*) and apricot pits and seeds (*Prunus armeniaca*) were purchased from The Agri-Food Cooperatives of Castilla La Mancha (Hellín, Albacete).

Prior to any treatment, fresh samples, received during the campaign period corresponding to the year 2022, were air-dried at 40 °C (Digitheat oven, J.P Selecta®, Abrera, Barcelona, Spain) for 24 h, and then stored at room temperature until use.

For compositional analysis, the stones of the *Prunus* fruits studied were separated manually, using a hammer, into shell and seed. The seeds were then crushed in an ultra-centrifugal grinder (Retsh™ ZM200, Haan, Alemania) and sieved with a stainless-steel sieve to particle sizes below 1 mm. Seed samples were stored in clear plastic zip-lock bags until analysis.

3.3. *Nutritional Analysis of the Four Types of Fruit Seed of Prunus Family*

3.3.1. Determination of Seed-to-Whole Stone Ratio

The percentage in weight of seeds in relation to the stone was determined by weighing 25 stones and their respective seeds on a 0.0001 g precision digital analytical balance (Precisa Series 290, Dietikon, Switzerland) for each of the *Prunus* varieties.

3.3.2. Determination of Moisture Content

The moisture content of the seeds was determined according to the standard procedure AOAC 925.10 [67], with slight modifications. Approximately 2 g of seed sample was weighed on a dried crucible and introduced in an oven at 105 °C for 2 h and 30 min until a constant weight was obtained. After cooling, the crucible was weighed again and the free water content was calculated as sample weight loss and expressed as a percentage. It was determined as percentage in weight (mean ± standard deviation, n = 3).

3.3.3. Determination of Ash Content

For the determination of ash, AOAC 923.03 standard procedure was followed [68]. Briefly, a sample amount of 2 g was weighed on a clean and dry crucible, which was then placed in muffle furnace (J.P Selecta®, Abrera, Barcelona, Spain) at 550 °C for 4 h. The appearances of grey/white ash indicated the complete oxidation of all organic matter in the sample. Then, the crucible with the ash was cooled in the desiccator and weighed on a precision digital analytical balance (Precisa Series 290, Dietikon, Switzerland) until reaching a constant weight. Finally, the ash content was then calculated as a percentage in weight of dried sample and expressed as mean ± standard deviation (n = 3).

3.3.4. Determination of Fat Content

The total oil content in the samples was determined following an AOAC 960.39 procedure [69]. First, a Soxhelt extraction was carried out by placing 15 g of seed with a particle size of less than 1 mm into a cellulose cartridge (FILTER-LAB®, Darmstadt, Germany), within a collecting flask of 250 mL capacity (Mervilab S.A., Madrid, Spain) that was previously dried in an oven (Digitheat, J.P Selecta®, Abrera, Barcelona, Spain) at 105 °C for 2 h and weighed. The cellulose cartridge was inserted into the Soxhlet extractor body and 150 mL of *n*-hexane (seed-solvent ratio 1:10 (*w/v*)) was added to the collecting flask. *Prunus* seeds were then extracted under reflux at 69 °C for 6 h (6–8 cycles/h). Then, the solvent was removed using a rotary evaporator (Buchi™ Rotavapor™ R-100, Fisher Scientific, Hampton, VA, USA) at 69 °C, and the collecting flask with the extract was placed in a vacuum oven (Vaciotem-TV, digital, J.P Selecta®, Abrera, Barcelona, Spain) at 40 °C for 24 h. Finally, it was cooled in a desiccator for 30 min and weighed again. This procedure was carried out in triplicate. The oils were stored in airtight amber-colored glass bottles and kept at 4 °C prior to analysis. The percentage of fat was expressed as mean ± standard deviation (n = 3) on a dry basis.

3.3.5. Determination of Crude Fiber Content

The content of crude fiber in the different seed samples was assessed according to an official methodology described elsewhere [70]. For this purpose, approximately 2 g of defatted seed was weighed on a precision digital analytical balance and subjected to a boiling step for 30 min with 200 mL of 0.128 M H_2SO_4 solution. Then, the solution was filtered through a cotton filter to drain the acid and the solid residue was washed with hot distilled water and subjected to a further boiling for 30 min with 200 mL of 0.313 M NaOH solution. Following filtration through a cotton filter, the insoluble residue was dried in an oven (Digitheat, J.P Selecta®, Abrera, Barcelona, Spain) at 230 °C for 2 h and weighed, and subsequently placed in a muffle furnace (J.P Selecta®, Abrera, Barcelona, Spain) at 550 °C for 2 h. Finally, the crucible with the samples was cooled in the desiccator and weighed again. The crude fiber content was determined using the quotient of the difference in weight of the dry insoluble residue and the incinerated residue between the total mass of the dry seed. This test was performed in triplicate and expressed as mean ± standard deviation.

3.3.6. Determination of Protein Nitrogen Content

The protein content of the seed samples was determined using the Kjeldahl method [71]. Approximately 1 g of dried sample was added in digestion flask with 12 mL of concentrated H_2SO_4 and one Kjeldahl catalyst tablet (Merck, Darmstadt, Germany). The mixture was placed in the digestion module (VELP Scientifica, Usmate, Italy) at 410 °C for 1 h. After cooling, the digested mixture was placed in the steam distillation module (VELP Scientifica, Usmate, Italy) with 50 mL of 2% (w) boric acid, two drops of methyl red and one drop of methylene blue. The system was programmed to add 18 mL of 40% (w) NaOH in 12 s and the distillation process took place for 210 s. Finally, the distilled ammonia collective in the boric acid solution was titrated with 0.03 M H_2SO_4 solution until it turned green to violet. The procedure was carried out in triplicate and two blanks were also prepared. Finally, the protein content was estimated from the percentage of nitrogen using Equation (1), where the coefficient of 6.25 is the correction factor for this type of sample and "%N" is the percentage of nitrogen in the sample; and Equation (2) where "s" is the sample titration reading, "b" is the blank titration reading, "M" is the molarity of H_2SO_4 and "0.014" the milli equivalent weight of nitrogen.

$$\text{Proteinnitrogen}(\%) = 6.25 \times \%\text{N} \quad (1)$$

$$\text{N}(\%) = \frac{(\text{s} - \text{b}) \times 0.014 \times \text{M}}{\text{wt}_{\text{sample}}} \quad (2)$$

3.3.7. Determination of Total Carbohydrates

The carbohydrate content in *Prunus* seeds, expressed as the mean value of the weight percentage ± standard deviation (n = 3), was calculated by subtracting the sum of the percentage of moisture, ash, fat and protein nitrogen contents from 100% according to Ayoola et al. [72].

3.4. Physico-Chemical Characterization of Prunus Seed Oils

3.4.1. Determination of Oil Density

The density of oils was determined using a density meter (Anton Paar DMA 5000, Madrid, Spain) with an operative temperature of 25 °C. The tests were carried out in triplicate for each sample.

3.4.2. Determination of Fatty Acid Profile

The determination of fatty acid composition in the extracted oils was carried out using gas chromatography coupled to a FID detector (Agilent Technologies, 7820A, Santa

Clara, CA, USA), following the internal derivatization procedure to methyl esters proposed by Lee et al. [51]. Prior to the chromatographic analysis, the extracted oils (200 mg approximately) were freeze-dried (Sp Scientific, Warminster, PA, USA) at −50 °C and 150 mbar for 72 h. To synthesize fatty acid methyl esters (FAME), the fatty acids were incubated with 0.5 M sodium methoxide at 60 °C for 15 min, followed by extraction with acetyl chloride in methanol 1:10 (*v*/*v*) and incubation at 60 °C for 60 min. One milliliter of purified water, 1.5 mL of hexane and sodium sulphate was added to each sample, followed by a centrifugation step (4 °C, 1500 rpm for 5 min). One milliliter of the supernatant was used for subsequent analyses. Samples were evaporated in a Savant™ SPD131DDA SpeedVac™ concentrator (Thermo Fisher Scientific, Madrid, Spain) and resuspended in hexane (Thermo Fisher Scientific, Madrid, Spain) The chromatographic separation was achieved using a capillary chromatographic column (60 m × 250 μm × 0.25 μm) (Agilent Technologies DB-23 Ref 122-2362), helium as a carrier gas at 1 mL·min^{-1} flow rate and split injection mode (40:1). The detector temperature was set at 260 °C and the injector furnace temperature at 250 °C. The oven temperature gradient started at 100 °C for 2 min, after which the temperature increased by 8 °C/min to 145 °C. This condition was maintained for 20 min and then rose by 5 °C/min to 230 °C. Chromatograms were recorded and analyzed using EZChrom Elite compact 3.3.2. software (Agilent Technologies, Madrid, Spain).

The identification of the fatty acids was performed by comparing the retention time of the samples with that of the commercial standards (FAME 37 SUPELCO Ref CRM47885 + PUFA No. 3 Menhaden oil Ref 47085-U). For quantification, an internal standard calibration of response factors (RF) was performed as a way to correlate the ratio of areas between each FAME and the internal standard with the FAME concentration, using tridecanoic acid (C13:0) as internal standard (1 mg was added before methylation). To determine the relative amounts of each FAME present in the different samples, a response factor of 1 was set and the composition was expressed as a percentage (%) considering the individual area of each FAME and the total area (considering that 100% corresponds to the sum of all the areas of the determined analytes). Analyses were performed in duplicate.

3.4.3. Lipid Nutritional Quality Indexes

To estimate the nutritional value of the seed oils studied the total content of saturated (SFA), unsaturated (UFA), monounsaturated (MUFA) and polyunsaturated (PUFA) fatty acids, along with the lipid nutritional quality indexes related to the fatty acid profile and healthy fat consumption (the atherogenicity index (AI), thrombogenicity index (TI), hypocholesterolemic-hypercholesterolemic ratio (H/H) and desirable fatty acid (DFA) index) were calculated as defined elsewhere [24,25]:

$$\sum \text{SFA} = \text{C16:0} + \text{C17:0} + \text{C18:0} + \text{C20:0} + \text{C22:0} + \text{C24:0} \tag{3}$$

$$\sum \text{UFA} = \sum \text{MUFA} + \sum \text{PUFA} \tag{4}$$

$$\sum \text{MUFA} = \text{C16:1n7} + \text{C18:1n7c} + \text{C18:1n9c} \tag{5}$$

$$\sum \text{PUFA} = \text{C18:2n6c} + \text{C18:3n3} + \text{C20:1n9} \tag{6}$$

$$\text{DFA} = \sum \text{MUFA} + \sum \text{PUFA} + \text{C18:0} \tag{7}$$

$$\text{AI} = \frac{\text{C12:0} + 4(\text{C14:0}) + \text{C16:0}}{\sum \text{MUFA} + \sum \text{PUFA}} \tag{8}$$

$$\text{H/H} = \frac{\text{C18:1} + \sum \text{PUFA}}{\text{C14:0} + \text{C16:0}} \tag{9}$$

$$TI = \frac{C12:0 + C16:0 + C18:0}{(0.5 \sum MUFA) + (0.5 \times n6 \sum PUFA) + (3 \times n3 \sum PUFA) \times \left(\frac{n3 \sum PUFA}{n6 \sum PUFA}\right)} \quad (10)$$

where n3∑PUFA stands for the sum of omega-3 polyunsaturated fatty acids, n6∑PUFA is the sum of omega-6 polyunsaturated fatty acids, C16:0 corresponds to palmitic acid, C16:1n7 is palmitoleic acid, C17:0 is margaric acid, C18:0 is stearic acid, C18:1n7c is cis-vaccenic acid, C18:1n9c is oleic acid, C18:2n6c is linoleic acid, C18:3n3 is α-linolenic acid, C20:0 is arachidic acid, C20:1n9 is 11-eicosenoic acid, C22:0 is behenic acid and C24:0 is lignoceric acid.

Finally, the n6/n3 fatty acid ratio, which is related to a healthy diet, was calculated according to the equation proposed by Asha et al. [73].

3.4.4. Determination of the Antioxidant Capacity of Seed Oils

The antioxidant activity of *Prunus* seed oils was measured as DPPH free-radical scavenging capacity, following the methodology proposed by Fratianni et al. [38], which was slightly modified. Briefly, 30 μL of eight methanolic working solutions (0–30 μL) prepared using dilution from oil solutions (448–850 mg·mL^{-1}, DMSO) were mixed with 270 μL of 6×10^{-5} M DPPH methanolic solution in 96-well microplate. The final solutions were stored in the dark at room temperature and under shaking (300 rpm) for 60 min. The absorbance was then measured at 515 nm using a Thermo Scientific Multiskan GO spectrophotometer. Finally, the oil concentrations were plotted against DPPH remaining percentages and the results were expressed as IC_{50} values, i.e., the concentration of sample required to inhibit 50% the initial DPPH concentration. The assay was performed in duplicate and Trolox standard was used as positive control.

3.4.5. Evaluation of the Antioxidant Stability of Seed Oils

The antioxidant activity of *Prunus* seed oils was monitored for 22 days to determine the oxidative stability of the evaluated oils using the DPPH method described in Section 3.4.4.

For this purpose, the IC_{100}, i.e., the minimum oil concentration that completely reduced the initial DPPH absorbance at 515 nm, was determined over the storage time (24 h and 22 days). The former was estimated as the initial concentration of antioxidant agents present in the oils and the data obtained were fitted to first-order kinetics, according to Equation (11), where "$ln_{c.antioxidants}$" is the logarithm of the antioxidants present in the oils during storage time, "ln_{C0}" is the logarithm of IC_{100} value, "k" is the velocity constant and "t" corresponds to the storage time.

Thus, from the logarithmic calibration fits, the mean degradation time, known as the time in which the initial concentration of antioxidants is halved, was calculated for the different *Prunus* seed oils.

$$ln_{c.antioxidants} = ln_{C0} - kt \quad (11)$$

3.5. Statistical Analysis

Statistical analysis was performed using the Statgraphics 19 software package (Statgraphics Technologies Inc., Rockville, MD, USA). Data were statistically analyzed using multivariate and univariate analysis of variance (ANOVA), principal component analysis (PCA) and Pearson correlation analysis. Significant differences between determinations were evaluated using Fisher's least significant difference (LSD) test at 95% confidence level (p-value < 0.05).

4. Conclusions

This study focuses on the valorization of peach, apricot, plum and cherry seed agri-food waste based on the extraction of seed oil and its characterization in terms of fatty acid content, antioxidant activity and oxidative stability.

Prunus seeds presented high added value due to their remarkable fat (30–38%, w), crude fiber (7–24%, w), protein (10–35%, w) and carbohydrate (13–25%, w) contents. The main components of interest of the seeds were the seed oils. The high content of unsaturated fatty acids in the oils, such as oleic (48.6–72.7%) and linoleic acid (16.4–39.3%), and their adequate heart-healthy indexes make their potential use in the food and nutraceutical industry feasible, either as food supplements or nutraceuticals. In addition, the outstanding antioxidant activity (IC_{50} = 30–35 mg·mL^{-1}) and the high oxidative stability during 1–22 days of storage of the oils, especially the plum seed oil, opens new applications in the cosmetic industry as an active ingredient in antioxidant cosmetics.

Supplementary Materials: The following supporting information can be downloaded at: https://www.mdpi.com/article/10.3390/molecules28207045/s1, Figure S1: Chromatogram of the standard mixture FAME 37 component SUPELCO Ref CRM47885 using GC-FID; Figure S2: Chromatogram of the standard mixture PUFA No. 3 Menhaden oil Ref 47085-U using GC-FID; Figure S3: Chromatogram of plum seed oil using GC-FID and Figure S4: Chromatogram of cherry seed oil using GC-FID.

Author Contributions: Conceptualization, S.R.-B., E.G.-M., N.R.-C., M.E.L.-G. and R.M.; methodology, S.R.-B., E.G.-M., N.R.-C., M.E.L.-G., B.G.-S. and R.M.; software, S.R.-B., E.G.-M., N.R.-C. and M.E.L.-G.; validation, S.R.-B., E.G.-M., N.R.-C., M.E.L.-G. and R.M.; formal analysis, S.R-B. and E.G.-M.; investigation, S.R.-B.; resources, E.G.-M., N.R.-C., M.E.L.-G. and R.M.; data curation, S.R.-B., E.G.-M., N.R.-C. and M.E.L.-G.; writing—original draft preparation, S.R.-B., E.G.-M., N.R.-C. and M.E.L.-G.; writing—review and editing, S.R.-B., E.G.-M., N.R.-C. and M.E.L.-G.; visualization, S.R.-B., E.G.-M., N.R.-C., M.E.L.-G., B.G.-S. and R.M.; supervision, S.R.-B., E.G.-M., N.R.-C., M.E.L.-G., B.G.-S. and R.M.; project administration. E.G.-M., N.R.-C., M.E.L.-G. and R.M.; funding acquisition, R.M. All authors have read and agreed to the published version of the manuscript.

Funding: This research was funded by the Ministry of Science and Innovation, the state research agency and the European Union NextGenerationEU/PRTR [project TED2021-129917B-I00].

Institutional Review Board Statement: Not applicable.

Informed Consent Statement: Not applicable.

Data Availability Statement: The data presented in this study are available on request from the corresponding author.

Acknowledgments: The authors are grateful to the Analysis Service Unit facilities of ICTAN for the chromatography analysis. This work was supported by the Complutense University through a research staff contract in the "Investigo programme" (CT36/22-30-UCM-INV).

Conflicts of Interest: The authors declare no conflict of interest.

Sample Availability: Samples of the compounds are available from the authors.

References

1. Djilas, S.; Čanadanović-Brunet, J.; Ćetković, G. By-Products of Fruits Processing as a Source of Phytochemicals. *Chem. Ind. Chem. Eng. Q.* **2009**, *15*, 191–202. [CrossRef]
2. Oreopoulou, V.; Tzia, C. Utilization of Plant By-Products for the Recovery of Proteins, Dietary Fibers, Antioxidants, and Colorants. *Util. By-Prod. Treat. Waste Food Ind.* **2007**, *3*, 209–232.
3. Redondo, D.; Arias, E.; Oria, R.; Venturini, M.E. Thinned Stone Fruits Are a Source of Polyphenols and Antioxidant Compounds. *J. Sci. Food Agric.* **2017**, *97*, 902–910. [CrossRef] [PubMed]
4. Chauhan, C.; Dhir, A.; Akram, M.U.; Salo, J. Food Loss and Waste in Food Supply Chains. A Systematic Literature Review and Framework Development Approach. *J. Clean. Prod.* **2021**, *295*, 126438. [CrossRef]
5. Tsegaye, B.; Jaiswal, S.; Jaiswal, A.K. Food Waste Biorefinery: Pathway towards Circular Bioeconomy. *Foods* **2021**, *10*, 1174. [CrossRef]
6. Mohamed, D.A.; Hamed, I.M.; Mohammed, S.E. Utilization of Grape and Apricot Fruits By-Products as Cheap Source for Biologically Active Compounds for Health Promotion. *Egypt. J. Chem.* **2021**, *64*, 2037–2045. [CrossRef]
7. Lazos, E.S. Composition and Oil Characteristics of Apricot, Peach and Cherry Kernel. *Grasas Aceites* **1991**, *42*, 127–131. [CrossRef]

8. Actualización, Ú. Boletín Fruta de Hueso. Resumen Campaña 2023 Inicio Producción Y Superficie Nacional-Avances ABRIL 2023. 2023. Available online: https://www.mapa.gob.es/es/agricultura/temas/producciones-agricolas/6_2023boletinfrutadehueso20234deoctubre2023_tcm30-661078.pdf (accessed on 10 July 2023).
9. Natić, M.; Zagorac, D.D.; Ćirić, I.; Meland, M.; Rabrenović, B.; Akšić, M.F. Cold Pressed Oils from Genus Prunus. In *Cold Press Oils: Green Technology, Bioactive Compounds, Functionality, and Applications*; Academic Press: Cambridge, MA, USA, 2020; pp. 637–658. [CrossRef]
10. Lara, M.V.; Bonghi, C.; Famiani, F.; Vizzotto, G.; Walker, R.P.; Drincovich, M.F. Stone Fruit as Biofactories of Phytochemicals With Potential Roles in Human Nutrition and Health. *Front. Plant Sci.* **2020**, *11*, 562252. [CrossRef]
11. Rudke, C.R.M.; Zielinski, A.A.F.; Ferreira, S.R.S. From Biorefinery to Food Product Design: Peach (*Prunus persica*) By-Products Deserve Attention. *Food Bioprocess Technol.* **2022**, *16*, 1197–1215. [CrossRef] [PubMed]
12. Górnaś, P.; Rudzińska, M.; Raczyk, M.; Mišina, I.; Soliven, A.; Segliņa, D. Composition of Bioactive Compounds in Kernel Oils Recovered from Sour Cherry (*Prunus cerasus* L.) by-Products: Impact of the Cultivar on Potential Applications. *Ind. Crops Prod.* **2016**, *82*, 44–50. [CrossRef]
13. Fidelis, M.; De Moura, C.; Kabbas, T.; Pap, N.; Mattila, P.; Mäkinen, S.; Putnik, P.; Kovačević, D.B.; Tian, Y.; Yang, B.; et al. Fruit Seeds as Sources of Bioactive Compounds: Sustainable Production of High Value-Added Ingredients from by-Products within Circular Economy. *Molecules* **2019**, *24*, 3854. [CrossRef] [PubMed]
14. Kumari, N.; Radha; Kumar, M.; Puri, S.; Zhang, B.; Rais, N.; Pundir, A.; Chandran, D.; Raman, P.; Dhumal, S.; et al. Peach (*Prunus persica* (L.) Batsch) Seeds and Kernels as Potential Plant-Based Functional Food Ingredients: A Review of Bioactive Compounds and Health-Promoting Activities. *Food Biosci.* **2023**, *54*, 102914. [CrossRef]
15. Khalil, M.N.A.; Farghal, H.H.; Farag, M.A. Outgoing and Potential Trends of Composition, Health Benefits, Juice Production and Waste Management of the Multi-Faceted Grapefruit Citrus X Paradisi: A Comprehensive Review for Maximizing Its Value. *Crit. Rev. Food Sci. Nutr.* **2022**, *62*, 935–956. [CrossRef] [PubMed]
16. Kumar, S.P.J.; Prasad, S.R.; Banerjee, R.; Agarwal, D.K.; Kulkarni, K.S.; Ramesh, K.V. Green Solvents and Technologies for Oil Extraction from Oilseeds. *Chem. Cent. J.* **2017**, *11*, 9. [CrossRef] [PubMed]
17. Eikani, M.H.; Golmohammad, F.; Homami, S.S. Extraction of Pomegranate (*Punica granatum* L.) Seed Oil Using Superheated Hexane. *Food Bioprod. Process* **2012**, *90*, 32–36. [CrossRef]
18. Maszewska, M.; Florowska, A.; Dłużewska, E.; Wroniak, M.; Marciniak-Lukasiak, K.; Zbikowska, A. Oxidative Stability of Selected Edible Oils. *Molecules* **2018**, *23*, 1746. [CrossRef] [PubMed]
19. Arbex, A.K.; Bizarro, V.R.; Santos, J.C.S.; Araújo, L.M.M.; de Jesus, A.L.C.; Fernandes, M.S.A.; Salles, M.M.; Rocha, D.R.T.W.; Marcadenti, A. The Impact of the Essential Fatty Acids (EFA) in Human Health. *Open J. Endocr. Metab. Dis.* **2015**, *5*, 98–104. [CrossRef]
20. Kaseke, T.; Opara, U.L.; Fawole, O.A. Fatty Acid Composition, Bioactive Phytochemicals, Antioxidant Properties and Oxidative Stability of Edible Fruit Seed Oil: Effect of Preharvest and Processing Factors. *Heliyon* **2020**, *6*, e04962. [CrossRef]
21. Lichtenstein, A.H.; Appel, L.J.; Brands, M.; Carnethon, M.; Daniels, S.; Franch, H.A.; Franklin, B.; Kris-Etherton, P.; Harris, W.S.; Howard, B.; et al. Diet and Lifestyle Recommendations Revision 2006: A Scientific Statement from the American Heart Association Nutrition Committee. *Circulation* **2006**, *114*, 82–96. [CrossRef]
22. Parodi, P.W. Has the Association between Saturated Fatty Acids, Serum Cholesterol and Coronary Heart Disease Been over Emphasized? *Int. Dairy J.* **2009**, *19*, 345–361. [CrossRef]
23. Hashempour-Baltork, F.; Torbati, M.; Azadmard-Damirchi, S.; Savage, G.P. Chemical, Rheological and Nutritional Characteristics of Sesame and Olive Oils Blended with Linseed Oil. *Adv. Pharm. Bull.* **2018**, *8*, 107–113. [CrossRef]
24. Ahmad, N.; Manzoor, M.F.; Shabbir, U.; Ahmed, S.; Ismail, T.; Saeed, F.; Nisa, M.; Anjum, F.M.; Hussain, S. Health Lipid Indices and Physicochemical Properties of Dual Fortified Yogurt with Extruded Flaxseed Omega Fatty Acids and Fibers for Hypercholesterolemic Subjects. *Food Sci. Nutr.* **2020**, *8*, 273–280. [CrossRef] [PubMed]
25. Santos-Silva, J.; Mendes, I.A.; Portugal, P.V.; Bessa, R.J.B. Effect of Particle Size and Soybean Oil Supplementation on Growth Performance, Carcass and Meat Quality and Fatty Acid Composition of Intramuscular Lipids of Lambs. *Livest. Prod. Sci.* **2004**, *90*, 79–88. [CrossRef]
26. Kaya, C.; Kola, O. Some Characteristics and Fatty Acids Composition of Wild Apricot (*Prunus pseudoarmeniaca* L.) Kernel Oil. *Artic. Asian J. Chem.* **2008**, *20*, 2597–2602.
27. Stryjecka, M.; Michalak, M.; Cymerman, J.; Kiełtyka-Dadasiewicz, A. Comparative Assessment of Phytochemical Compounds and Antioxidant Properties of Kernel Oil from Eight Sour Cherry (*Prunus cerasus* L.) Cultivars. *Molecules* **2022**, *27*, 696. [CrossRef] [PubMed]
28. Lee, J.M.; Chung, H.; Chang, P.S.; Lee, J.H. Development of a Method Predicting the Oxidative Stability of Edible Oils Using 2,2-Diphenyl-1-Picrylhydrazyl (DPPH). *Food Chem.* **2007**, *103*, 662–669. [CrossRef]
29. Grosshagauer, S.; Steinschaden, R.; Pignitter, M. Strategies to Increase the Oxidative Stability of Cold Pressed Oils. *LWT* **2019**, *106*, 72–77. [CrossRef]
30. Szterk, A.; Roszko, M.; Sosińska, E.; Derewiaka, D.; Lewicki, P.P. Chemical Composition and Oxidative Stability of Selected Plant Oils. *JAOCS J. Am. Oil Chem. Soc.* **2010**, *87*, 637–645. [CrossRef]
31. Bozan, B.; Temelli, F. Chemical Composition and Oxidative Stability of Flax, Safflower and Poppy Seed and Seed Oils. *Bioresour. Technol.* **2008**, *99*, 6354–6359. [CrossRef] [PubMed]

32. Redondo-Cuevas, L.; Castellano, G.; Torrens, F.; Raikos, V. Revealing the Relationship between Vegetable Oil Composition and Oxidative Stability: A Multifactorial Approach. *J. Food Compos. Anal.* **2018**, *66*, 221–229. [CrossRef]
33. Fox, N.J.; Stachowiak, G.W. Vegetable Oil-Based Lubricants-A Review of Oxidation. *Tribol. Int.* **2007**, *40*, 1035–1046. [CrossRef]
34. Wettasinghe, M.; Shahidi, F. Scavenging of Reactive-Oxygen Species and DPPH Free Radicals by Extracts of Borage and Evening Primrose Meals. *Food Chem.* **2000**, *70*, 17–26. [CrossRef]
35. Patras, A.; Brunton, N.P.; Tiwari, B.K.; Butler, F. Stability and Degradation Kinetics of Bioactive Compounds and Colour in Strawberry Jam during Storage. *Food Bioprocess Technol.* **2011**, *4*, 1245–1252. [CrossRef]
36. Al-Bachir, M. Compositions and Microbial Properties of Gamma Irradiated Apricot (*Prunus armeniaca* L.) Kernel. *J. Stress Physiol. Biochem.* **2021**, *17*, 79–87.
37. Farag, M.A.; Bahaa Eldin, A.; Khalifa, I. Valorization and Extraction Optimization of Prunus Seeds for Food and Functional Food Applications: A Review with Further Perspectives. *Food Chem.* **2022**, *388*, 132955. [CrossRef]
38. Fratianni, F.; d'Acierno, A.; Ombra, M.N.; Amato, G.; De Feo, V.; Ayala-Zavala, J.F.; Coppola, R.; Nazzaro, F. Fatty Acid Composition, Antioxidant, and in Vitro Anti-Inflammatory Activity of Five Cold-Pressed Prunus Seed Oils, and Their Anti-Biofilm Effect Against Pathogenic Bacteria. *Front. Nutr.* **2021**, *8*, 775751. [CrossRef] [PubMed]
39. Lykke, A.M.; Gregersen, S.B.; Padonou, E.A.; Bassolé, I.H.N.; Dalsgaard, T.K. Potential of Unconventional Seed Oils and Fats from West African Trees: A Review of Fatty Acid Composition and Perspectives. *Lipids* **2021**, *56*, 357–390. [CrossRef] [PubMed]
40. Grancieri, M.; Martino, H.S.D.; Gonzalez de Mejia, E. Chia Seed (*Salvia hispanica* L.) as a Source of Proteins and Bioactive Peptides with Health Benefits: A Review. *Compr. Rev. Food Sci. Food Saf.* **2019**, *18*, 480–499. [CrossRef]
41. Yangilar, F. The Application of Dietary Fibre in Food Industry: Structural Features, Effects on Health and Definition, Obtaining and Analysis of Dietary Fibre: A Review. *J. Food Nutr. Res.* **2013**, *1*, 13–23.
42. Andreasen, M.F.; Landbo, A.K.; Christensen, L.P.; Hansen, A.; Meyer, A.S. Antioxidant Effects of Phenolic Rye (*Secale cereale* L.) Extracts, Monomeric Hydroxycinnamates, and Ferulic Acid Dehydrodimers on Human Low-Density Lipoproteins. *J. Agric. Food Chem.* **2001**, *49*, 4090–4096. [CrossRef] [PubMed]
43. Davidson, M.H.; McDonald, A. Fiber: Forms and Functions. *Nutr. Res.* **1998**, *18*, 617–624. [CrossRef]
44. Ashraf, C.M.; Iqbal, S.; Ahmed, D. Nutritional and Physicochemical Studies on Fruit Pulp, Seed and Shell of Indigenous *Prunus persica*. *J. Med. Plants Res.* **2011**, *5*, 3917–3921.
45. Shariatifar, N.; Pourfard, I.M.; Khaniki, G.J.; Nabizadeh, R.; Akbarzadeh, A.; Nejad, A.S.M. Mineral Composition, Physico-Chemical Properties and Fatty Acids Profile of *Prunus armeniaca* Apricot Seed Oil. *Asian J. Chem.* **2017**, *29*, 2011–2015. [CrossRef]
46. Usenik, V.; Fabčič, J.; Štampar, F. Sugars, Organic Acids, Phenolic Composition and Antioxidant Activity of Sweet Cherry (*Prunus avium* L.). *Food Chem.* **2008**, *107*, 185–192. [CrossRef]
47. Shukla, R.K.; Prajapati, K.; Shukla, A.; Singh, R. Evaluation of Nutritive Value, Phytochemical Screening, Total Phenolic Content and in-Vitro Antioxidant Activity of the Seed of *Prunus domestica* L. *Plant Sci. Today* **2021**, *8*, 830–835. [CrossRef]
48. El-Aal, M.H.A.; Hamza, M.A.; Rahma, E.H. In Vitro Digestibility, Physico-Chemical and Functional Properties of Apricot Kernel Proteins. *Food Chem.* **1986**, *19*, 197–211. [CrossRef]
49. Savic, I.; Gajic, I.S.; Gajic, D. Physico-Chemical Properties and Oxidative Stability of Fixed Oil from Plum Seeds (*Prunus domestica* Linn.). *Biomolecules* **2020**, *10*, 294. [CrossRef] [PubMed]
50. Neagu, A.-A.; Niţa, I.; Botez, E.; Geaca, S. A Physico-Chemical Study for Some Edible Oils Properties. *Analele Univ. Ovidius Constanta Ser. Chim.* **2014**, *24*, 121–126. [CrossRef]
51. Lee, M.R.F.; Tweed, J.K.S.; Kim, E.J.; Scollan, N.D. Beef, Chicken and Lamb Fatty Acid Analysis—A Simplified Direct Bimethylation Procedure Using Freeze-Dried Material. *Meat Sci.* **2012**, *92*, 863–866. [CrossRef]
52. Zhang, H.; Wang, Z.; Liu, O. Development and Validation of a GC-FID Method for Quantitative Analysis of Oleic Acid and Related Fatty Acids. *J. Pharm. Anal.* **2015**, *5*, 223–230. [CrossRef] [PubMed]
53. ATİK, İ.; Şevik, R.; Karasu, S. Soğuk Press Kiraz (*Prunus avium*) Çekirdeği Yayının Fizikokimyasal Özellikleri, Yağ Asidi, Sterol, Tokoferol ve Fenolik Bileşen Karakterizasyonu. *Eur. J. Sci. Technol.* **2019**, *17*, 959–965. [CrossRef]
54. Perifanova-Nemska, M.; Delinska, N.; Dimitrova, E. Chemical Characteristics of Soap with Using Plum Kernel Oil (*Prunus domestica* L.). In Proceedings of the 2022 8th International Conference on Energy Efficiency and Agricultural Engineering, EE and AE 2022, Ruse, Bulgaria, 30 June–2 July 2022; Institute of Electrical and Electronics Engineers Inc.: Piscataway, NJ, USA, 2022.
55. Sales-Campos, H.; Reis de Souza, P.; Crema Peghini, B.; Santana da Silva, J.; Ribeiro Cardoso, C. An Overview of the Modulatory Effects of Oleic Acid in Health and Disease. *Mini-Rev. Med. Chem.* **2013**, *13*, 201–210. [CrossRef] [PubMed]
56. Stark, A.H.; Crawford, M.A.; Reifen, R. Update on Alpha-Linolenic Acid. *Nutr. Rev.* **2008**, *66*, 326–332. [CrossRef]
57. Djoussé, L.; Matthan, N.R.; Lichtenstein, A.H.; Gaziano, J.M. Red Blood Cell Membrane Concentration of Cis-Palmitoleic and Cis-Vaccenic Acids and Risk of Coronary Heart Disease. *Am. J. Cardiol.* **2012**, *110*, 539–544. [CrossRef] [PubMed]
58. de Souza, C.O.; Valenzuela, C.A.; Baker, E.J.; Miles, E.A.; Rosa Neto, J.C.; Calder, P.C. Palmitoleic Acid Has Stronger Anti-Inflammatory Potential in Human Endothelial Cells Compared to Oleic and Palmitic Acids. *Mol. Nutr. Food Res.* **2018**, *62*, 322. [CrossRef] [PubMed]
59. Stryjecka, M.; Kiełtyka-Dadasiewicz, A.; Michalak, M.; Rachoń, L.; Głowacka, A. Chemical Composition and Antioxidant Properties of Oils from the Seeds of Five Apricot (*Prunus armeniaca* L.) Cultivars. *J. Oleo Sci.* **2019**, *68*, 729–738. [CrossRef] [PubMed]

60. Saldaña y Hernández, M.I.; Gómez-Álvarez, R.; Rivera-Cruz, M.d.C.; Álvarez-Solís, J.D.; Pat-Fernández, J.M.; Ortiz-García, C.F. The Influence of Organic Fertilizers on the Chemical Properties of Soil and the Production of *Alpinia purpurata*. *Cienc. Investig. Agrar.* **2014**, *41*, 215–224. [CrossRef]
61. Lutterodt, H.; Slavin, M.; Whent, M.; Turner, E.; Yu, L. Fatty Acid Composition, Oxidative Stability, Antioxidant and Antiproliferative Properties of Selected Cold-Pressed Grape Seed Oils and Flours. *Food Chem.* **2011**, *128*, 391–399. [CrossRef] [PubMed]
62. Rokosik, E.; Dwiecki, K.; Siger, A. Nutritional Quality and Phytochemical Contents of Cold Pressed Oil Obtained from Chia, Milk Thistle, Nigella, and White and Black Poppy Seeds. *Grasas Aceites* **2020**, *71*, e368. [CrossRef]
63. Lamine, M.; Mliki, A.; Mlikia, A. Genetic Diversity and Salt Tolerance in Barley Germplasm: Physiological, Biochemical & Molecular Characterization View Project Citrus Waste Valorization View Project Nutritional Quality Perceptions through Fatty Acid Profiling, Health Lipid Indices and Antioxidant Potentialities. *Open J. Nutr. Food Sci.* **2021**, *3*, 1015.
64. Nawirska-Olszańska, A.; Kita, A.; Biesiada, A.; Sokół-ŁEtowska, A.; Kucharska, A.Z. Characteristics of Antioxidant Activity and Composition of Pumpkin Seed Oils in 12 Cultivars. *Food Chem.* **2013**, *139*, 155–161. [CrossRef] [PubMed]
65. Nayak, A.; Bhushan, B.; Rosales, A.; Turienzo, L.R.; Cortina, J.L. Valorisation Potential of Cabernet Grape Pomace for the Recovery of Polyphenols: Process Intensification, Optimisation and Study of Kinetics. *Food Bioprod. Process* **2018**, *109*, 74–85. [CrossRef]
66. Nederal, S.; Škevin, D.; Kraljić, K.; Obranović, M.; Papeša, S.; Bataljaku, A. Chemical Composition and Oxidative Stability of Roasted and Cold Pressed Pumpkin Seed Oils. *JAOCS J. Am. Oil Chem. Soc.* **2012**, *89*, 1763–1770. [CrossRef]
67. Association of Official Analytical Chemists (AOAC). *AOAC Method 925.10 (Air Oven Method) for Moisture in Flour*, 17th ed.; AOAC International: Gaithersburg, MD, USA, 2000.
68. Association of Official Analytical chemists (AOAC). *Official Methods of the AOAC, Methods 923.03, 920.85, 920.87, 978.10, 950.46*, 17th ed.; AOAC international: Gaithersburg, MD, USA, 2003.
69. Association of Official Analytical Chemists (AOAC). *Method 960.39*, 17th ed.; AOAC International: Gaithersburg, MD, USA, 2000.
70. Horwitz, W. *AOAC Official Method 962.09. Fiber (Crude) in Animal Feed and Pet Food*, 16th ed.; AOAC International: Gaithersburg, MD, USA, 2000.
71. AOAC. *Official Method 920.87—Protein (Total) in Flour, Final Action*, 17th ed.; AOAC International: Gaithersburg, MD, USA, 1995.
72. Ayoola, P.; Adeyeye, A. Chemical Evaluation of Food Value of Groundnut (*Arachi hypogaea*) Seeds. *Am. J. Food Nutr.* **2012**, *2*, 55–57. [CrossRef]
73. Asha, K.K.; Anandan, R.; Mathew, S.; Lakshmanan, P.T. Biochemical Profile of Oyster Crassostrea Madrasensis and Its Nutritional Attributes. *Egypt. J. Aquat. Res.* **2014**, *40*, 35–41. [CrossRef]

molecules

MDPI

Article

Assessment of the Use of Common Juniper (*Juniperus communis* L.) Foliage following the Cascade Principle

Irene Mediavilla [1,*], Raquel Bados [1], Lillian Barros [2,3], Virginie Xavier [2,3], Tiane C. Finimundy [2,3], Tania C. S. P. Pires [2,3], Sandrina A. Heleno [2,3], Ricardo C. Calhelha [2,3], Joana S. Amaral [2,3], Andrea Maria Rizzo [4], David Casini [4], Giacomo Lombardi [4], David Chiaramonti [4], Miguel Cámara [5], Ana Suárez [5], Tomás Ardid [5] and Luis Saúl Esteban [1]

1 Centre for the Development of Renewable Energies—Centre for Energy, Environmental and Technological Research, CEDER-CIEMAT, Autovía de Navarra A-15, Salida 56, 42290 Lubia, Spain; raquel.bados@ciemat.es (R.B.); luis.esteban@ciemat.es (L.S.E.)

2 Centro de Investigação de Montanha (CIMO), Instituto Politécnico de Bragança, Campus de Santa Apolónia, 5300-253 Bragança, Portugal; lillian@ipb.pt (L.B.); virginie.xavier@ipb.pt (V.X.); tiane@ipb.pt (T.C.F.); tania.pires@ipb.pt (T.C.S.P.P.); sheleno@ipb.pt (S.A.H.); calhelha@ipb.pt (R.C.C.); jamaral@ipb.pt (J.S.A.)

3 Laboratório Associado para a Sustentabilidade e Tecnologia em Regiões de Montanha (SusTEC), Instituto Politécnico de Bragança, Campus de Santa Apolónia, 5300-253 Bragança, Portugal

4 Renewable Energy Consortium for Research and Demonstration, RE-CORD, Viale J. F. Kennedy, 182, 50038 Scarperia e San Piero, Italy; andreamaria.rizzo@re-cord.org (A.M.R.); david.casini@re-cord.org (D.C.); giacomo.lombardi@re-cord.org (G.L.); david.chiaramonti@polito.it (D.C.)

5 TOLSA, Calle Núñez de Balboa, 51, 28001 Madrid, Spain; mcamara@tolsa.com (M.C.); asuarez@tolsa.com (A.S.); tardid@tolsa.com (T.A.)

* Correspondence: irene.mediavilla@ciemat.es; Tel.: +34-975281013

Abstract: *Juniperus communis* L. is a species commonly grown in regions of the Northern Hemisphere, and is a good candidate to be cultivated in marginal lands. Plants coming from a pruning performed in a natural population located in Spain were used to assess the yield and quality of different products obtained following the cascade principle. A total of 1050 kg of foliage biomass were crushed, steam-distilled, and separated into fractions to produce biochar and absorbents for the pet industry using pilot plants. The obtained products were analysed. The essential oil, with a yield of 0.45% dry basis and a qualitative chemical composition similar to that described for the berries in international standards or monographs, showed antioxidant activity with promising CAA results (inhibition of 89% of the cell's oxidation). However, regarding antibacterial and antifungal activities, it only inhibited the growth of microorganisms at the maximum concentration tested, 2.5%. Concerning the hydrolate, it did not show bioactivity. Regarding the biochar, whose yield was 28.79% dry basis, interesting results were obtained for its characterisation as a possible soil improver for agronomic purposes (PFC 3(A)). Finally, promising results were obtained regarding the use of common juniper as absorbent, taking into account the physical characterisation and odour control capacity.

Keywords: absorbent; bioactivity; biochar; essential oil; hydrolate

1. Introduction

A sustainable and circular European bioeconomy is needed to deal with global challenges such as climate change, land and ecosystem degradation, and a growing population. In this sense, modernisation and strengthening of the EU industrial base through the creation of new value chains and greener, more cost-effective industrial processes are of particular importance [1]. However, the production of new biobased products from vegetal biomass entails the use of land, which is a finite and scarce resource, and competition with food production or other necessities such as preservation of habitats, regeneration of ecosystems, or sequestration of carbon, can happen [2]. Then, the production of biomass on abandoned, unused, or severely degraded land (also referred to as marginal land) [3] could be a way to overcome a wide range of land-use challenges [2].

The main objective of the BeonNAT project is to create added-value biobased products within the concept of biorefinery, growing underused tree and shrub species in marginal lands. The BeonNAT biorefinery encompasses refining lignocellulosic biomass into intermediate outputs to be processed into a spectrum of biobased marketable products (vegetal extracts, essential oils, bioplastics, biochar, active carbon, absorbents for pets, particleboard, and pulp for paper), and bioenergy. Prior to the use of cultivated species, different tests are carried out with wild biomass in order to study the different processes and the quality and application of the products obtained. One of the species selected within the project is *Juniperus communis* L. It is an evergreen, perennial, long-lived coniferous plant which has the largest range of any woody plant in the cool temperate geographical regions of the Northern Hemisphere, from the Arctic south, in mountains, to around a latitude of 30° north in Europe, Asia, and North America [4]. It grows in poor soils and harsh environments, being drought- and cold-tolerant, although it requires a minimum of a year's water precipitation. In its southern distribution area, it can tolerate shade and can be found in the understorey of many forests. Moreover, common juniper can grow on acidic sandy or calcareous soils and favours free-draining soils and rocky outcrops.

Nowadays, the berry cones of *J. communis* and their essential oils are recognised by the European Pharmacopoeia. Berry cones are traditionally well known by folk medicine [5] and different studies on their essential oil have shown its strong antibacterial, antifungal, antiviral, antioxidant, and anti-inflammatory properties [4,6,7]. Some differences have been found between the essential oil of *J. communis* berry cones and leaves with regard to essential oil yield and composition [4,8,9], and most of the studies related to the bioactivity of *J. communis* essential oils have been focused on the oil coming from the berry cones. However, some studies have shown antioxidant and insecticidal properties for the essential oil obtained from the leaves and foliage of this species [10–12], but more research work is needed to study the bioactivity of this essential oil in order to know more information about its bactericidal and antifungal activities and complementary studies considering its antioxidant capacity.

After the steam distillation process, different byproducts are obtained, such as distilled vegetal biomass, distillation wastewater, and hydrolate. The distilled vegetal biomass is used as fuel to produce process heat or for composting in some industrial installations. However, other uses, such as extracts [13–15] or bio-oil [16] production, are being investigated with different species. To the authors' knowledge, alternative uses of distilled *J. communis* have not been studied, and the production of new green products, such as biochar and absorbent pellets for the pet industry, is proposed in this work.

Although juniper pyrolysis has been traditionally used to produce tar for different purposes such as gluing materials, waterproofing decoration, medicine, and cosmetics [17], no investigation has been found concerning the production of biochar, which is an interesting product from the point of view of soil improver for agronomic purposes and as strategic solution for carbon capture and storage.

Regarding the absorbents for the pet industry, the cat litter market is nowadays led by minerals, more specifically by clays—such as bentonite, sepiolite, and attapulgite—due to their high absorption and odour control capacity. However, a new biodegradable, eco-friendly mindset is surfacing in consumers and pushing cat litter manufacturers to enlarge their products on offer. The most known and sold product in this matter is wood pellets, which are made of sawdust obtained from heat-treated wood waste to remove toxins, oils, and allergens. Although wood pellets are well known for their high absorption capacity, they disintegrate in contact with liquid and, in principle, do not present a specific structure (as mineral do) to retain bad-odour-causing molecules and, consequently, ammoniacal odours can be detected [18]. Even so, other types of vegetal/plant-based fibres, such as those obtained after *J. communis* distillation, may be more efficient in odour control and capable of retaining or neutralising bad odour molecules.

On the other hand, hydrolate is a product of condensation after the essential oil isolation procedure. It is a colloidal suspension composed of a continuous phase, the distilled water, and a dispersed phase, which is an emulsion of essential oil droplets (usually below 1 g/L) and water-soluble components, namely, oxygen-containing compounds [19,20]. Hydrolates are easy to obtain, being formed in high amounts in the essential oil industry and, considering sustainability, there is a growing interest in giving added value to this byproduct. They have been historically used in traditional medicine in Mediterranean countries, as refreshing drinks and flavourings [21], and in cosmetics [22]. Additionally, investigations focused on their composition and biological properties have recently demonstrated their antimicrobial [21] and antioxidant [22] activities. Regarding the *J. communis* hydrolate, very few authors have published studies on its bioactivity, such as Oral et al. [23] who studied its antibacterial capacity. Considering the high amounts of hydrolate obtained during the steam distillation process, the study of possible uses of that hydrolate is important to complement the studies carried out on the essential oil.

Finally, the distillation wastewater results from condensation of some of the steam passing through the biomass, and it is collected at the bottom of the container. Currently, it is not a usable product and is released as a waste product. Very few studies have been carried out on its possible applications [19,24].

The objective of this work is to assess the yield and quality of different products obtained from *Juniperus communis*, such as essential oil, hydrolate, biochar, and absorbents, following the cascade principle.

2. Results and Discussion

2.1. Conditioning of Biomass and Steam Distillation

All the biomass collected was shredded at 20 mm and a sample was separated in order to analyse its moisture content, which was 42.5%.

Two samples of 400 kg of shredded material were distilled in the pilot plant described in Section 3.3 and the average essential oil yield was 0.45% (standard deviation: 0.035), expressed in weight percentage of dry essential oil referred to dry juniper. This value was of the same order of magnitude as those obtained in a previous work with *J. communis* collected in May 2018 and June 2020 in an area next to the area considered in this work and distilled in a plant with a capacity of 30 L [11]. However, the yields reported for *J. communis* foliage distillation in other studies [25–29] are variable (0.05–2.43%), although these results were obtained on a laboratory scale using a Clevenger apparatus with steam distillation or hydrodistillation and are not comparable to the tests considered in the present work.

Concerning the hydrolate and distillation wastewater production, the byproduct yields were 35.9% (standard deviation: 4.9) for hydrolate and 35.8% (standard deviation: 7.2) for wastewater, expressed in weight percentage of byproduct referred to dry juniper biomass.

After the distillation, the distilled biomass was air-dried, reaching a moisture content of 10.3%, and it was separated into three fractions using a sieving (4 mm) and blowing step. Two tests using 200 kg of air-dried distilled biomass each were performed, obtaining the following results, expressed as average value in weight percentage (wet basis): 11.9% (standard deviation: 0.42) of biomass from blowing, 54.6% (standard deviation: 1.04) of biomass < 4 mm from sieving, and 33.5% (standard deviation: 1.46) of biomass > 4 mm from sieving. Figure 1 shows some pictures of the biomass fractions obtained.

After the separation process, the fine fraction, composed of the biomass from blowing and the biomass with size below 4 mm obtained after sieving, corresponded to 66.5%, and the coarse fraction, composed of the biomass with size above 4 mm obtained after sieving, was 33.5% of the total biomass distilled. Taking into account the cascade defined in this work (Figure 2), pelletisation of the fine fraction was carried out, whereas milling at 8 mm of the coarse fraction was performed prior to pyrolysation.

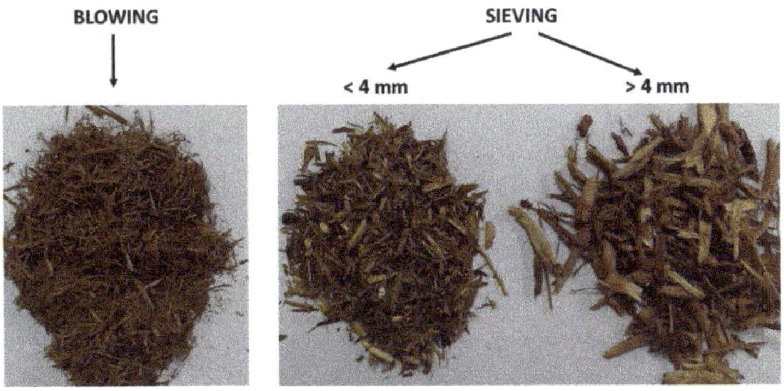

Figure 1. Biomass fractions obtained after the separation process.

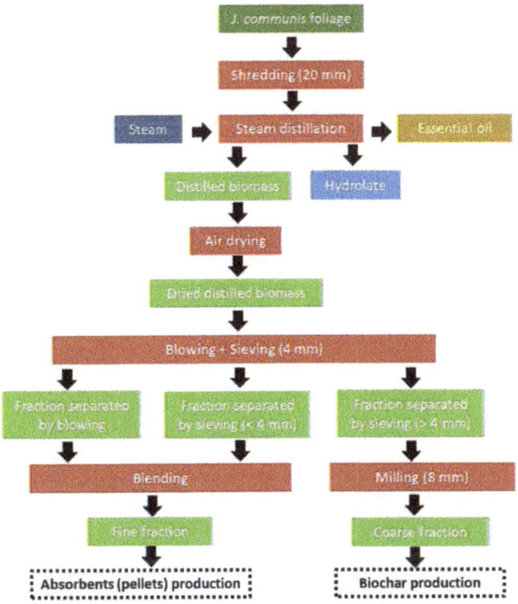

Figure 2. Block diagram of the biomass conditioning process and cascading.

2.2. Essential Oil and Hydrolate Composition

The essential oils obtained in the two steam distillation tests were blended and analysed using GC–MS. All the components identified and their quantification using the relative area percentage can be found in Mediavilla et al. [30], while Table 1 shows only the main compounds detected (>5%) in addition to those included in the European Pharmacopoeia for *Juniperus communis* berries essential oil and the standard ISO 8897:2010.

Table 1. Chemical composition of the *J. communis* essential oil.

Compound	Rt (min)	LRI [a]	LRI [b]	Relative % [c]
α-Pinene	14.05	928	932	18 ± 2
Sabinene	16.11	968	969	11 ± 1
β-Pinene	16.24	970	974	1.69 ± 0.02
Myrcene	17.08	986	988	5.9 ± 0.4
α-Phellandrene	17.70	998	1002	2.2 ± 0.1
Limonene	19.00	1023	1025	16 ± 2
Terpinen-4-ol	26.54	1172	1174	3.6 ± 0.1
Bornyl acetate	31.72	1281	1284	0.29 ± 0.05
β-Caryophyllene	37.72	1416	1417	2.2 ± 0.3
cis-Thujopsene	38.22	1428	1429	5.1 ± 0.5
Humulene	39.15	1451	1452	1.5 ± 0.2
Germacrene D	40.28	1478	1480	1.8 ± 0.3

[a] LRI: linear retention index determined on a DB-5 MS fused silica column relative to a series of n-alkanes (C8–C40). [b] LRI: linear retention index reported in the literature [31]. [c] Relative % is given as average ± standard deviation.

The characterisation of the analysed essential oil showed that monoterpene hydrocarbons were the most abundant compounds (68.1%), followed by sesquiterpene hydrocarbons (21.5%), oxygenated monoterpenes (5.7%), and, finally, oxygenated sesquiterpenes (0.8%). The main compounds (>5%) were four monoterpene hydrocarbons, namely, α-pinene (18%), limonene (16%), sabinene (11%), and myrcene (5.9%), and one sesquiterpene hydrocarbon, i.e., cis-thujopsene (5.1%). Comparing the obtained composition with the limits considered by the European Pharmacopoeia and the standard ISO 8897:2010, both referred to *J. communis* berries, it can be observed that the composition of the foliage essential oil shown in this work was close to meeting the limits. However, it can be noted that α-pinene was slightly below the limit (20.0% in the European Pharmacopoeia and 25.0% in the ISO standard), limonene was higher than the limit (12.0% in the European Pharmacopoeia and 8.0% in the ISO standard), and α-phellandrene (2.2%) was higher than the limit considered by the European Pharmacopoeia (1.0%). Comparing this characterisation with that obtained in a previous study of steam distillation of *J. communis* foliage collected in Spain, it can be observed that the distribution of percentages among the different component groups was similar, although with higher contents of sabinene and lower contents of limonene and myrcene [11]. Taking into account that the composition of *J. communis* essential oil changes throughout the year [27,32], being also affected by the proportion of leaves and berries contained in the sample distilled [8–10], more studies are required. They should comprise different locations and collecting periods to establish if the essential oil obtained from steam distillation of the foliage could fulfil the limits set out for the berries essential oil as described in the European Pharmacopoeia and/or the standard ISO 8897:2010.

The hydrolates obtained in the two steam distillation tests were blended and extracted, obtaining a yield of 0.18% (*w*/*w*). Afterwards, the extracted fraction was analysed using GC–MS. The components identified and their quantification using the relative area percentage are shown in Table 2.

The analysed hydrolate showed a qualitative and quantitative profile different from that of the essential oil since it contained mainly oxygenated monoterpenes. In the hydrolate, terpinen-4-ol was the most abundant compound (58%), followed by α-terpineol (10%). All the remaining identified compounds represented less than 5% of the total composition. Despite appearing in low amounts, some of the compounds were identified only in the hydrolate, probably due to their higher solubility in the aqueous phase since those were mainly small-weight alcohols and ketones.

Table 2. Chemical composition of *J. communis* hydrolate (oil fraction extracted).

Compound	Rt (min)	LRI [a]	LRI [b]	Relative % [c]
2-Hexenal	10.14	848	846	0.089 ± 0.002
3-Hexen-1-ol	10.27	851	850	0.89 ± 0.02
2-Hexen-1-ol	10.82	863	859	0.219 ± 0.02
1-Hexanol	10.93	865	863	0.34 ± 0.03
α-Pinene	14.06	929	932	0.73 ± 0.04
Camphene	14.80	943	946	0.20 ± 0.02
1-Octen-3-ol	16.52	976	974	0.27 ± 0.03
β-Myrcene	17.12	988	988	0.14 ± 0.01
α-Terpinene	18.79	1020	1014	0.1281 ± 0.004
p-Cymene	19.01	1024	1020	0.55 ± 0.01
Limonene	19.12	1026	1025	0.44 ± 0.03
γ-Terpinene	21.29	1068	1054	0.28 ± 0.02
trans-Linalool oxide	22.12	1084	1084	0.18 ± 0.01
Linalool	23.78	1117	1095	1.4 ± 0.1
2-p-Menthen-1-ol	24.01	1122	1118	0.165 ± 0.003
α-Campholenal	24.47	1131	1122	0.17 ± 0.01
trans-p-Mentha-2,8-dien-1-ol	24.67	1135	1133	2.8 ± 0.1
trans-Pinocarveol	24.94	1141	1135	3.2 ± 0.1
Sabinaketone	25.75	1157	1154	0.152 ± 0.002
BorneoL	26.05	1163	1165	0.9 ± 0.1
p-Mentha-1,5-dien-8-ol	26.08	1163	1166	0.67 ± 0.03
Terpinen-4-ol	26.69	1176	1174	58 ± 2
Cryptone	26.99	1182	1185	3.7 ± 0.1
α-Terpineol	27.27	1187	1186	10 ± 1
Myrtenol	27.54	1193	1194	0.83 ± 0.04
cis-Verbenone	28.12	1205	1204	3.0 ± 0.2
trans-Carveol	28.6	1215	1215	1.3 ± 0.1
Citronellol	29.03	1224	1223	0.48 ± 0.01
cis-Carveol	29.15	1227	1226	0.3 ± 0.2
Carvone	29.76	1240	1239	0.43 ± 0.03
Piperitone	30.25	1250	1249	0.27 ± 0.02
Phellandral	31.22	1271	1273	0.15 ± 0.02
p-Cymen-7-ol	31.95	1286	1289	0.45 ± 0.01
β-Elemene	36.53	1388	1389	0.10 ± 0.01
β-Caryophyllene	37.75	1416	1417	0.139 ± 0.003
cis-Thujopsene	38.25	1428	1429	0.346 ± 0.005
β-cadiene	42.01	1521	1520	0.138 ± 0.002
Oplopanone	49.97	1745	1739	0.21 ± 0.01
Total identified				95.14%
Monoterpene hydrocarbons				2.78%
Oxygen-containing monoterpenes				89.1%
Sesquiterpene hydrocarbons				0.9%
Others				1.54%
Not identified				5.64%

[a] LRI: linear retention index determined on a DB-5 MS fused silica column relative to a series of n-alkanes (C8–C40). [b] LRI: linear retention index reported in the literature [31]. [c] Relative % is given as average ± standard deviation.

2.3. Bioactivity of Essential Oil and Hydrolate

With regard to the antioxidant activity, the essential oil presented an EC50 of 1.14 ± 0.09 mg/mL in the reducing power assay (positive control: Trolox = 41 μg/mL) and inhibited 89% of the cells' oxidation in the CAA assay. Similar to the hydrolate, the essential oil also presented hepatotoxicity at a concentration of 179 ± 9 μg/mL. In all the bioactive assays performed, the hydrolate did not present activity at the higher concentration tested (2000 μg/mL), neither antioxidant nor antimicrobial activity, which is possibly explained by the high dilution factor of these products. Still, the hydrolate presented some hepatotoxicity (219 ± 13 μg/mL).

The antibacterial activity of the essential oil was tested in a concentration range from 2.5% (v/v) to 0.039% (v/v) and the clinical bacteria were not sensitive at the highest concentration tested (Table 3). Better results were obtained against the foodborne bacteria (Table 4) since the Gram-negative *S. enterica* and the Gram-positive *B. cereus* were inhibited by the *J. communis* essential oil at the highest concentration tested 2.5% (v/v). The essential oil at 2.5% (v/v) was also able to inhibit the growth of the two tested fungi (Table 5).

Table 3. Antibacterial activity of *J. communis* essential oil obtained by steam distillation (clinical bacteria). MIC and MBC values (% v/v).

			Controls					
	J. communis		**Ampicillin**		**Imipenem**		**Vancomycin**	
			20 mg/mL		**1 mg/mL**		**1 mg/mL**	
Clinical Bacteria	**MIC**	**MBC**	**MIC**	**MBC**	**MIC**	**MBC**	**MIC**	**MBC**
Gram-negative bacteria								
Escherichia coli	>2.5	>2.5	<0.15	<0.15	<0.0078	<0.0078	n.t	n.t.
Klebsiella pneumoniae	>2.5	>2.5	10	20	<0.0078	<0.0078	n.t	n.t.
Morganella morganii	>2.5	>2.5	20	>20	<0.0078	<0.0078	n.t	n.t.
Proteus mirabilis	>2.5	>2.5	<0.15	<0.15	<0.0078	<0.0078	n.t	n.t.
Pseudomonas aeruginosa	>2.5	>2.5	>20	>20	0.5	1	n.t.	n.t.
Gram-positive bacteria								
Enterococcus faecalis	>2.5	>2.5	<0.15	<0.15	n.t.	n.t.	<0.0078	<0.0078
Listeria monocytogenes	>2.5	>2.5	<0.15	<0.15	<0.0078	<0.0078	n.t	n.t.
MRSA	>2.5	>2.5	<0.15	<0.15	n.t.	n.t.	0.25	0.25

MIC: minimum inhibitory concentration; MBC: minimum bactericidal concentration; MRSA: methicillin-resistant *Staphylococcus aureus*; n.t.: not tested.

Table 4. Antibacterial activity of *J. communis* essential oil obtained by steam distillation (foodborne bacteria).

			Controls					
	J. communis		**Streptomycin**		**Methicillin**		**Ampicillin**	
	(% v/v)		**1 mg/mL**		**1 mg/mL**		**20 mg/mL**	
Food Bacteria	**MIC**	**MBC**	**MIC**	**MBC**	**MIC**	**MBC**	**MIC**	**MBC**
Gram-negative bacteria								
Enterobacter cloacae	>2.5	>2.5	0.007	0.007	n.t.	n.t	0.15	0.15
Escherichia coli	>2.5	>2.5	0.01	0.01	n.t.	n.t.	0.15	0.15
Pseudomonas aeruginosa	>2.5	>2.5	0.06	0.06	n.t.	n.t.	0.63	0.63
Salmonella enterica	2.5	>2.5	0.007	0.007	n.t.	n.t.	0.15	0.15
Yersinia enterocolitica	>2.5	>2.5	0.007	0.007	n.t.	n.t.	0.15	0.15
Gram-positive bacteria								
Bacillus cereus	2.5	>2.5	0.007	0.007	n.t.	n.t.	n.t.	n.t.
Listeria monocytogenes	>2.5	>2.5	0.007	0.007	n.t.	n.t.	0.15	0.15
Staphylococcus aureus	>2.5	>2.5	0.007	0.007	0.007	0.007	0.15	0.15

MIC: minimum inhibitory concentration; MBC: minimum bactericidal concentration; n.t. not tested.

Table 5. Antifungal activity of *J. communis* essential oil obtained by steam distillation.

	J. communis (% *v*/*v*)		Ketoconazole 1 mg/mL	
Fungi	**MIC**	**MFC**	**MIC**	**MFC**
Aspergillus brasiliensis	2.5	>2.5	0.06	0.125
Aspergillus fumigatus	2.5	>2.5	0.5	1

MIC: minimum inhibitory concentration; MFC: minimum fungicidal concentration.

According to Borges et al. [33], the concentration of α-pinene is directly related with antibacterial properties. Comparing the results obtained by Xavier et al. [34], the oil of the same species obtained in the same region showed α-pinene as the major compound, in concentrations about twice as high, and consequently results with greater antibacterial potential. Gonçalves et al. [35] found that the essential oil derived from *J. communis* biomass displayed potent inhibitory activity against *E. coli*, with concentrations of 1.25–2.5 mg/mL. However, no notable inhibitory activities were observed against other Gram-negative bacteria, including *P. mirabilis*, *K. pneumoniae*, *P. aeruginosa*, and *M. morganii*. There was a slight activity against *L. monocytogenes* and methicillin-resistant *S. aureus*. Dumitrescu et al. [36] discovered that commercially available essential oils of *J. communis* were active against *E. coli* and *S. aureus*, but not *P. aeruginosa*. The MIC values for various *Aspergillus* species ranged from 11 to 14 mg/mL. Meanwhile, the essential oil from *J. communis* berries, as per Cavaleiro et al. [37], showed an MIC of 10 μL/mL against *A. fumigatus*. As for antioxidant activity, Gonçalves et al. [35] stated that the essential oils tested exhibited the ability to scavenge ferric species (0.47 and 1.11 mM $FeSO_4 \cdot 7H_2O$). When compared to Xavier et al. [34], the oil from the same species in the same region demonstrated an EC_{50} of 1.35 ± 0.20 mg/mL with reducing power assay and $68.79 \pm 3.34\%$ oxidation inhibition with CAA assay. The essential oil also showed hepatoxicity (212.03 ± 23.26 ug/mL). Jakubczyk et al. [22] found that juniper hydrolate contained 2 292.98 μM Fe(II)/L, while other plants' hydrolates had higher antioxidant potential depending on the species, origin, part of the plant, and preservation method used. The juniper essential oil and hydrolate may possess bioactive properties depending on various factors. However, caution must be exercised while using them due to their potential toxicity towards liver human cell lines.

2.4. Pyrolysis and Biochar Characterisation

The coarse fraction obtained after the separation of distilled juniper biomass (Figure 2) was pyrolysed in the pilot scale plant described in Section 3.6, and a biochar yield of 28.79% by dry weight was obtained. Biochar mass yield (the solid fraction resulted by the thermochemical conversion of biomass through the pyrolysis process) depends strictly on the feedstock characteristics, the plant used, and the process parameters chosen (heating rates, maximum temperature, and residence times) [38,39]. SPYRO pilot plant, through the slow pyrolysis process, maximises the mass yield of high-quality char (commonly about 30% by dry weight), while minimising the production of liquid and gaseous products.

The biochar produced showed a total carbon content of 87.8% *w*/*w* d.b. and a fixed carbon content of 78.4% *w*/*w* d.b. As reported by Leng et al. [40], biochar fixed carbon is closely related to stable C content. Moisture content was 1.8% *w*/*w* w.b., and volatile matter and ash content resulted, respectively, in 13.0 and 8.7% *w*/*w* d.b. Fixed carbon content and H/C molar ratio indicate a good degree of carbonisation and stability for the biochar obtained [40,41]. H/C molar ratio values fluctuate depending on the feedstock and the process used; generally, materials with low H/C molar ratio represent products with higher stability and resistance to degradation, similar to in this case, where the molar H/C ratio resulted in 0.35.

The complete set of proximate and ultimate analysis, elements, and organic pollutants content can be found in Appendix A (respectively, in Table A1, Table A2, and Table A3), as well as the SEM pictures (Figure A1). Biochar porosity analysis can be found in Table A4 in

Appendix A, both using BET methodology and mercury porosimetry for the specific surface area and pore volume evaluation. In particular, results with the mercury porosimeter show a volume porosity of 66% and a specific volume intrusion of 1.59 cm^3/g in the range of meso- and macroporosity.

The biochar water-holding capacity test at 0.01 bar resulted in 141.6% w/w wet basis. According to Usevičiūtė and Baltrėnaitė-Gedienė [42], wood-based biochars have a wide range of sorption capacity values, mainly related to the feedstock characteristics and to the conversion process, commonly comprising about 1 to about 3 mL/g; the biochar obtained from *J. communis* showed a water-holding capacity of 1.41 mL/g.

The high carbon content, resistant to thermochemical and biological degradation, and only marginally subject to mineralisation by microorganisms [40,43], coupled with the water-holding ability that resulted, represent interesting results for the application of the product obtained as an effective soil improver for agronomic purposes and, at the same time, a potential innovative carbon capture and storage strategic solution (as indicated in the IPCC report released in 2019 [44]. The modifications to Annexes II, III, and IV of the EU Reg. 2019/1009 for fertilising products included the possibility to classify pyrolysis solid residue (biochar) as Component Material Category n.14 (CMC 14). In the Tables 6 and 7 are presented the compliance of the biochar produced with CMC 14 threshold and the Product Function Category n.3A (PFC 3A) that permits characterisation of the product as a soil improver.

Table 6. Biochar compliance with EU regulation n.2019/1009 for fertilising products, as CMC 14.

Parameter	CMC14 Threshold	*J. communis* Biochar
PAH16 (mg/kg d.b.)	<6.0	1.36
PCDD/F (ng $_{\text{WHO toxicity equivalents}}$/kg d.b.)	<20.0	<1.0
PCB non-dioxin-like (mg/kg d.b.)	<0.8	0.001
Cl^- (g/kg d.b.)	<30.0	0.02
Tl (mg/kg d.b.) *	<2.0	<1.0
H/C_{ORG} molar ratio **	<0.7	0.356

d.b.: Dry basis; * Reg. (EU) 2019/1009: with pyrolysis additives > 5% of loaded fresh mass; ** Reg. (EU) 2019/1009: on dry and ash-free fraction for material with a C_{ORG} content < 50%.

Table 7. Biochar compliance with EU regulation n.2019/1009 for fertilising products, as PFC 3(A).

Parameter	PFC 3(A) Threshold	*J. communis* Biochar
Organic carbon (% w/w d.b.)	>7.5	87.3
Dry matter (% w/w d.b.)	>20.0	98.2
Cadmium (mg/kg d.b.)	<2.0	0.4
Hexavalent chromium (mg/kg d.b.)	<2.0	<0.2
Mercury (mg/kg d.b.)	<1.0	<0.1
Nickel (mg/kg d.b.)	<50.0	b.d.l.
Lead (mg/kg d.b.)	<120.0	b.d.l.
Inorganic arsenic (mg/kg d.b.)	<40.0	<0.2 (as Total As)
Copper (mg/kg d.b.)	<300.0	57.0
Zinc (mg/kg d.b.)	<800.0	9.0
Salmonella spp. (CFU/25 g)	absent	n.a.
Escherichia coli or Enterococcaceae (CFU/g)	<1000	n.a.

% w/w: % Weight/weight; d.b.: dry basis; CFU: colony-forming units; b.d.l.: below detection limit; n.a.: not available.

2.5. Pelletisation and Absorbent Pellets Characterisation

The fine fraction obtained after the separation of distilled juniper biomass (Figure 2) was pelletised with a moisture content of 12.8%. Concerning the pelletisation process, a specific mass flow of 7.6 kg of dry matter per hour and per kW of drive power and a specific energy of 78 kWh per t of dry matter were obtained. When comparing these values with previous works carried out in a pilot plant to produce solid biofuels, the specific mass flow was higher (27%) than the values obtained with a shrub biomass (*Genista cinerascens* L.) [45] and pine sawdust [46], and the specific energy was lower (34%). These values show that the yield of pelletisation of the fine fraction of *J. communis* separated following the process described in Section 3.2 is higher than the value corresponding to a biomass typically used to produce solid biofuels, such as pine sawdust, or a shrub biomass, such as *G. cinerascens*. This fact could be due to the higher bark content of the fine fraction obtained after the separation process (see Figure 1), since some authors have demonstrated that a higher bark content increases pellet production [47,48].

Regarding the use of these pellets as cat litter, the analysis results can be found in Table 8.

Table 8. Physical–chemical characterisation of *J. communis* pellets as cat litter and reference values.

Parameter	Absorbing Plant-Based Cat Litter Feasibility Reference Values	*J. communis* Pellets
Appearance	Clear colours usually related to hygiene sensation	Spotted dark brown cylindrical particles
Dry particle size distribution (mm)	1.0–8.0	5.6–6.3
Moisture content (% w/w, w.b.)	Max. 14.0	10.5
Dust content (a.u.)	As low as possible	7
Bulk density (g/L) (w.m.)	450–650	465
Water absorption (% w/w, w.b.)	>180	267
Durability (%w/w, w.b.)	>95.0	88.9
Ammonia absorption (NH_3 ppm) (4 h)	As low as possible	0

% w/w: % Weight/weight; w.b.: wet basis; a.u.: arbitrary units; w.m: wet matter.

In terms of appearance (Figure 3), the analysed *J. communis* pellets showed well-defined cylindrical shape and darker colour (reddish dark brown with cream–yellowish spots) than that of the wood pellets mostly found in the market. Concerning the results of dry particle size distribution, the pellets were sized between the limits considered as reference. Moreover, it must be noted that the particle size distribution was homogeneous (5.6–6.3 mm), and this fact makes the product more attractive for consumers.

Moisture content, bulk density, and water absorption capacity showed values included in the limits considered as reference. Therefore, the *J. communis* pellets are stable from the point of view of their moisture content, lightweight, and highly absorbent, characteristics demanded in the market for pet absorbents.

Regarding the dust content, although traditional litters of mineral origin can reach values up to 50 u.a., commercial plant-based cat litter is not usually dusty, with values around 8–14 a.u. Consequently, the result obtained with *J. communis* pellets (7 a.u.) was satisfactory.

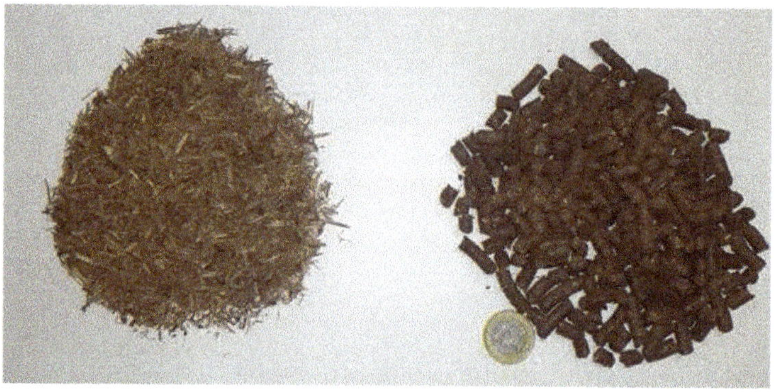

Figure 3. Appearance of *J. communis* material before and after the pelletisation process.

Durability evaluates the resistance of pellets to repeated beating (transport and handling) and, ideally, in the case of cat litter pellets, it should be higher than 95.0%. However, the *J. communis* pellets analysed showed a durability of 88.9% and, consequently, improving this parameter would be worthy. It must be noted that mechanical durability not only depends on the biomass used but also on the die compression used during the pelletisation process [46]. Then, although this parameter does not fulfil the limits considered as reference, it could be improved through setting the pelletisation process parameters.

Finally, the odour control result, expressed as the NH_3 concentration that is not retained/neutralised by the material and measured 4 h after the addition of aged real cat urine, was 0 ppm, compared with 16 ppm, which was measured with commercial wood pellets. Consequently, the *J. communis* pellets analysed have very high deodorising capacity.

3. Materials and Methods

3.1. Vegetal Material

Natural populations of *Juniperus communis* in Spain are shown in Figure 4. One of these populations, located in a mountain area in Spain (Barriomartín; UTM coordinates: 30T 545081; 4649553), was selected. This location has an altitude of 1407 m (a.s.l.) and its vegetation is mainly composed of forest and heath. Regarding the marginality of the site, predominantly poor substrate and low rooting depth can be highlighted.

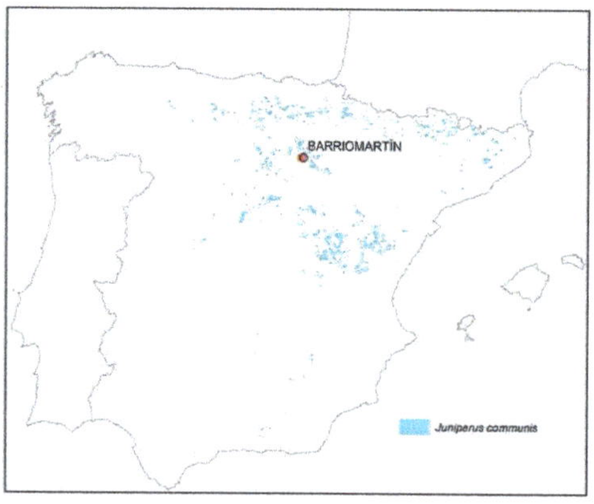

Figure 4. Distribution of natural populations of *J. communis* in Spain (based on MFE25 [49] and MFE200 [50]).

A sample of 1050 kg of foliage (50% of male plants and 50% of female plants) coming from plants with stem diameter below 50 mm was collected on 6 and 7 April 2021. The objective of using plants with this stem diameter was to reproduce the pruning process in a plantation of this species, since common juniper has good response to trimming.

3.2. Conditioning of Biomass

The collected foliage biomass was crushed (20 mm) using a shredder (90 kW, slow-rotating single-shaft type). The freshly ground biomass was distilled in a steam distillation pilot plant and the distilled biomass was air-dried at temperature below 40 °C and was separated into two fractions by means of a sieving and blowing step (0.37 kW, gyratory-reciprocating motion screener). The sieve used had a mesh of 4 mm, and a fine fraction composed of the particles with size below 4 mm and blown particles and a coarse fraction composed of the particles with a size above 4 mm were obtained. Finally, the coarse fraction was milled in a hammer mill (11 kW) at 8 mm. Subsamples were taken along the process to determine the moisture content in an oven at 105 °C until they reached a constant weight, following the standard ISO 18134-2:2017. Figure 2 shows the different steps followed.

3.3. Steam Distillation

A steam distillation pilot plant described in a previous work [30] was used to distil the *J. communis* biomass. Two batch distillations of 400 kg each were performed with a duration of 6 h (time was measured from the moment the first drop of distillate fell). The duration of the tests was defined considering that the quantity of essential oil obtained in the last 1.5 h was below 5% of the total essential oil obtained during the whole process. The essential oil samples were weighed and dried using anhydrous sodium sulphate and, after filtration, stored at 4 °C until further analysis. The oil yield for each sample was calculated as a percentage (w/w) on a biomass dry weight basis.

The hydrolate and the residual water obtained during the distillation process were weighed. A sample of hydrolate was separated and stored at 4 °C until further analysis. The hydrolate and residual water yields were calculated as a percentage (w/w) on a biomass dry weight basis.

3.4. Essential Oil and Hydrolate Characterisation: Chemical Composition

One sample of essential oil was obtained, blending the two samples of essential oil produced in the steam distillation tests, and it was analysed by gas chromatography–mass spectrometry (GC–MS) on a Shimadzu GC-2010 Plus chromatograph equipped with AOC-20iPlus automatic injector (Shimadzu, Canby, OR, USA) and an SH-RXi fused-silica column (30 m × 0.25 mm i.d., film thickness 0.25 μm; Shimadzu, Canby, OR, USA) according to the conditions described by Spréa et al. [51].

One sample of hydrolate was obtained, blending the two samples of hydrolate produced in the steam distillation tests, and it was analysed by GC–MS under the same conditions. The hydrolate (15 mL) was extracted using liquid–liquid extraction with organic solvents. Two cycles of diethyl ether (15 mL) and 3 cycles of hexane (15 mL) were performed. Anhydrous sodium sulphate was added to guarantee that no water from the hydrolate remained in the organic fraction. The extracted fraction was filtered and evaporated until dry. The remaining fraction was diluted in 2 mL of hexane (HPLC grade), filtered with syringe filter, and stored in the freezer until further analysis.

3.5. Essential Oil and Hydrolate Characterisation: Bioactive Evaluation

Both essential oil and hydrolate were evaluated for their antimicrobial activity, antioxidant activity, and hepatotoxicity.

3.5.1. Antimicrobial Activity

The antibacterial activity of *J. communis* essential oil and hydrolate was evaluated against clinical isolates, foodborne bacteria, and fungal species. The clinical isolates were obtained from patients hospitalized in various departments at the northeastern local health unit (Bragança, Portugal) and Hospital Center of Trás-os-Montes and Alto Douro (Vila Real, Portugal). Five Gram-negative bacteria, *Escherichia coli* (isolated from urine), *Proteus mirabilis* (isolated from wound exudate), *Klebsiella pneumoniae* (isolated from urine), *Pseudomonas aeruginosa* (isolated from expectoration), and *Morganella morganii* (isolated from urine), and three Gram-positive bacteria, *Enterococcus faecalis* (isolated from urine), *Listeria monocytogenes* (isolated from cerebrospinal fluid), and methicillin-resistant *Staphylococcus aureus* (MRSA) (isolated from expectoration), were tested. Concerning the food contaminants, the essential oil and hydrolate were tested against five Gram-negative bacteria, namely, *Enterobacter cloacae* (ATCC 49741), *Escherichia coli* (ATCC 25922), *Pseudomonas aeruginosa* (ATCC 9027), *Salmonella enterica* subsp. (ATCC 13076), and *Yersinia enterocolitica* (ATCC 8610), and three Gram-positive bacteria, namely, *Bacillus cereus* (ATCC 11778), *Listeria monocytogenes* (ATCC 19111), and *Staphylococcus aureus* (ATCC 25923).

Additionally, the essential oil and hydrolate were also tested against two fungi: *Aspergillus brasiliensis* and *Aspergillus f*umigatus. *A. brasiliensis* is a common fungal species found in various environments, including soil, food, and indoor settings, such as industrial plants. Although it is a frequent food contaminant, it rarely causes human illness. In contrast, *A. fumigatus* can colonize the upper respiratory tract of individuals with asthma, causing severe symptoms, reduced lung function, and occasionally resulting in severe diseases.

Food strains and fungal species were purchased at Frilabo, Porto, Portugal.

The antimicrobial activity was evaluated through the broth microdilution method, based on the methodology described by Falcão et al. [6] and later adapted to a microdilution method by Xavier et al. [34].

3.5.2. Antioxidant Activity

The antioxidant capability of the essential oil and hydrolate was determined using the reducing power (RP) [52] and the cellular antioxidant activity (CAA) [53] assays. All human or animal cell lines used in this manuscript were commercially available and were purchased from different authorized cell line resources, including the German Collection of Microorganisms and Cell Cultures (DSMZ) and the European Collection of Authenticated Cell Cultures (ECCAC). In order to maintain high scientific standards, all procedures were performed according to the best practices observed in the Guidance on Good Cell Culture Practice (GCCP). The efficacy of the antioxidant treatments was subsequently measured by the percentage reduction in fluorescence for CAA measurement at an excitation wavelength of 485 nm.

3.5.3. Hepatotoxicity

The hepatotoxicity of the essential oil was performed following a sulforhodamine B (SRB) assay previously described by the authors [54].

3.6. *Pyrolysis and Biochar Characterisation*

The coarse fraction obtained after the conditioning of the distilled biomass (Figure 2) was pyrolysed using an innovative pilot plant composed of a continuous auger-type pyrolysis reactor (SPYRO) and by an in-series condensation unit. SPYRO is designed to process up to 3 kg/h of biomass and can be operated up to 600 °C. The rotating speed of the reactor screw can be easily adjusted to vary the solids residence time, from few minutes up to 1 h. A total of 4220 g of wet feedstock were processed with an average heating rate of 17.8 °C/min and a residence time of about 30 min at the maximum pyrolysis process temperature of 550 °C (slow pyrolysis process). The charcoal was collected by gravity in a sealed vessel, while volatiles were separated into a pyrolysis liquid that was collected in glass bottles, and an off-gas stream composed of permanent gas.

The biochar obtained was characterised in terms of proximate and ultimate analysis, elements content, organic pollutants, conductivity, specific surface area, pH, and water-holding capacity at 0.01 bar (results are presented in Appendix A). Biochar sample was also analysed using a scanning electron microscopy.

The moisture, ash, and volatile matter contents were analysed using a Leco Thermogravimetric Analyser TGA 701. The moisture content was measured at 105 °C following the UNI EN ISO 18134-2 standard, the ash content was measured at 550 °C according to UNI EN ISO 18122, and the volatile matter at 900 °C according to UNI EN ISO 18123. The fixed carbon was calculated according to UNI EN 1860-2. The total carbon (C), hydrogen (H), and nitrogen (N) contents were analysed in a Leco TruSpec CHN analyser according to UNI EN ISO 16948.

The sulphur and chlorine contents were analysed by ion chromatography according to UNI EN ISO 16994 in a Metrohm 883 Basic IC Plus.

The inorganic carbon content was measured according to the current Italian decree n.7276, addition n.13 of the 31 May 2006 (Dietrich–Fruhling calcimeter); and the organic carbon was calculated as the difference between the total (CHN) and the inorganic carbon.

The water-holding capacity of the biochar was determined according to Italian D.M. 1 August 1997 Method 5, which refers to soil physical analysis, and adjusted to be suitable for biochar analysis.

Microelement and macroelement contents were analysed through an ICP (Agilent 4200 MP-AES, Santa Clara, CA, USA), previously calibrated with a multielemental standard solution. For the former mineralisation step, 0.05 g of biochar were weighed and 3 mL of H_2O_2 and 8 mL of HNO_3 were added, then the samples were mineralised in a Milestone Start D Microwave Digestor System. At the end of the step, HNO_3 at 1% concentration was added to the collected mineralised samples, reaching 20 mL in volume, and then the solutions were analysed in the ICP.

The concentration of toxic metals, such as Cd, As, Hg, and Tl were analysed according to EN 13657 + EN ISO 7294, while Cr VI was analysed according to EPA 3060 A + EPA 7196. Other harmful compounds (PAH, polychlorinated biphenyls, dibenzodioxins and dibenzofurans) were analysed, respectively, through EPA 3540 C + EPA 3630 C + EPA 8270 E for PAHs, EPA 1668 C for polychlorinated biphenyls, and EPA 1613 B for polychlorinated dibenzodioxins and dibenzofurans.

The biochar specific surface area was determined according Brunauer–Emmett–Teller method (BET), by N_2 adsorption isotherms, in a Quantachrome NOVA 2200E instrument. All measurements were performed on 60 mg of samples preliminarily dried at 200 °C for 48 h and then degassed under vacuum (200 °C for 24 h). Meso- and macroporosity, in terms of specific surface area and pore volume, were investigated using a Micromeritics AutoPore V 9600 mercury porosimeter.

The pH was measured according to UNI EN ISO 10390 in 0.1 M of $CaCl_2$ (1:5 *v*/*v*) through a Metrohm 827 pH meter.

Electrical conductivity was determined according to ISO 11265 using a Thermo Scientific (Waltham, MA, USA) COND6+ conductivity meter after water extraction and filtration.

Finally, the SEM experiment was conducted using a Thermo Scientific Phenom XL G2. Measurements were conducted on uncoated samples.

3.7. Pelletisation and Absorbent Pellets Characterisation

Finally, the fine fraction obtained after the biomass conditioning (Figure 2) was used to produce pellets in a small pilot plant. The pellet press, KAHL 14-175, is a flat-die machine with dosing hopper and variable speed. With an engine of 3 kW, this press can produce 20–40 kg pellets/h. The flat die used has a diameter of 175 mm, holes with 6 mm of diameter, and a die compression (length of the inlet cone + straight channel of the hole) of 28 mm. Two rollers with a width of 15 mm and rotating speed between 0.5 and 0.8 m/s force the material to move through the flat die.

With the objective of producing high-quality pellets and optimising the operation of the pellet press with stable power demand and low vibration, the flows of water and biomass fed to the machine were modified. Once these conditions were achieved, the steady state was reached and it was maintained for 40 min. Once the pellets were cooled down, they were manually sieved with a 3.15 mm sieve in order to simulate an industrial process removing the fines content.

Two process variables were recorded in the pelletisation tests: the specific mass flow, which is expressed in kg of dry matter per hour and per kW of drive power, and the specific energy, which is expressed in kWh per t of dry matter. In the calculation of the specific mass flow, the mass of pelletised material, in kg of dry matter, is divided by the time used to pelletise it, expressed in hours, and by the power of the pellet press, which is 3 kW. On the other hand, the specific energy is calculated, considering the active electric energy required to pelletise the material, divided by the mass of pellets obtained, expressed in t of dry matter.

Since the final use of the obtained pellets is as absorbent cat litter, the following characteristics were determined:

- Appearance. This is visually determined by observing and writing down all the particularities referring to the nature of the sample: colour, particle size distribution, structure, and porosity of the particles, as well as dust generation, possible blend of raw materials, and possible additives presence.
- Dry particle size distribution (method based on UNE 22-162 and ISO 2591-1). This is the relative percentage of different size particles conforming a product. This trial is performed by dry-sifting throughout a series of standardised screens, and calculation of the percentage of material that remains on each screen.
- Moisture content (own method). This provides information on the quantity of water naturally contained in the sample, and this test is carried out by means of a halogen moisture analyser (Mettler Toledo, HG53, Columbus, OH, USA) at a temperature of 145 °C.
- Dust content (own method). This parameter measures the dust cloud generated by the cat litter when pouring the material in terms of the cloud's height and time that it takes to disappear. A sample is placed in a funnel at a known distance from the ground and dropped. From the moment that the sample ends, the time needed for dissipating the cloud of dust generated is measured. Moreover, the density and height reached by the dust cloud are also assessed and the final result is obtained in arbitrary units.
- Bulk density (method based on AFNOR NFT 73-405, UNE 55-516-89, ISO 697 and BS 3762). This is calculated by dividing the mass of pellets confined by a certain volume.
- Water absorption (method based on AFNOR NF V 19-002). This is determined by means of the Westinghouse method, which tests the static water absorption capacity of the vegetal pellets when fully immersed and wet until saturation.
- Durability (own method). This parameter determines the resistance to pellet breakage and fines generation. It is measured by the durability index, which represents the pellet that remains intact after shaking 500 g at 50 rpm for 10 min in a Pfost tumbling box.
- Ammonia absorption capacity (own method). This is calculated using a rapid laboratory method for punctually assessing the deodorising capacity of cat litter against ammoniacal odours from urine. The technique is based on the use of suitably defrosted aged urine, which is mixed with the litter, allowing absorption. After 4 h, ammonia release is measured as NH_3 gas concentration (ppm), combined with olfactory perception. For measuring ammonia, a Dräger Accuro model gas detector pump combined with control tubes for ammonia determination (type ammonia 5/a) and 500 mL bottles with cap are used. The results are expressed as follows:
    - High deodorant capacity: when no unpleasant odour is observed and the concentration of NH_3 emitted by the sample is less than 5 ppm.
    - Medium deodorant capacity: when a slight odour of urine is perceived and the concentration of NH_3 emitted is between 5 and 70 ppm.

- Low deodorant capacity: when a clear smell of urine is perceived and the concentration of NH_3 emitted is between 70 and 210 ppm.
- No deodorant capacity: when the intense smell of urine is annoying and the concentration of NH_3 emitted by the sample is greater than 210 ppm.

4. Conclusions

Common juniper obtained from pruning seems to be an appropriate raw material to produce essential oil, biochar, and absorbents following the cascade principle, which could be an incentive to grow this species or to increase its forest management. Yields of 0.45% and 35.9% on dry weight were obtained for essential oil and hydrolate, respectively, while the distilled biomass was separated into two fractions, dedicated to biochar (33.5%) and absorbents (66.5%) production.

To the best of our knowledge, this work describes for the first time the chemical composition of common juniper foliage hydrolate, evidencing oxygenated monoterpenes as the major group of compounds. The essential oil showed antioxidant activity with promising CAA results. From all the tested bacteria, the essential oil only showed bacteriostatic action against *S. enterica* and *B. cereus* at the maximum concentration tested; furthermore, it was able to inhibit the growth of the two tested fungi. In general, the qualitative chemical composition of the essential oil obtained from juniper foliage was similar to that described for the berries in the European Pharmacopoeia and the standard ISO 8897:2010; however, it did not comply with all criteria described for the berries essential oil since the amounts of limonene, α-pinene, and α-phellandrene were not in the value range described. Considering that the chemical composition can vary with several factors such as climate, soil, and plant sex, among others, more research is needed to determine whether the essential oil extracted from the foliage of *J. communis* might meet the requirements set for the berries essential oil as described in the international standards or monographs.

Thanks to the thermochemical conversion of 33.5% of the distilled biomass (10.3% moisture content) through a slow pyrolysis pilot unit, it was possible to obtain, with a mass yield of 28.79% on dry weight, a quality biochar with a high stable carbon content. The water retention value of 1.42 mL/g resulted as coherent with the total intrusion volume resulted in the range of meso- and macroporosity. This property coupled with the high recalcitrant carbon content of the biochar represent interesting results for the potential application of this product as an effective soil improver for agronomic purposes and, at the same time, a potential innovative strategic solution for carbon capture and storage. The complete characterisation of the sample shows its compliance with EU legislation for fertilising products as a soil improver, PFC 3(A).

Finally, concerning the use of common juniper as absorbent, high yield was obtained during pelletisation (7.6 kg of dry matter per hour and per kW of drive power and 78 kWh per t of dry matter). Moreover, considering the use of these pellets as cat litter, appropriate values regarding moisture content, bulk density, water absorption, dust content, and odour control were obtained, resulting in a very interesting product for this purpose. However, pellets durability should be improved in order to meet the requirements established for this kind of product, and, consequently, further investigation on the pelletisation process is needed.

Author Contributions: Conceptualization, I.M., L.B., D.C. (David Casini), D.C. (David Chiaramonti), A.S., T.A. and L.S.E.; data curation, D.C. (David Casini), G. L., A.S. and T.A.; formal analysis, V.X., T.C.F., J.S.A., R.C.C., T.C.S.P.P., D.C. (David Casini), G.L., M.C., A.S. and T.A.; funding acquisition: L.S.E.; investigation, I.M., R.B., V.X., T.C.F., S.A.H., J.S.A., R.C.C., T.C.S.P.P., L.B., D.C. (David Casini), G.L., M.C., A.S. and T.A.; methodology, I.M., R.B., V.X., T.C.F., J.S.A., R.C.C., T.C.S.P.P., L.B., A.M.R., D.C. (David Casini), G.L., M.C. and A.S.; project administration: D.C. (David Casini), T.A. and L.S.E.; resources, L.B., A.M.R., D.C. (David Chiaramonti), M.C., A.S., T.A. and L.S.E.; supervision, I.M, S.A.H., L.B., A.M.R., D.C. (David Chiaramonti), A.S. and L.S.E.; validation, I.M., A.M.R., D.C. (David Casini), G.L., A.S. and T.A.; writing—original draft, I.M., V.X., T.C.F., D.C. (David Casini) and T.A.;

writing—review and editing, I.M., S.A.H., J.S.A., R.C.C., L.B., A.M.R., D.C. (David Casini), A.S., T.A. and L.S.E. All authors have read and agreed to the published version of the manuscript.

Funding: This work was carried out within the BeonNAT project, which received funding from the Bio Based Industries Joint Undertaking (JU) under grant agreement No 887917 BeonNAT. The JU receives support from the European Union's Horizon 2020 research and innovation programme and the Bio Based Industries Consortium.

Institutional Review Board Statement: The animal study protocol was approved by the Comissão de Ética do Instituto Politécnico de Bragança No. 62/2021, 29/11/2021.

Informed Consent Statement: Not applicable.

Data Availability Statement: Not applicable.

Acknowledgments: The authors are also thankful to the Foundation for Science and Technology (FCT, Portugal) for financial support through national funds FCT/MCTES (PIDDAC) to CIMO (UIDB/00690/2020 and UIDP/00690/2020) and SusTEC (LA/P/0007/2020); L. Barros, R. Calhelha, and S. Heleno (CEECIND/00831/2018) thank the national funding by FCT, P.I., through the institutional and individual scientific employment program-contract for their contract.

Conflicts of Interest: The authors declare no conflict of interest. The funders had no role in the design of the study; in the collection, analyses, or interpretation of data; in the writing of the manuscript; or in the decision to publish the results.

Sample Availability: Samples of the compounds are not available from the authors.

Abbreviations

a.u.	arbitrary units
a.s.l.	above sea level
b.d.l.	below detection limit
CAA	cellular antioxidant activity
CFU	colony forming units
CMC	component material category
CORG	organic carbon
d.b.	dry basis
GI50	extract concentration that provides 50% of cell growth inhibition
IPCC	Intergovernmental Panel on Climate Change
LRI	linear retention index
MBC	minimum bactericidal concentration
MFC	minimum fungicidal concentration
MIC	minimum inhibitory concentration
MRSA	Methicillin-resistant *Staphylococcus aureus*
n.a.	not available
n.t.	not tested
PAH	polycyclic aromatic hydrocarbon
PCDD/F	polychlorinated-p-dioxins and furans
PFC	product function category
RP	reducing power
v/*v*	volume/volume
w.b.	wet basis
w.m	wet matter
w/*w*	weight/weight

Appendix A

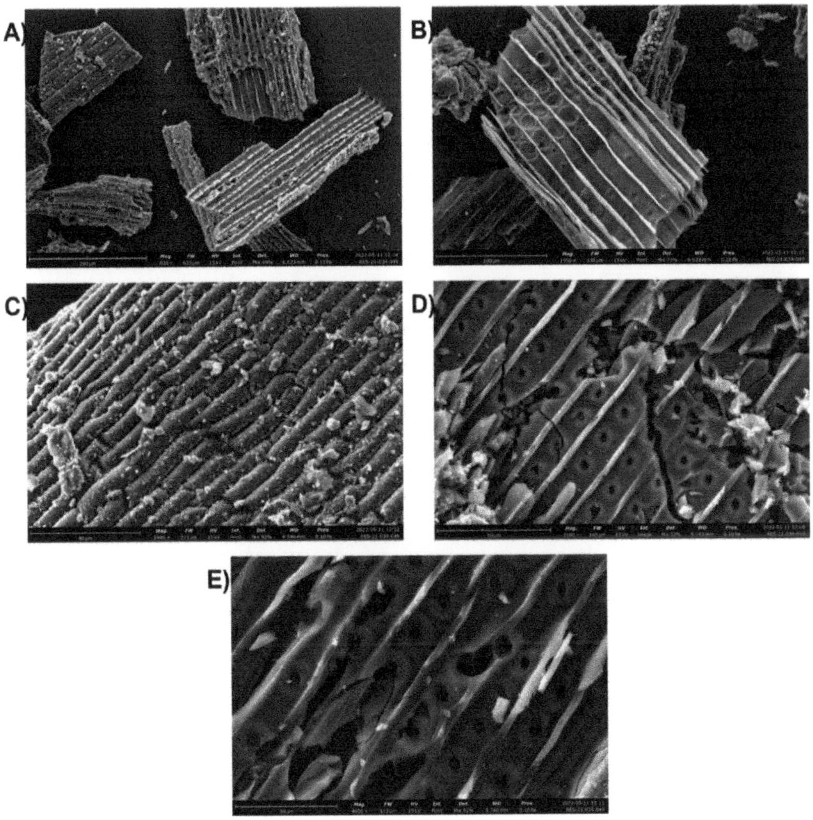

Figure A1. *J. communis* biochar analysed through SEM. (**A**) 200 µm view. (**B**) 100 µm view. (**C**) 80 µm view. (**D**) 50 µm view. (**E**) 30 µm view.

Table A1. Characterisation of *J. communis* biochar—proximate and ultimate analyses.

Parameter	Result	Unit of Measure
Moisture	1.80	% *w*/*w*, a.r.
Ashes	8.65	% *w*/*w*, d.b.
Volatiles	12.98	% *w*/*w*, d.b.
Fixed Carbon	78.37	% *w*/*w*, d.b.
C	87.76	% *w*/*w*, d.b.
H	2.61	% *w*/*w*, d.b.
N	0.74	% *w*/*w*, d.b.
Cl	0.02	% *w*/*w*, d.b.
S	0.03	% *w*/*w*, d.b.
Inorganic C	0.49	% *w*/*w*, d.b.
pH	7.5	
Conductivity	395.1	µS/cm

% *w*/*w*: % Weight/weight; a.r.: as received; d.b.: dry basis.

Table A2. Characterisation of *J.communis* biochar—Elements content.

Parameter	Result	Unit of Measure
Al	265	mg/kg d.b.
B	b.d.l.	mg/kg, d.b.
Ba	88	mg/kg, d.b.
Ca	15,455	mg/kg, d.b.
Co	b.d.l.	mg/kg, d.b.
Cr	b.d.l.	mg/kg, d.b.
Cu	57	mg/kg, d.b.
Fe	241	mg/kg, d.b.
K	7035	mg/kg, d.b.
Li	b.d.l.	mg/kg, d.b.
Mg	1666	mg/kg, d.b.
Mn	422	mg/kg, d.b.
Mo	b.d.l.	mg/kg, d.b.
Na	1543	mg/kg, d.b.
Ni	b.d.l.	mg/kg, d.b.
P	b.d.l.	mg/kg, d.b.
Pb	b.d.l.	mg/kg, d.b.
Si	514	mg/kg, d.b.
Ti	26	mg/kg, d.b.
V	b.d.l.	mg/kg, d.b.
Zn	9	mg/kg, d.b.
Cr VI	<0.2	mg/kg, d.b.
Cd	0.40	mg/kg, d.b.
As	<2	mg/kg, d.b.
Hg	<0.1	mg/kg, d.b.
Tl	<1	mg/kg, d.b.

d.b.: Dry basis.

Table A3. Characterisation of *J. communis* biochar—Organic pollutants.

Parameter	Result	Unit of Measure
	PAH	
NAPHTALENE	<0.05	mg/kg, d.b.
ACENAPHTHYLENE	<0.05	mg/kg, d.b.
ACENAFTENE	<0.05	mg/kg, d.b.
FLUORENE	<0.05	mg/kg, d.b.
PHENANTHRENE	0.43	mg/kg, d.b.
ANTHRACENE	0.10	mg/kg, d.b.
FLUORANTHENE	0.21	mg/kg, d.b.
PYRENE	0.24	mg/kg, d.b.
BENZO(A)ANTHRACENE	0.08	mg/kg, d.b.
CRISENE	0.07	mg/kg, d.b.
BENZO(B + J + K)FLUORANTHENE	0.05	mg/kg, d.b.
BENZO(E)PYRENE	<0.05	mg/kg, d.b.
BENZO(A)PYRENE	0.05	mg/kg, d.b.
PERILENE	<0.05	mg/kg, d.b.
INDENO(1,2,3,CD)PYRENE	<0.05	mg/kg, d.b.
DIBENZO(AH)ANTHRACENE	<0.05	mg/kg, d.b.
BENZO(GHI)PERILENE	<0.05	mg/kg, d.b.
DIBENZO(A,L)PYRENE	<0.05	mg/kg, d.b.
DIBENZO(A,I)PYRENE	<0.05	mg/kg, d.b.
DIBENZO(A,E)PYRENE	<0.05	mg/kg, d.b.
DIBENZO(A,H)PYRENE	<0.05	mg/kg, d.b.
SUM PAH	1.36	mg/kg, d.b.

Table A3. *Cont.*

Parameter	Result	Unit of Measure
Polychlorinated Dibenzodioxins and Polychlorinated Dibenzofurans		
2,3,7,8 TETRA CDD	<1	ng/kg, d.b.
1,2,3,7,8 PENTA CDD	<5	ng/kg, d.b.
1,2,3,4,7,8 ESA CDD	<5	ng/kg, d.b.
1,2,3,6,7,8 ESA CDD	<5	ng/kg, d.b.
1,2,3,7,8,9 ESA CDD	<5	ng/kg, d.b.
1,2,3,4,6,7,8 EPTA CDD	<5	ng/kg, d.b.
OCTA CDD	<10	ng/kg, d.b.
2,3,7,8 TETRA CDF	<1	ng/kg, d.b.
1,2,3,7,8 PENTA CDF	<5	ng/kg, d.b.
2,3,4,7,8, PENTA CDF	<5	ng/kg, d.b.
1,2,3,4,7,8 ESA CDF	<5	ng/kg, d.b.
1,2,3,6,7,8 ESA CDF	<5	ng/kg, d.b.
2,3,4,6,7,8 ESA CDF	<5	ng/kg, d.b.
1,2,3,7,8,9 ESA CDF	<5	ng/kg, d.b.
1,2,3,4,6,7,8 EPTA CDF	<5	ng/kg, d.b.
1,2,3,4,7,8,9 EPTA CDF	<5	ng/kg, d.b.
OCTA CDF	<10	ng/kg, d.b.
Equivalent Toxicity according to WHO-TEQ	<1	ng WHO-TEQ/kg d.b.
Polychlorinated Biphenyls		
T3CB-28	0.00027	mg/kg, d.b.
T4CB-52	0.00023	mg/kg, d.b.
P5CB-95	0.00008	mg/kg, d.b.
P5CB-101	0.00010	mg/kg, d.b.
P5CB-99	0.00003	mg/kg, d.b.
P5CB-110	0.00008	mg/kg, d.b.
P5CB-118	0.00006	mg/kg, d.b.
H6CB-151	<0.0001	mg/kg, d.b.
H6CB-149	0.00003	mg/kg, d.b.
H6CB-146	<0.0001	mg/kg, d.b.
H6CB-153	0.00006	mg/kg, d.b.
H6CB-138	0.00004	mg/kg, d.b.
H6CB-128	<0.0001	mg/kg, d.b.
H7CB-187	<0.0001	mg/kg, d.b.
H7CB-183	<0.0001	mg/kg, d.b.
H7CB-177	<0.0001	mg/kg, d.b.
H7CB-180	<0.0001	mg/kg, d.b.
H7CB-170	<0.0001	mg/kg, d.b.
SUM PCB	0.00101	mg/kg, d.b.
WHO-PCB (dioxin-like)		
T4CB-77	<0.0001	ng/kg, d.b.
T4CB-81	<0.0001	ng/kg, d.b.
P5CB-105	0.00	ng/kg, d.b.
P5CB-114	<0.0001	ng/kg, d.b.
P5CB-118	<0.0001	ng/kg, d.b.
P5CB-123	<0.0001	ng/kg, d.b.
P5CB-126	<0.0001	ng/kg, d.b.
H6CB-156	<0.0001	ng/kg, d.b.
H6CB-157	<0.0001	ng/kg, d.b.
H6CB-167	<0.0001	ng/kg, d.b.
H6CB-169	<0.0001	ng/kg, d.b.
H7CB-189	<0.0001	ng/kg, d.b.
Equivalent Toxicity according to WHO-TEQ	<0.01	ng WHO-TEQ/kg, d.b.

d.b.: Dry basis.

Table A4. Characterisation of *J. communis* biochar—Porosity and water sorption capacity.

Parameter	Result	Unit of Measure
BET and DFT analysis results for micro-mesopore range		
Specific surface area (BET)	61	m^2/g
Specific pore volume (DFT)	0.04	cm^3/g
Mercury porosimeter analysis results for meso-macropore range		
Specific surface area	40	m^2/g
Specific intrusion volume	1.59	cm^3/g
Porosity	66.5	%
Water-holding capacity results		
Water specific retention	1.42	ml_{H2O}/g_{CHAR}

References

1. European Commission. Directorate-General for Research and Innovation, 2018. A Sustainable Bioeconomy for Europe: Strengthening the Connection between Economy, Society and the Environment: Updated Bioeconomy Strategy, Publications Office. Available online: https://data.europa.eu/doi/10.2777/478385 (accessed on 5 April 2023).
2. Muscat, A.; de Olde, E.M.; Candel, J.J.L.; de Boer, I.J.M.; Ripoll-Bosch, R. The promised land: Contrasting frames of marginal land in the European Union. *Land Use Policy* **2022**, *112*, 105860. [CrossRef]
3. Singh, A.; Chistensen, T.; Panoutsou, C. Policy review for biomass value chains in the European bioeconomy. *Glob. Transit.* **2021**, *3*, 13–42. [CrossRef]
4. Loziene, K.; Venskutonis, P.R. Chapter 56: Juniper (*Juniperus communis* L.) oils. In *Essential Oils in Food Preservation, Flavor and Safety*; Preedy, V.R., Ed.; Elsevier: Amsterdam, The Netherlands, 2016; pp. 495–500. [CrossRef]
5. Pandey, S.; Tiwari, S.; Kumar, A.; Niranjan, A.; Chand, J.; Lehri, A.; Chauhan, P.S. Antioxidant and anti-aging potential of Juniper berry (*Juniperus communis* L.) essential oil in Caenorhabditis elegans model system. *Ind. Crops Prod.* **2018**, *120*, 113–122. [CrossRef]
6. Falcão, S.; Bacém, I.; Igrejas, G.; Rodrigues, P.J.; Vilas-Boas, M.; Amaral, J.S. Chemical composition and antimicrobial activity of hydrodistilled oil from juniper berries. *Ind. Crops Prod.* **2018**, *124*, 878–884. [CrossRef]
7. Höferl, M.; Stoilova, I.; Schmidt, E.; Wanner, J.; Jirovetz, L.; Trifonova, D.; Krastev, L.; Krastanov, A. Chemical composition and antioxidant properties of juniper berry (*Juniperus communis* L.) essential oil. Action of the essential oil on the antioxidant protection of Saccharomyces cerevisiae model organism. *Antioxidants* **2014**, *3*, 81–98. [CrossRef]
8. Butkienė, R.; Nivinskienė, O.; Mockutė, D. Differences in the essential oils of the leaves (needles), unripe and ripe berries of *Juniperus communis* L. growing wild in Vilnius district (Lithuania). *J. Essent. Oil Res.* **2006**, *18*, 489–494. [CrossRef]
9. Orav, A.; Koel, M.; Kailas, T.; Müürisepp, M. Comparative analysis of the composition of essential oils and supercritical carbon dioxide extracts from the berries and needles of Estonian juniper (*Juniperus communis* L.). In Proceedings of the 5th Conference by Nordic Separation Science Society, Tallinn, Estonia, 26–29 August 2009; Volume 2, pp. 161–167. [CrossRef]
10. Emami, S.A.; Javadi, B.; Hassanzadeh, M.K. Antioxidant activity of the essential oil of different parts of *Juniperus communis* subsp. *hemisphaerica and Juniperus oblonga. Pharm. Biol.* **2007**, *45*, 769–776. [CrossRef]
11. Mediavilla, I.; Guillamón, E.; Ruiz, A.; Esteban, L.S. Essential oils from residual foliage of forest tree and shrub species: Yield and antioxidant capacity. *Molecules* **2021**, *26*, 3257. [CrossRef]
12. Semerdjieva, I.; Zheljazkov, V.D.; Radoukova, T.; Dincheva, I.; Piperkova, N.; Maneva, V.; Astatkie, T.; Kacániová, M. Biological activity of essential oils of four juniper species and their potential as biopesticides. *Molecules* **2021**, *26*, 6358. [CrossRef]
13. Alves-Ferreira, J.; Duarte, L.C.; Lourenco, A.; Roseiro, L.B.; Fernandes, M.C.; Pereira, H.; Carvalheiro, F. Distillery residues from *Cistus ladanifer* (rockrose) as feedstock for the production of added-value phenolic compounds and hemicellulosic oligosaccharides. *Bioenergy Res.* **2019**, *12*, 347–358. [CrossRef]
14. Ortiz de Elguea-Culebras, G.; Melero Bravo, E.; Sánchez-Vioque, S. Potential sources and methodologies for the recovery of phenolic compounds from distillation residues of Mediterranean aromatic plants. An approach to the valuation of by-products of the essential oil market—A review. *Ind. Crops Prod.* **2022**, *175*, 114261. [CrossRef]
15. Tsimogiannis, D.; Choulitoudi, E.; Bimpilas, A.; Mitropoulo, G.; Kourkoutas, Y.; Oreopoulou, V. Exploitation of the biological potential of *Satureja thymbra* essential oil and distillation by-products. *J. Appl. Res. Med. Aromat. Plants* **2017**, *4*, 12–20. [CrossRef]
16. Abu Bakar, M.S.; Ahmed, A.; Jeffery, D.M.; Hidayat, S.; Sukri, R.S.; Mahlia, T.M.I.; Jamil, F.; Khurrum, M.S.; Inayat, A.; Moogi, S.; et al. Pyrolysis of solid waste residues from Lemon Myrtle essential oil extraction for bio-oil production. *Bioresour. Technol.* **2020**, *318*, 123913. [CrossRef] [PubMed]
17. Ninich, O.; Et-tahir, A.; Kettani, K.; Ghanmi, M.; Aoujdad, J.; El Antry, S.; Ouajdi, M.; Satrani, B. Plant sources, techniques of production and uses of tar: A review. *J. Ethnopharmacol.* **2022**, *285*, 114889. [CrossRef] [PubMed]
18. Cliff, M.; Heymann, H. Physical and sensory characteristics of cat litter. *Sens. Stud.* **1991**, *6*, 255–266. [CrossRef]
19. Zheljazkov, V.D.; Astatkie, T. Effect of residual distillation water of 15 plants and three plant hormones on Schotch spearmint (*Mentha* × *gracilis* Sole). *Ind. Crops Prod.* **2011**, *33*, 704–709. [CrossRef]

20. Tavares, C.S.; Gameiro, J.A.; Roseiro, L.B.; Figueiredo, A.C. Hydrolates: A review on their volatiles composition, biological properties and potential uses. *Phytochem. Rev.* **2022**, *21*, 1661–1737. [CrossRef]
21. D'Amato, S.; Serio, A.; Chaves López, C.; Paparella, A. Hydrosols: Biological activity and potential as antimicrobials for food applications. *Food Control* **2018**, *86*, 126–137. [CrossRef]
22. Jakubczyk, K.; Tuchowska, A.; Janda-Milczarek, K. Plant hydrolates—Antioxidant properties, chemical composition and potential applications. *Biomed. Pharmacother.* **2021**, *142*, 112033. [CrossRef]
23. Oral, N.; Vatansever, L.; Güven, A.; Gülmez, M. Antibacterial activity of some Turkish plant hydrosols. *Kafkas Üniv. Vet. Fak. Derg.* **2008**, *14*, 205–209.
24. Mielnik, M.B.; Sem, S.; Egelandsdal, B.; Skrede, G. By-products from herbs essential oil production as ingredient in marinade for turkey thighs. *LWT* **2008**, *41*, 93–100. [CrossRef]
25. Angioni, A.; Barra, A.; Russo, M.; Coroneo, V.; Dessi, S.; Cabras, P. Chemical composition of the essential oils of Juniperus from ripe and unripe berries and leaves and their antimicrobial activity. *J. Agric. Food Chem.* **2003**, *51*, 3073–3078. [CrossRef] [PubMed]
26. Koundal, R.; Kumar, A.; Thakur, S.; Agnihotri, V.; Chand, G.; Singh, R. Seasonal variation in phytochemicals of essential oil from Juniperus communis needles in western Himalaya. *J. Essent. Oil Res.* **2015**, *27*, 406–411. [CrossRef]
27. Raal, A.; Kanut, M.; Orav, A. Annual variation of yield and composition of the essential oil of common juniper (*Juniperus communis* L.) branches from Estonia. *Balt. For.* **2010**, *16*, 50–56.
28. Radoukova, T.; Zheljazkov, V.; Semerdjieva, I.; Dincheva, I.; Stoyanova, A.; Kacaniova, M.; Markovic, T.; Radanovic, D.; Astatkie, T.; Salamon, I. Differences in essential oil yield, composition, and bioactivity of three juniper species from Eastern Europe. *Ind. Crops Prod.* **2018**, *124*, 643–652. [CrossRef]
29. Rostaefar, A.; Hassani, A.; Sefidkon, F. Seasonal variations of essential oil content and composition in male and female plants of *Juniperus communis* L. ssp. *hemisphaerica growing wild in Iran. J. Essent. Oil Res.* **2017**, *29*, 357–360. [CrossRef]
30. Mediavilla, I.; Bados, R.; Barros, L.; Xavier, V.; Finimundy, T.C.; Amaral, J.S.; Rizzo, A.M.; Casini, D.; Lombardi, G.; Cámara, M.; et al. Assessment of the use of common juniper (*Juniperus communis* L.) foliage following the cascade principle: Essential oil, absorbents and biochar. In Proceedings of the 30th European Biomass Conference and Exhibition, Online, 9–12 May 2022; pp. 1035–1041. [CrossRef]
31. Adams, R. *Identification of Essential Oil Components by Gas Chromatography/Mass Spectrometry*, 4th ed.; Allured Publishing Corporation: Carol Stream, IN, USA, 2007.
32. Falasca, A.; Caprari, C.; De Felice, V.; Fortini, P.; Saviano, G.; Zollo, F.; Iorizzi, M. GC-MS analysis of the essential oils of *Juniperus communis* L. berries growing wild in the Molise region: Seasonal variability and in vitro antifungal activity. *Biochem. Syst. Ecol.* **2016**, *69*, 166–175. [CrossRef]
33. Borges, M.F.D.A.; Lacerda, R.D.S.; Correia, J.P.D.A.; de Melo, T.R.; Ferreira, S.B. Potential antibacterial action of α-Pinene. *Med. Sci. Forum* **2022**, *12*, 11. [CrossRef]
34. Xavier, V.; Finimundy, T.C.; Heleno, S.A.; Amaral, J.S.; Calhelha, R.C.; Vaz, J.; Pires, T.C.S.P.; Mediavilla, I.; Esteban, L.S.; Ferreira, I.C.F.R.; et al. Chemical and bioactive characterization of the essential oils obtained from three Mediterranean plants. *Molecules* **2021**, *26*, 7472. [CrossRef]
35. Gonçalves, A.C.; Flores-Félix, J.D.; Coutinho, P.; Alves, G.; Silva, L.R. Zimbro (*Juniperus communis* L.) as a promising source of bioactive compounds and biomedical activities: A review on recent trends. *Int. J. Mol. Sci.* **2022**, *23*, 3197. [CrossRef]
36. Dumitrescu, E.; Muselin, F.; Dumitrescu, C.S.; Orasan-Alic, S.A.; Moruzi, R.F.; Doma, A.O.; Mohamed, E.A.; Cristina, R.T. *Juniper communis* L. essential oils from Western Romanian Carpathians: Bio-structure and effective antibacterial activity. *Appl. Sci.* **2022**, *12*, 2949. [CrossRef]
37. Cavaleiro, C.; Pinto, E.; Goncalves, M.J.; Salgueiro, L. Antifungal activity of *Juniperus* essential oils against dermatophyte, *Aspergillus* and *Candida* strains. *J. Appl. Microbiol.* **2006**, *100*, 1333–1338. [CrossRef] [PubMed]
38. Al-Rumaihi, A.; Shahbaz, M.; Mckay, G.; Mackey, H.; Al-Ansari, T. A review of pyrolysis technologies and feedstock: A blending approach for plastic and biomass towards optimum biochar yield. *Renew. Sustain. Energy Rev.* **2022**, *167*, 112715. [CrossRef]
39. Laird, D.A.; Brown, R.C.; Amonette, J.E.; Lehmann, J. Review of the pyrolysis platform for coproducing bio-oil and biochar. *Biofuel Bioprod. Biorefin.* **2009**, *3*, 547–562. [CrossRef]
40. Leng, L.; Huang, H.; Li, H.; Li, J.; Zhou, W. Biochar stability assessment methods: A review. *Sci. Total Environ.* **2019**, *647*, 210–222. [CrossRef]
41. Budai, A.; Zimmerman, A.R.; Cowie, A.L.; Webber, J.B.W.; Singh, B.P.; Glaser, B.; Masiello, C.A.; Andersson, D.; Shields, F.; Lehmann, J.; et al. Biochar Carbon Stability Test Method: An Assessment of Methods to Determine Biochar Carbon Stability. International Biochar Initiative. 20 September 2013. Available online: https://www.biochar-international.org/wp-content/uploads/2018/06/IBI_Report_Biochar_Stability_Test_Method_Final.pdf (accessed on 5 April 2023).
42. Usevičiūtė, L.; Baltrėnaitė-Gedienė, E. Dependence of pyrolysis temperature and lignocellulosic physical-chemical properties of biochar on its wettability. *Biomass Convers. Biorefin.* **2021**, *11*, 2775–2793. [CrossRef]
43. Lehmann, J.; Stephen, J. *Biochar for Environmental Management: Science, Technology and Implementation*, 2nd ed.; Routledge: London, UK, 2015. [CrossRef]
44. IPCC. *Appendix 4: Method for Estimating the Change in Mineral Soil Organic Carbon Stocks from Biochar Amendments: Basis for Future Methodological Development, 2019 Refinement to the 2006 IPCC Guidelines for National Greenhouse Gas Inventories*; IPCC: Geneva, Switzerland, 2019.

45. Mediavilla, I.; Borjabad, E.; Fernández, M.J.; Ramos, R.; Pérez, P.; Bados, R.; Carrasco, J.E.; Esteban, L.S. Biofuels from broom clearings: Production and combustion in commercial boilers. *Energy* **2017**, *141*, 1845–1856. [CrossRef]
46. Mediavilla, I.; Esteban, L.S.; Carrasco, J.E. Optimisation of pine sawdust pelletisation conditions. In Proceedings of the 18th European Biomass Conference and Exhibition, Lyon, France, 3–7 May 2010; pp. 1598–1602.
47. Bradfield, J.; Levi, M.P. Effect of species and wood to bark ratio on pelleting of southern woods. *For. Prod. J.* **1984**, *34*, 61–63.
48. Filbakk, T.; Jirjis, R.; Nurmi, J.; Hoibo, O. The effect of bark content on quality parameters of Scots pine (*Pinus sylvestris* L.) pellets. *Biomass Bioenergy* **2011**, *35*, 3342–3349. [CrossRef]
49. MAPAMA. Dirección General de Desarrollo Rural, 2018. MFE25. Mapa Forestal de España. Available online: https://www.miteco.gob.es/es/cartografia-y-sig/ide/descargas/biodiversidad/mfe.aspx (accessed on 5 April 2023).
50. Ministerio de Medio Ambiente, y Medio Rural y Marino. Dirección General de Medio Natural y Política Forestal, 1997. MFE200. Mapa Forestal de España. Available online: https://www.miteco.gob.es/es/biodiversidad/servicios/banco-datos-naturaleza/informacion-disponible/mfe200_descargas.aspx/ (accessed on 5 April 2023).
51. Spréa, R.M.; Fernandes, A.; Finimundy, T.C.; Pereira, C.; Alves, M.J.; Calhelha, R.C.; Canan, C.; Barros, L.; Amaral, J.S.; Ferreira, I.C.F.R. Lovage (*Levisticum officinale* W.D.J. Koch) roots: A source of bioactive compounds towards a circular economy. *Resources* **2020**, *9*, 81. [CrossRef]
52. Kostić, M.; Smiljković, M.; Petrović, J.; Glamočlija, J.; Barros, L.; Ferreira, I.C.F.R.; Ćirić, A.; Soković, M. Chemical, nutritive composition and a wide range of bioactive properties of honey mushroom *Armillaria mellea* (Vahl: Fr.) Kummer. *Food Funct.* **2017**, *8*, 3239–3249. [CrossRef] [PubMed]
53. Wolfe, K.L.; Kang, C.; He, X.; Dong, M.; Zhang, Q.; Liu, R.H. Cellular antioxidant activity of common fruits. *J. Agric. Food Chem.* **2008**, *56*, 8418–8426. [CrossRef] [PubMed]
54. Vichai, V.; Kirtikara, K. Sulforhodamine B colorimetric assay for cytotoxicity screening. *Nat. Protoc.* **2006**, *1*, 1112–1116. [CrossRef] [PubMed]

MDPI AG
Grosspeteranlage 5
4052 Basel
Switzerland
Tel.: +41 61 683 77 34

Molecules Editorial Office
E-mail: molecules@mdpi.com
www.mdpi.com/journal/molecules

www.ingramcontent.com/pod-product-compliance
Lightning Source LLC
Chambersburg PA
CBHW061516210926
51850CB00008B/1936
9783725864300